Revision Notes for the FRCEM Primary

SECOND EDITION

EDITED BY

Dr Mark Harrison
Consultant in Emergency Medicine
Northumbria Healthcare NHS Trust, UK

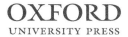

OXFORD
UNIVERSITY PRESS

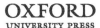

Great Clarendon Street, Oxford, OX2 6DP,
United Kingdom

Oxford University Press is a department of the University of Oxford.
It furthers the University's objective of excellence in research, scholarship,
and education by publishing worldwide. Oxford is a registered trade mark of
Oxford University Press in the UK and in certain other countries

© Oxford University Press 2017

The moral rights of the authors have been asserted

First Edition Published in 2011
Second Edition Published in 2017

Published in the United States of America by Oxford University Press
198 Madison Avenue, New York, NY 10016, United States of America

British Library Cataloguing in Publication Data

Data available

Library of Congress Control Number: 2016951477

ISBN 978-0-19-876587-5

To Andreja, who always believes.
And to Luka and Tilen, who make everything worthwhile.

Contents

Abbreviations

5HT	serotonin	**BNF**	British National Formulary
πGC	oncotic pressure in glomerular capillary	**BP**	blood pressure
		BPH	benign prostatic hypertrophy
ABC	airway, breathing, circulation	**BTS**	British Thoracic Society
ABCDE	airway, breathing, circulation, disability, environment	**CA**	carbonic anhydrase
		cAMP	cyclic adenosine monophosphate
ABG	arterial blood gas	**CBF**	cerebral blood flow
ACE	angiotensin-converting enzyme	**CBM**	cerebellum
Ach	acetylcholine	**CCF**	congestive cardiac failure
ACS	acute coronary syndrome	**CCK**	cholecystokinin
ACTH	adrenocorticotrophic hormone	**CD**	collecting duct
ADH	antidiuretic hormone	**CF**	cystic fibrosis
ADP	adenosine diphosphate	**cGMP**	cyclic guanosine monophosphate
AF	atrial fibrillation	**CI**	confidence interval
AGE	arterial gas embolism	**CICR**	calcium-induced calcium release
AIDS	acquired immunodeficiency syndrome	**CK**	creatine kinase
		CMRO$_2$	cerebral metabolic rate for oxygen
ALT	alanine aminotransferase	**CN**	cranial nerve
AMI	acute myocardial infarction	**CNS**	central nervous system
AMP	adenosine monophosphate	**CO**	cardiac output
ANA	antinuclear antibody	**COHb**	carboxyhaemoglobin
ANF	antinuclear factor	**COMT**	catechol-O-methyltransferase
ANP	atrial natriuretic peptide	**COPD**	chronic obstructive pulmonary disease
ANS	autonomic nervous system		
AP	action potential	**COX**	cyclooxygenase
APTT	activated partial thromboplastin time	**CPG**	central pattern generator
		CPP	cerebral perfusion pressure
ARDS	acute/adult respiratory distress syndrome	**CPR**	cardiopulmonary resuscitation
		CRH	corticotrophin-releasing hormone
ASIS	anterior superior iliac spine	**CRP**	C-reactive protein
AST	aspartate aminotransferase	**CSF**	cerebrospinal fluid
ATP	adenosine triphosphate	**CSU**	catheter-specimen urine
AUC	area under the curve	**CT**	computed tomography
AV	atrioventricular	**CTL**	cytotoxic T lymphocyte
AVA	arteriovenous anastomosis	**CTZ**	chemoreceptor trigger zone
AVN	atrioventricular node	**CV**	cardiovascular
BBB	blood–brain barrier	**CVA**	cerebrovascular accident
BCG	bacillus Calmette–Guérin	**CVC**	central venous catheter
bd	twice daily	**CVP**	central venous pressure
BDZ	benzodiazepine	**CVS**	cardiovascular system
BM	blood glucose (Boehringer Mannheim)	**CXR**	chest X-ray
		DAG	diacylglycerol

DCI	decompression illness	**GCS**	Glasgow Coma Score
DCS	decompression sickness	**GDP**	guanosine diphosphate
DCT	distal convoluted tubule	**GFR**	glomerular filtration rate
DHEA	dehydroepiandrosterone	**GH**	growth hormone
DI	diabetes insipidus	**GI**	gastrointestinal
DIC	disseminated intravascular	**GIP**	gastric inhibitory peptide
	coagulation	**GORD**	gastro-oesophageal reflux disease
DKA	diabetic ketoacidosis	**GTN**	glyceryl trinitrate
DM	diabetes mellitus	**GTP**	guanosine triphosphate
DMT1	divalent metal transporter 1	**HAV**	hepatitis A virus
DNA	deoxyribonucleic acid	**Hb**	haemoglobin
DO$_2$	oxygen delivery	**HbF**	fetal haemoglobin
DP	distal phalanx	**HbO$_2$**	oxyhaemoglobin
DPG	diphosphoglycerate	**HBV**	hepatitis B virus
DRG	dorsal respiratory group	**HCl**	hydrochloric acid
DSCT	dorsal spinocerebellar tract	**HCV**	hepatitis C virus
DT	diphtheria and tetanus toxoids	**HDL**	high-density lipoprotein
	(vaccine)	**HDN**	haemolytic disease of the
DTP	diphtheria, pertussis, and tetanus		newborn
	(vaccine)	**HIB**	*Haemophilus influenzae* type b
DVT	deep vein thrombosis	**HIT**	heparin-induced
EABV	effective arterial blood volume		thrombocytopenia
EC	excitation–contraction	**HIV**	human immunodeficiency virus
ECF	extracellular fluid	**HLA**	human leucocyte antigen
ECG	electrocardiogram	**HMG CoA**	3-hydroxy-3-methylglutaryl
ED	emergency department		coenzyme A
EDHF	endothelium-derived	**HONK**	hyperosmolar hyperglycaemic
	hyperpolarizing factor		non-ketotic coma
EDV	end-diastolic volume	**HPIV**	human parainfluenza virus
EEG	electroencephalography	**HPV**	human papilloma virus
ELISA	enzyme-linked	**HR**	heart rate
	immunosorbent assay	**HSV**	herpes simplex virus
ENaC	epithelial Na$^+$ channel	**IBS**	irritable bowel syndrome
EPO	erythropoietin	**IC**	inspiratory capacity
EPSP	excitatory postsynaptic potential	**ICU**	intensive care unit
ER	endoplasmic reticulum	**ICF**	intracellular fluid
ERP	effective refractory period	**ICP**	intracranial pressure
ERV	expiratory reserve volume	**Ig**	immunoglobulin
ESBL	extended-spectrum	**IHG**	ischaemic heart disease
	beta-lactamase	**IL**	interleukin
ESR	erythrocyte sedimentation rate	**IM**	intramuscular
ESV	end-systolic volume	**IN**	intranasal
FBC	full blood count	**INR**	international normalized ratio
FC	flexor carpii	**IP3**	inositol triphosphate
FDP	flexor digitorum profundus	**IPJ**	interphalangeal joint
FDS	flexor digitorum superficialis	**IPSP**	inhibitory postsynaptic potential
FEV$_1$	forced expiratory volume in	**IRDS**	infant respiratory distress
	1 second		syndrome
FFP	fresh frozen plasma	**IRV**	inspiratory reserve volume
FH	family history	**ISA**	intrinsic sympathomimetic activity
FPL	flexor pollicis longus	**ITP**	idiopathic thrombocytopenic
FRC	functional residual capacity		purpura
FSH	follicle-stimulating hormone	**ITU**	intensive therapy unit
FVC	forced vital capacity	**IV**	intravenous
GABA	γ-aminobutyric acid	**IVC**	inferior vena cava
GBS	Guillain–Barré syndrome	**IVDU**	intravenous drug use/user

IVU	intravenous urogram	NPV	negative predictive value
JG	juxtaglomerular	NSAID	non-steroidal anti-inflammatory drug
JVP	jugular venous pressure		
K_{CO}	carbon monoxide transfer coefficient	N&V	nausea and vomiting
		OCP	oral contraceptive pill
LAD	left anterior descending	od	once daily
LBBB	left bundle branch block	OD	overdose
LCST	lateral corticospinal tract	ODC	oxyhaemoglobin dissociation curve
LDH	lactate dehydrogenase	PBS	hydrostatic pressure in Bowman's space
LDL	low-density lipoprotein		
LFT	liver function test	PCI	percutaneous coronary intervention
LGN	lateral geniculate nucleus		
LH	luteinizing hormone	PCO_2	partial pressure of carbon dioxide
LIF	left iliac fossa	PCR	polymerase chain reaction
LMN	lower motor neuron	PCT	proximal convoluted tubule
LMWH	low-molecular-weight heparin	PCWP	pulmonary capillary wedge pressure
LoH	loop of Henle		
LOS	lipooligosaccharide	PE	pulmonary embolism
LP	lumbar puncture	PEA	pulseless electrical activity
LSTT	lateral spinothalamic tract	PEFR	peak expiratory flow rate
LV	left ventricle/ventricular	PGC	hydrostatic pressure in glomerular capillary
LVF	left ventricular failure		
MAC	membrane attack complex	PG	prostaglandin
MALT	mucosa-associated lymphatic tissue	PGI2	prostacyclin
		PHI	peptide histadine-isoleucine
MAO	monoamine oxidase	PICA	posterior inferior cerebellar artery
MAOI	monoamine oxidase inhibitor	PID	pelvic inflammatory disease
MAP	mean arterial pressure	PIP2	phosphatidylinositol 4,5-bisphosphate
MC	metacarpal		
MCPJ	metacarpophalangeal joint	PKA	protein kinase A
MH	malignant hyperthermia	PLC	phospholipase C
MI	myocardial infarction	PMC	premotor cortex
MMR	measles, mumps, and rubella (vaccine)	PMN	polymorphonuclear neutrophil
		PO	orally
MN	motor neuron	PO_2	partial pressure of oxygen
MP	middle phalanx	PP	proximal phalanx
MRI	magnetic resonance imaging	PPI	proton pump inhibitor
MRSA	methicillin-resistant *Staphylococcus aureus*	PPV	positive predictive value
		PR	per rectum
MS	multiple sclerosis	PRG	pontine respiratory group
MSU	mid-stream urine	PRN	as needed
NAAT	nucleic acid antigen test	PT	proximal tubule
NADPH	nicotinamide adenine dinucleotide phosphate	PTH	parathyroid hormone
		PUO	pyrexia of unknown origin
NAPQI	N-acetyl P-amino-benzoquinone imine	PVR	pulmonary vascular resistance
		qds	four times daily
NDF	net driving force	RA	rheumatoid arthritis
NE	norepinephrine	RANKL	receptor activator for nuclear factor κB-ligand
NET	neutrophil extracellular trap		
NICE	National Institute for Health and Care Excellence	RAAS	renin–angiotensin–aldosterone system
NK	natural killer (cell)	R_{aw}	airway resistance
NMJ	neuromuscular junction	RBBB	right bundle branch block
NMS	neuroleptic malignant syndrome	RBC	red blood cell
NO	nitric oxide	RBF	renal blood flow
NOS	nitric oxide synthase	RCA	right coronary artery

RCT	randomized controlled trial	**TCA**	tricyclic antidepressant
RF	rheumatoid factor	**tds**	three times daily
RICE	rest, ice, compress, and elevate	**TENS**	transcutaneous electronic nerve stimulation
RIF	right iliac fossa		
RNA	ribonucleic acid	**TF**	tissue factor
RPF	renal plasma flow	**TFT**	thyroid function test
RR	respiratory rate	**TGF**	tubuloglomerular feedback
RSI	rapid sequence induction	**TIA**	transient ischaemic attack
RSV	respiratory syncytial virus	**TLC**	total lung capacity
RUQ	right upper quadrant	**TL$_{CO}$**	carbon monoxide transfer factor
RV	residual volume	**Tm**	transport maximum
SA	sinoatrial	**TMJ**	temporomandibular joint
SAN	sinoatrial node	**TNF**	tumour necrosis factor
SAP	systemic arterial pressure	**TOE**	transoesophageal echocardiography
SC	subcutaneous		
SD	standard deviation	**TPA**	tissue (type) plasminogen activator
SIADH	syndrome of inappropriate antidiuretic hormone (hypersecretion)		
		TRH	thyroid-releasing hormone
		TSH	thyroid-stimulating hormone
SIGN	Scottish Intercollegiate Guidelines Network	**TXA2**	thromboxane A2
		UC	ulcerative colitis
SIRS	systemic inflammatory response syndrome	**U&E**	urea and electrolytes
		UMN	upper motor neuron
SL	sublingual	**URTI**	upper respiratory tract infection
SLE	systemic lupus erythematosus	**USS**	ultrasound scan
SMA	supplementary motor area	**UTI**	urinary tract infection
SO$_2$	oxygen saturation	**V$_A$**	alveolar volume
SpO$_2$	percentage of Hb saturated with oxygen	**VC**	vital capacity
		VmC	vomiting centre
SSRI	selective serotonin reuptake inhibitor	**V$_D$**	dead space volume
		VF	ventricular fibrillation
STD	sexually transmitted disease	**VHF**	viral haemorrhagic fever
STI	sexually transmitted infection	**VIP**	vasoactive intestinal polypeptide
STT	spinothalamic tract	**VRG**	ventral respiratory group
SV	stroke volume	**VSCT**	ventral spinocerebellar tract
SVR	systemic vascular resistance	**VSD**	ventricular septal defect
SVT	supraventricular tachycardia	**V$_T$**	tidal volume
t$_{1/2}$	half-life	**VT**	ventricular tachycardia
T1DM	type 1 diabetes mellitus	**VWF**	von Willebrand factor
T2DM	type 2 diabetes mellitus	**VZV**	varicella zoster virus
T3	triiodothyronine	**WBC**	white blood cell
T4	thyroxine	**WCC**	white cell count
TB	tuberculosis	**WPW**	Wolff–Parkinson–White (syndrome)
TBG	thyroxine binding globulin		

First edition contributors

Dr Naveed Azam
General Practitioner (Locum)
Northern Deanery, UK

Dr Daniel Alexander Bearn
ST6 Emergency Medicine
Northern Deanery, UK

Dr Gordon G Boyle
Specialty Registrar
Health Education North East, UK

Dr Mark Harrison
Consultant in Emergency Medicine
Northumbria Healthcare NHS Trust, UK

Lt Col Paul Hunt
Military Consultant and Defence Lecturer in
Emergency Medicine
Defence Medical Group (North), UK

Dr Ellie Kitcatt
Retrieval Registrar
Careflight Medical Services, Australia

Dr Steven Land
Speciality Doctor
Newcastle upon Tyne Hospital NHS Trust, UK

Mr Alister T Oliver
Consultant in Emergency Medicine
Northumbria Healthcare NHS Trust, UK

Dr Matthew Oliver
Advanced Trainee, Emergency Department
Royal Prince Alfred Hospital, Sydney, Australia

Mr Piers Page
Orthopaedic Registrar & Honorary Clinical Lecturer
in Orthopaedic and Trauma Surgery
Frimley Park Hospital, UK & Brighton and Sussex
Medical School, UK

Dr James Taylor
Consultant Emergency Medicine
Queen Elizabeth Hospital, Gateshead, UK

Metka Štrukelj
For providing artwork

SECTION A

ANATOMY

Upper limb

CONTENTS

1.1 Pectoral region

1.1.1 Muscles

- Pectoralis major:
  - From:
    - Sternum
    - Upper 6 costal cartilages
    - Medial ½ clavicle
  - To: anterior axillary fold (lateral humerus)
  - Actions:
    - Adduction of arm
    - Flexion of arm
    - Medial rotation of arm
  - Nerve supply: C5–T1 =
    - Medial pectoral nerve
    - Lateral pectoral nerve
- Pectoralis minor:
  - From: ribs 3–5
  - To: coracoid process of scapula
  - Actions:
    - Depresses tip of shoulder
    - Stabilizes scapula
  - Nerve supply: C8–T1 =
    - Medial pectoral nerve
    - Lateral pectoral nerve
- Trapezius:
  - From:
    - Occipital protuberance
    - Cervical and thoracic vertebrae

- To:
  - Spine of scapula
  - Lateral $\frac{1}{3}$ clavicle
- Actions:
  - Elevates, retracts, and rotates scapula
  - Braces shoulder backwards
- Nerve supply: CN XI = spinal accessory nerve
- Latissimus dorsi:
  - From:
    - T6–L5 spines
    - Iliac crest (thoracolumbar fascia)
  - To: intertubercle groove of humerus
  - Actions:
    - Adduction of arm
    - Medial rotation of arm
    - Raises body towards arms in climbing
  - Nerve supply: C6 + C7 = thoracodorsal nerve
- Serratus anterior:
  - From: lateral surface of ribs 1–8
  - To: medial border of scapula
  - Actions:
    - Rotates scapula (helps abduction)
    - Protracts scapula
    - Holds scapula against thoracic wall
  - Nerve supply: C6 + C7 = long thoracic nerve

1.1.2 Joints

- Sterno-clavicular joint:
  - Fibro-cartilage with articular discs
  - Stability due to ligaments
  - Allows pectoral movements
- Acromio-clavicular joint:
  - As for sterno-clavicular joint
  - Easily dislocated after a fall due to transmission of force and rupture of *acromio-clavicular* ligament and *coraco-clavicular* ligament, making the acromion appear inferior to clavicle and more prominent.

1.2 Axilla

1.2.1 Muscles

- Subscapularis:
  - From: subscapular fossa
  - To: lesser tubercle of humerus
  - Actions:
    - Medial rotation of arm
    - Adduction of arm
  - Nerve supply: C5–7 = subscapular nerves

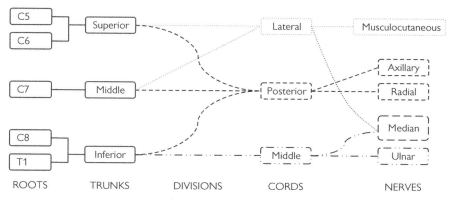

Figure A.1.1 Schematic of brachial plexus

- Teres major:
  - From: lower angle of scapula
  - To: intertubercular sulcus of humerus
  - Actions:
    - Adduction of arm
    - Medial rotation of arm
  - Nerve supply: C6 + C7 = lower subscapular nerve

1.2.2 Contents

- The axilla transmits the neurovascular bundle from the neck to the upper limbs.
- Axillary artery:
  - From: subclavian artery at lateral border of 1st rib
  - To: brachial artery at inferior border of teres major
  - Supplies: circumflex humeral arteries
  - Other: split in 3 by pectoralis minor (number of parts = number of branches in each part)
- Brachial plexus:
  - See Figure A.1.1 for diagram of brachial plexus
  - Potential for damage due to position of plexus in axilla
  - Waiter's tip:
    - Superior plexus injury
    - Separation of neck from shoulder
  - Claw hand:
    - Inferior plexus injury
    - Sudden pull of arm superiorly

1.3 Breast

- Base of breast:
  - Ribs 2–6
  - Lateral edge of sternum
  - Midaxillary line
- Axillary tail: extends laterally under pectoralis

- Lymph drainage:
  - Based upon quadrants of breast
  - Lateral ½:—axillary nodes:
    - Anterior (75%)
    - Central
    - Apical
    - Lateral
  - Medial ½—*parasternal nodes*
  - Other sites:
    - Posterior intercostals nodes
    - Infraclavicular nodes
    - Supraclavicular nodes
  - Minor pathways—important in metastatic spread of malignancy:
    - Opposite breast
    - Anterior abdominal wall
- Chest drains:
  - Insertion site: 5th intercostal space (note this is higher in late pregnancy)
  - Midaxillary line (just lateral to base of the breast)

1.4 Shoulder

1.4.1 Muscles

- Supraspinatus:
  - Actions: initiates abduction of arm
  - Nerve supply: C4–6 = suprascapular nerve
- Infraspinatus:
  - Actions: lateral rotation of arm
  - Nerve supply: C4–6 = suprascapular nerve
- Teres minor:
  - Actions: lateral rotation of arm
  - Nerve supply: C5 + C6 = axillary nerve
- Deltoid:
  - Actions:
    - Ant. flexion and medial rotation of arm
    - Mid. abduction
    - Post. extension and lateral rotation of arm
  - Nerve supply: C5 + C6 = axillary nerve

1.4.2 Movements

- Flexion:
  - 0–90°
  - Pectoralis major
  - Deltoid (anterior)
- Extension:
  - 0–45°
  - Teres major
  - Latissimus dorsi
  - Deltoid (posterior)

- Internal rotation:
  - 0–40°
  - Pectoralis major
  - Latissimus dorsi
  - Teres major
  - Deltoid (anterior)
  - Subscapularis
- External rotation:
  - 0–55°
  - Infraspinatus
  - Teres minor
  - Deltoid (posterior)
- Adduction:
  - 0–45°
  - Pectoralis major
  - Latissimus dorsi
- Abduction:
  - 0–180°
  - Supraspinatus
  - Deltoid (all)
  - Trapezius (rotates scapula)
  - Serratus anterior (rotates scapula)

1.4.3 Shoulder joint

- The shoulder joint is a synovial 'ball and socket' joint allowing multi-axial movement.
- Ligamentous stability by:
  - Glenohumeral ligaments—anterior reinforcement
  - Coraco-humeral ligament—superior reinforcement
  - Coraco-acromial ligament—superior protection
- Coraco-acromial arch:
  - Contains:
    - Supraspinatus tendon insertion
    - Subacromial bursa (does *not* communicate with shoulder joint)
  - Inflammation causes a *painful arc* with limited abduction (60–120°)
  - Muscular stability—*rotator cuff*:
    - Subscapularis (anterior)
    - Supraspinatus (superior)
    - Infraspinatus (posterior)
    - Teres minor (posterior)

1.5 The anterior arm

1.5.1 Muscles

- Coracobrachialis:
  - Actions:
    - Flexion of upper arm
    - Adduction of arm
  - Nerve supply: C5–7 = musculocutaneous nerve

- Brachialis:
  - Actions: flexion of forearm
  - Nerve supply: C5 + C6 = musculocutaneous nerve
- Biceps:
  - Actions:
    - Flexion of forearm
    - Supination of forearm
  - Nerve supply: C5 + C6 = musculocutaneous nerve
  - Others:
    - Brachial pulse felt medial to biceps tendon
    - Median nerve just medial to pulse

1.5.2 Brachial artery

- Commences at *inferior border of teres major* as a continuation of the *axillary artery* and ends by bifurcating into the *radial* and *ulnar arteries* at the level of the *neck of radius* (see Figure A.1.2).
- Lies anterior to triceps and initially medially to humerus before moving anteriorly.
- *Brachial pulse* is felt by pressing laterally at a point medial to the bicipital tendon.
- Accompanied along its course by deep veins of the arm (venae comitantes).
- Branches:
  - Profunda brachii: near origin, winds behind humerus with radial nerve in spiral groove to anastamosis at elbow
  - Muscular artery
  - Nutrient artery: supplies the humerus
  - Ulnar collateral: superior and inferior. Accompanies *ulnar nerve* to anastamosis at elbow

1.5.3 Nerves

- Median nerve:
  - Arises from medial and lateral cords of brachial plexus just lateral to axillary artery

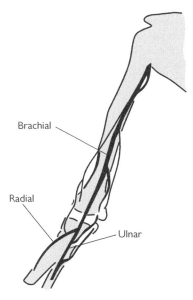

Brachial

Radial

Ulnar

Figure A.1.2 Brachial artery

- ■ Crosses brachial artery medially in the mid-arm
- ■ In cubital fossa lies medially to brachial artery medial to bicipital tendon
- ● Musculocutaneous nerve:
  - ■ Supplies skin of lateral forearm
  - ■ Nerve of flexor component of arm:
    - ● Coracobrachialis
    - ● Brachialis
    - ● Biceps brachii
- ● Ulnar nerve:
  - ■ Passes down medial aspect of arm and runs *posterior* to medial epicondyle
- ● Intercostobrachial nerve:
  - ■ Supplies medial glenoid skin
- ● Medial cutaneous nerve:
  - ■ Of arm: supplies skin on medial side of arm
  - ■ Of forearm: supplies skin on medial side of forearm

1.5.4 Lymph nodes

- ● Supratrochlear:
  - ■ Position: lies subcutaneously above the medial epicondyle
  - ■ Drains:
    - ● Ulnar side of forearm
    - ● Ulnar side of hand
  - ■ To: lymph passes to lateral group of axillary nodes
- ● Infraclavicular:
  - ■ Position: lies in delto-pectoral groove (under mid-clavicle)
  - ■ Drains: radial side of upper limb
  - ■ To: lymph passes to apical group of axillary nodes

1.6 The posterior arm

1.6.1 Muscles

- ● Triceps:
  - ■ Actions: extension of forearm
  - ■ Nerve supply: C6–8 = radial nerve

1.6.2 Radial nerve

- ● Runs with *profunda brachii artery* between long and medial head of triceps into *posterior* compartment, and lays on *spiral groove of humerus* at midpoint. Here it moves *anterior* and passes over the lateral epicondyle.
- ● Due to the fact that it lies in spiral groove, it is susceptible to damage with *humeral shaft fractures*.
- ● It innervates the triceps, causing extension of the forearm.

1.6.3 Elbow joint

- ● This is a synovial hinge joint.
- ● Bony articulations:
  - ■ Humeral capitulum → radial head
  - ■ Trochlea of humerus → trochlear notch of ulna
- ● Ligaments (see Figure A.1.3):
  - ■ Lateral collateral: fan-like on radial side from epicondyle
  - ■ Medial collateral: 3 bands to coranoid process on ulna

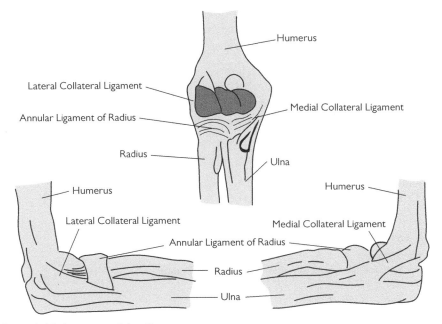

Figure A.1.3 Ligaments of the elbow

- Annular:
  - A loop attached to radial notch of ulna
  - Surrounds head of radius
  - *Allows radial rotation*
- Movements:
  - Flexion (140°):
    - Biceps
    - Brachialis
    - Brachioradialis
  - Extension (0°):
    - Triceps
  - Pronation (90°):
    - Pronator teres
    - Pronator quadratus
  - Supination (90°):
    - Biceps (inserts on radial tuberosity)
    - Supinator
    - Extensor pollicis longus + brevis
- The medial border of the trochlea is greater than the lateral border. This creates the *carrying angle*—the slight lateral angle made between arm and forearm when elbow is extended. If this in increased pathologically then there is a risk of *ulnar nerve palsy*.

1.7 The anterior forearm

1.7.1 Muscles

Figure A.1.4 shows the muscles of the forearm.

- *All* originate from medial humeral epicondyle.

- Pronator teres:
  - Actions: pronation of forearm
  - Nerve supply: C6 + C7 = median nerve
- Flexor carpi radialis:
  - Actions:
    - Flexion of wrist
    - Abduction of hand
  - Nerve supply: C6 + C7 = median nerve
- Flexor digitorum superficialis:
  - Actions: flexion of MP, PP, and wrist
  - Nerve supply: C7–T1 = median nerve
- Palmaris longus:
  - Actions: flexion of wrist
  - Nerve supply: C7 + C8 = median nerve
- Flexor carpi ulnaris:
  - Actions:
    - Flexion of wrist
    - Adduction of hand
  - Nerve supply: C7 + C8 = ulnar nerve
- Flexor digitorum profundus:
  - Actions: flexion of DP + wrist
  - Nerve supply: C8 + T1 = median + ulnar nerve
- Flexor pollicis longus:
  - Actions: flexion of DP + PP of thumb
  - Nerve supply: C8 + T1 = median nerve
- Pronator quadratus:
  - Actions: pronation of forearm
  - Nerve supply: C8 + T1 = median nerve
- (The radial nerve only supplies *extensors* except brachioradialis.)

1.7.2 Arteries

- The *brachial artery* bifurcates into the *radial* and *ulnar arteries* at the neck of the radius.
- Radial artery:
  - Begins in the cubital fossa
  - Passes inferolaterally deep to brachioradialis
  - In distal forearm it lies on anterior surface of radius
  - Pulse felt at wrist *lateral to tendon of flexor carpi radialis*
- Ulnar artery:
  - Begins in cubital fossa
  - Passes deep and descends on FDP with the ulnar nerve
  - Pulse felt at wrist *lateral to tendon of flexor carpi ulnaris*
  - 1st branch (just distal to bifurcation) = *common interosseous artery*

1.7.3 Wrist anastamoses

- Palmar carpal arch:
  - From: radial and ulnar arteries
  - Located: at distal radioulnar joint
  - Supplies: deep palmar arch
- Dorsal carpal arch:
  - From: radial and ulnar arteries
  - Located: over carpal bones
  - Supplies: dorsal MC arteries

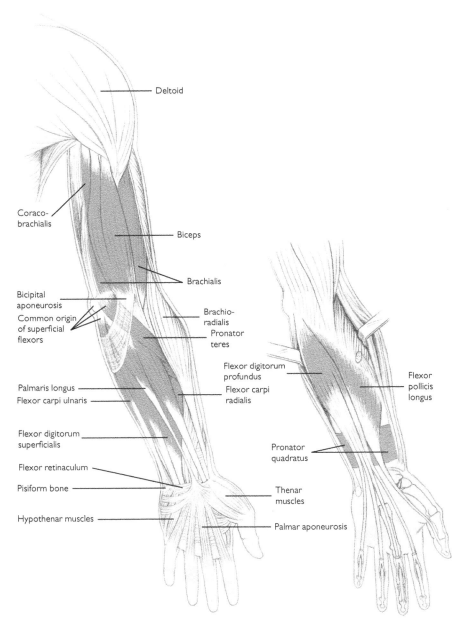

Deltoid

Coraco-
brachialis

Biceps

Brachialis

Bicipital
aponeurosis

Common origin
of superficial
flexors

Brachio-
radialis

Pronator
teres

Flexor digitorum
profundus

Palmaris longus

Flexor carpi ulnaris

Flexor carpi
radialis

Flexor digitorum
superficialis

Flexor retinaculum

Pisiform bone

Hypothenar muscles

Pronator
quadratus

Thenar
muscles

Palmar aponeurosis

Flexor
pollicis
longus

Figure A.1.4 (a) Superficial flexor muscles of arm and forearm. (b) Deep flexor muscles of the forearm

Reproduced with permission from MacKinnon P, Morris J. (2005). *Oxford Textbook of Functional Anatomy*, Vol. 1. Oxford: Oxford University Press, © 2005.

1.7.4 Veins

- Deep veins: consist of venae comitantes (accompanying arteries).
- Superficial veins:
  - Cephalic vein:
    - From snuffbox along lateral to wrist
    - Anterolateral to forearm and arm
    - Follows deltopectoral groove to axillary vein
  - Basilic vein:
    - Medial aspect of wrist and forearm
    - Passes deep in mid-arm to axillary vein
  - Median cubital vein:
    - Communication between basilic and cephalic veins
    - In anterior elbow (cubital fossa)

1.7.5 Nerves

Figure A.1.5 shows the nerves of the forearm.

- Medial cutaneous nerve:
  - Supplies: skin of medial forearm
- Lateral cutaneous nerve:
  - Supplies: skin of distal ½ of lateral forearm
- Median nerve:
  - Lies: medial to brachial artery in cubital fossa
  - Passes: deep between 2 heads of pronator teres
  - Gives off: *anterior interosseous branch*, which supplies the *deep flexors* (FPL, pronator quadratus, FDP)
    - Passes: between FDS and FDP
    - Supplies: *all remaining flexors except FC ulnaris* (FC radialis, FDS, palmaris longus)
    - *Palmar cutaneous branch* just proximal to the wrist, which supplies *skin of thenar eminence* and passes superficial to flexor retinaculum (carpal tunnel) in midline
  - Injury (e.g. slit wrists):
    - Paralysis of thenar muscles and 1st 2 lumbricals
    - Loss of sensation over thumb and 2½ digits
- Ulnar nerve:
  - Lies: posterior to medial epicondyle at elbow
  - Passes: between 2 heads of carpi ulnaris to enter forearm
  - Supplies:
    - Flexor carpi ulnaris
    - FDP (½)
  - Continues: between these 2 muscles to lie lateral to tendon of FC ulnaris at wrist (medial to ulnar artery)
  - Passes: superficial to flexor retinaculum medially

1.7.6 Radioulnar joints

- Pronation:
  - Pronator teres
  - Pronator quadratus
- Supination:
  - Biceps (most powerful)
  - Supinator

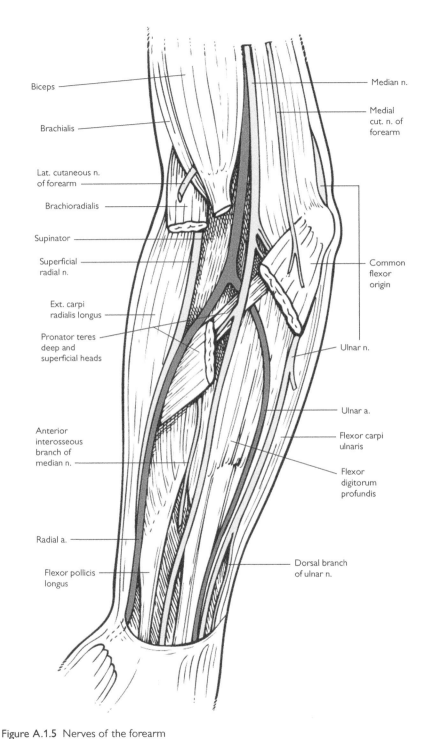

Biceps

Brachialis

Lat. cutaneous n.
of forearm

Brachioradialis

Supinator

Superficial
radial n.

Ext. carpi
radialis longus

Pronator teres
deep and
superficial heads

Anterior
interosseous
branch of
median n.

Radial a.

Flexor pollicis
longus

Median n.

Medial
cut. n. of
forearm

Common
flexor
origin

Ulnar n.

Ulnar a.

Flexor carpi
ulnaris

Flexor
digitorum
profundis

Dorsal branch
of ulnar n.

Figure A.1.5 Nerves of the forearm

Reproduced with permission from McLeod et al., (2012). *Principles and Practice of Regional Anaesthesia* (4 ed.).
Oxford: Oxford University Press, © 2012.

- Extensor pollicis longus
- Extensor pollicis brevis
- Rotation movements of radius and ulna are due to proximal and distal joints.

1.8 Posterior compartment of the forearm

1.8.1 Muscles

Figure A.1.6 shows the muscles in the posterior compartment of the forearm.

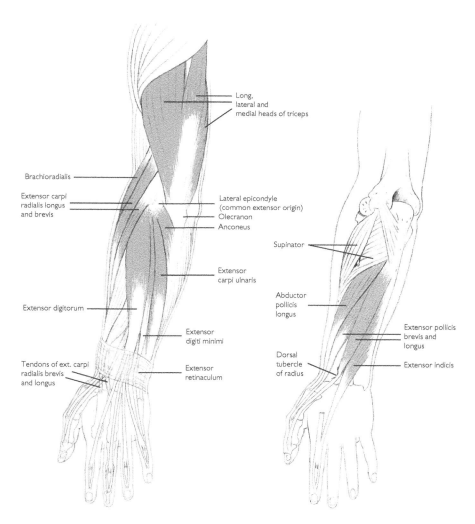

Figure A.1.6 (a) Superficial extensor muscles of arm and forearm. (b) Deep extensor muscles of the forearm

Reproduced with permission from MacKinnon P, Morris J. (2005). *Oxford Textbook of Functional Anatomy*, Vol. 1. Oxford: Oxford University Press, © 2005.

- Brachioradialis:
  - Actions: flexion of forearm
  - Nerve supply: C5–7 = radial nerve
- Extensor carpi radialis longus and extensor carpi radialis brevis:
  - Actions:
    - Extension of wrist
    - Abduction of hand
  - Nerve supply: C6–8 = radial nerve
- Extensor digitorum:
  - Actions:
    - Extension of MCPJ
    - Extension of wrist
  - Nerve supply: C7 + C8 = posterior interosseous nerve (from radial)
- Extensor carpi ulnaris:
  - Actions:
    - Extension of wrist
    - Adduction of hand
  - Nerve supply: C7 + C8 = posterior interosseous nerve
- Supinator:
  - Actions: supination
  - Nerve supply: C5 + C6 = radial nerve
- Abductor pollicis longus:
  - Actions:
    - Abduction of thumb
    - Extension of thumb
  - Nerve supply: C7 + C8 = posterior interosseous nerve
- Extensor pollicis longus:
  - Actions: extension of thumb at MCPJ and IPJ (DP)
  - Nerve supply: C7 + C8 = posterior interosseous nerve
- Extensor pollicis brevis:
  - Actions: extension of thumb at IPJ (PP)
  - Nerve supply: C7 + C8 = posterior interosseous nerve
- Extensor indicis:
  - Actions: extension of index finger
  - Nerve supply: C7 + C8 = Posterior interosseous nerve
- (The radial nerve only supplies *extensors* except brachioradialis (which is a flexor).)

1.8.2 Anatomical snuffbox

- See Figure A.1.7.
- Medial boundary:
  - Extensor pollicis longus
- Lateral boundary:
  - Extensor pollicis brevis
  - Abductor pollicis longus
- Bones palpable:
  - Trapezium
  - Scaphoid (tenderness here is a sign of fracture)

1.8.3 Extensor retinaculum

- This fascia lies over the wrist joint.
- Attachments:
  - Laterally: radius

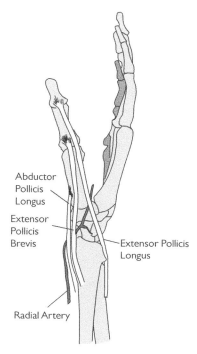

Abductor
Pollicis
Longus

Extensor
Pollicis
Brevis

Extensor Pollicis
Longus

Radial Artery

Figure A.1.7 Anatomical snuffbox

- Medially:
  - Styloid process of ulna
  - Pisiform
  - Triquetrium
- Contents:
  - Radial:
    - Abductor pollicis longus
    - Extensor pollicis brevis
    - Extensor carpi radialis longus
    - Extensor carpi radialis brevis
    - Extensor pollicis longus
    - Extensor digitorum
    - Extensor indicis
    - Extensor digiti minimi
  - Ulnar: extensor carpi ulnaris

1.9 Wrist and hand

1.9.1 Movements

- Flexion (80°):
  - Flexor digitorum profundus
  - Flexor pollicis longus
  - Flexor digitorum superficialis

- Flexor carpi radialis
- Flexor carpi ulnaris
- Palmaris longus
- Extension (80°):
  - Extensor indicis
  - Extensor digitorum
  - Extensor carpi radialis longus
  - Extensor carpi radialis brevis
  - Extensor carpi ulnaris
- Abduction:
  - Flexor carpi radialis
  - Extensor carpi radialis longus
  - Extensor carpi radialis brevis
- Adduction:
  - Flexor carpi ulnaris
  - Extensor carpi ulnaris

1.9.2 Palmar aponeurosis

- Structure:
  - A thick central layer of deep fascia attached to the distal border of the flexor retinaculum
  - *Triangle*-shaped from *palmaris longus* tendon to distally splitting into *4 slips* at the bones of the fingers with the fibrous flexor sheaths
- Function:
  - Protects underlying soft tissues and long flexor tendons

1.9.3 Flexor retinaculum

- Attachments:
  - Laterally =
    - Scaphoid
    - Trapezium
  - Medially =
    - Pisiform
    - Hook of hamate
- Thenar and hypothenar muscles arise from this on either end.
- No arteries or veins transmitted through due to risk of compression. *Ulnar artery and nerve pass over retinaculum therefore are outside of the carpal tunnel.*

1.9.4 Carpal tunnel

- Contains:
  - Separated tendons of FDS
  - Separated tendons of FDP
  - Flexor pollicis longus
  - Flexor carpi radialis
  - Median nerve (superficial)
  - See Figure A.1.8

1.9.5 Thenar eminence

- Abductor pollicis brevis:
  - Actions:
    - Abduction of thumb
    - Helps in opposition
  - Nerve supply: C8 + T1 = median nerve

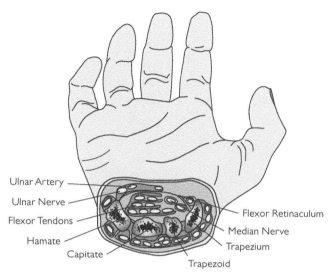

Figure A.1.8 Anatomy of carpal tunnel

- Flexor pollicis brevis:
  - Actions: flexion of PP of thumb
  - Nerve supply: C8 + T1 = median nerve
- Opponens pollicis:
  - Actions: opposition of thumb
  - Nerve supply: C8 + T1 = median nerve

1.9.6 Hypothenar eminence

Figure A.1.9 shows the superficial aspect of the palm.

- Abductor digiti minimi:
  - Actions: abduction of little finger
  - Nerve supply: C8 + T1 = ulnar nerve
- Flexor digiti minimi:
  - Actions: flexion of PP of little finger
  - Nerve supply: C8 + T1 = ulnar nerve
- Opponens digiti minimi:
  - Actions: opposition of little finger
  - Nerve supply: C8 + T1 = ulnar nerve

1.9.7 Palmar arches

- Deep:
  - Mainly radial, contribution from ulnar:
    - 3 palmar metacarpal arteries (middle, ring, little)
    - Princeps pollicis (thumb)
    - Radialis indicis (index)
- Superficial:
  - Contribution from radial, mainly ulnar:
    - 3 common palmar digital arteries (middle, ring, little)
    - Thenar muscles

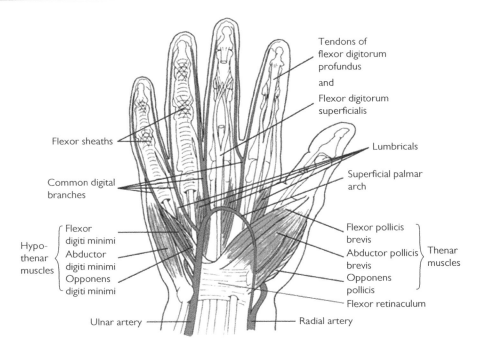

Figure A.1.9 Superficial aspect of palm

Reproduced with permission from MacKinnon P, Morris J. (2005). *Oxford Textbook of Functional Anatomy*, Vol. 1. Oxford: Oxford University Press, © 2005.

- Damage: profuse bleeding and due to dual supply need to compress brachial artery with a tourniquet.

1.9.8 Digital nerves

- Median nerve—supplies:
  - 1st and 2nd lumbricals
  - Cutaneous supply to palmar skin of thumb, index, middle and ½ ring fingers
  - *Recurrent branch* to thenar muscles (opponens pollicis, abductor pollicis brevis, flexor pollicis brevis)—this can be severed by minor laceration of thenar eminence causing paralysis of thumb
- Ulnar nerve—supplies:
  - Cutaneous supply to medial 1½ fingers
  - 3rd and 4th lumbricals
  - All dorsal interossei
  - Adductor pollicis
  - Hypothenar muscles (flexor digiti minimi, abductor digiti minimi, opponens digiti minimi)
- Digital nerves are *palmar terminal branches* of cutaneous supply and run down lateral aspect of each digit on both sides.

1.9.9 Lumbricals and interossei

- Lumbricals:
  - Origin: sides of tendons of FDP
  - Attachments: lateral extensor expansions of extensor digitorum and PP

- Nerve supply: C8 + T1 = ulnar (medial 2), median (lateral 2)
- Actions:
  - Flexion of MCPJ
  - Extension of IPJ
- Palmar interossei:
  - Origin: inside of MCP 2, 4, and 5
  - Nerve supply: C8 + T1 = ulnar nerve
  - Actions:
    - Assist lumbricals (flex MCPJ and extend IPJ)
    - Adduction of digits (not middle)
- Dorsal interossei:
  - Origin: between each 2 MCPJs (therefore 4)
  - Nerve supply: C8 + T1 = ulnar nerve
  - Actions:
    - Assist lumbricals
    - Abduction of digits (middle either way)
- Palmar ADduct, Dorsal ABduct = PAD-DAB

1.9.10 The flexor sheaths

- Digital flexor tendons lie within synovial sheaths to enable tendons to slide freely over each other during movement (see Figure A.1.10).
- Puncture wounds (e.g. rusty nail) can cause infection of synovial sheaths (= *tenosynovitis*) causing a swollen digit and *painful movement*.
- Index, middle, and ring finger have separate synovial sheaths, therefore infection usually confined in digit.

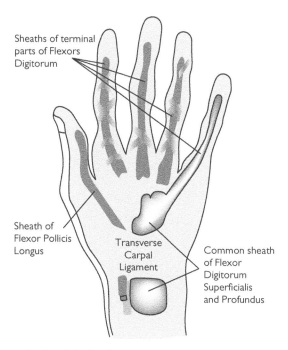

Figure A.1.10 Flexor sheaths of the hand

- If neglected, proximal end of sheath may rupture and allow infection to spread to the *midpalmar space*.
- Synovial sheaths of thumb and little finger are often continuous with the *common flexor synovial sheath* and infection may spread easily.

1.10 The digital attachments of the long tendons

1.10.1 Flexor tendons

- Flexor pollicis longus: base of DP of thumb.
- FDP: base of DP of all 4 fingers.
- FDS: either side of bodies of MP of all 4 fingers.
- Palmaris longus: becomes flexor retinaculum and palmar aponeurosis.

1.10.2 Extensor tendons

- Extensor pollicis longus: base of DP of thumb.
- Extensor pollicis brevis: base of PP of thumb.
- Abductor pollicis longus: base of 1st MC.
- Extensor digitorum: base of DP and MP of all 4 fingers via extensor expansion.
- Extensor digiti minimi: extensor expansion of little finger.
- Extensor indicis: extensor expansion of index finger.

1.11 Other aspects of upper limb anatomy

1.11.1 Dermatomes

See Figure A.1.11.

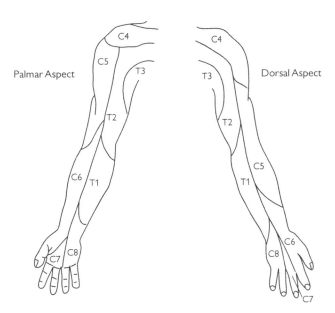

Figure A.1.11 Dermatomes of the upper limb

1.11.2 Innervation of muscles

- Shoulder:
  - Flexion:
    - Lateral and medial pectoral nerves (pec. major)
    - Musculocutaneous nerve (coracobrachialis)
    - Axillary nerve (deltoid)
  - Extension:
    - Lower subscapular nerve (teres major)
    - Thoracodorsal nerve (latissimus dorsi)
    - Axillary nerve (deltoid)
  - Internal rotation:
    - Lateral and medial pectoral nerves (pec. major)
    - Thoracodorsal nerve (latissimus dorsi)
    - Axillary nerve (deltoid)
    - Upper and lower subscapular nerves (teres major + subscapularis)
  - External rotation:
    - Suprascapular nerve (infraspinatus)
    - Axillary nerve (teres minor + deltoid)
  - Adduction:
    - Lateral and medial pectoral nerves (pec. major)
    - Thoracodorsal nerve (latissimus dorsi)
  - Abduction:
    - Suprascapular nerve (infraspinatus)
    - Axillary nerve (deltoid)
    - Accessory nerve (trapezius)
    - Long thoracic nerve (serratus anterior)
- Elbow:
  - Flexion:
    - Musculocutaneous nerve (biceps + brachialis)
    - Radial nerve (brachioradialis)
  - Extension:
    - Radial nerve (triceps)
  - Pronation:
    - Median nerve (pronator teres + pronator quadratus)
  - Supination:
    - Musculocutaneous nerve (biceps)
    - Radial nerve (supinator)
    - Posterior interosseous nerve (extensor pollicis longus + brevis)
- Wrist:
  - Flexion:
    - Median nerve (FDS + FDP + palmaris longus + flexor carpi radialis)
    - Anterior interosseous nerve (flexor pollicis longus)
    - Ulnar nerve (flexor carpi ulnaris)
  - Extension:
    - Posterior interosseous nerve (extensor indicis + digitorum + extensor carpi ulnaris)
    - Radial nerve (extensor carpi radialis longus + brevis)
  - Abduction:
    - Median nerve (flexor carpi radialis)
    - Radial nerve (extensor carpi radialis longus + brevis)

- Adduction:
  - Ulnar nerve (flexor carpi ulnaris)
  - Posterior interosseous nerve (extensor carpi ulnaris)

1.11.3 Injuries to nerves

- Brachial plexus:
  - Excessive downward traction of upper limbs (separation of head and neck), e.g. birth/RTA.
  - *Causes Erb's palsy* = C5 + C6 = *Waiter's tip* =
    - Pronation
    - Medial rotation
    - Wrist flexion (behind)
  - Excessive upward traction of upper limbs, e.g. fall and grab branch/birth.
  - *Causes Klumpke's palsy* = C8 + T1 =
    - Claw hand
    - Horner's syndrome
- Axillary nerve:
  - Caused by *surgical neck of humerus fracture or shoulder dislocation*
  - Motor effect: loss of deltoid abduction
  - Sensory effect: 'regimental badge' area of deltoid
- Radial nerve:
  - Caused by *humeral shaft fracture*
  - Motor effect: loss of forearm extensors (*wrist drop*)
  - Sensory effect: loss of anatomical snuffbox
- Ulnar nerve:
  - Caused by *medial epicondyle fracture* or *wrist laceration*
  - Motor effect:
    - (below elbow): *claw hand* of ring and little fingers
    - (above elbow): small muscle wasting
  - Sensory effect: loss of medial 1½ digits and hand
- Median nerve:
  - Caused by *carpal tunnel syndrome* or *wrist laceration*
  - Motor effect: weakness and wasting of thenar muscles
  - Sensory effect: loss of lateral palm and 2½ digits

Lower limb

CONTENTS

2.1 Anterior thigh

2.1.1 Superficial innervation

- Dermatomal pattern of innervation from L1 to L5 (see Figure A.2.1).

2.1.2 Superficial arteries

- Just after the femoral artery emerges from under the inguinal ligament, it gives off 4 cutaneous branches supplying the superficial tissues of the lower abdominal wall and perineum.

2.1.3 Superficial veins

- The great saphenous vein:
  - Arises: medial end of dorsal venous arch on the foot
  - Passes:
    - Anterior to medial malleolus along anteromedial aspect of the calf
    - Migrates posteriorly to a hand's-breadth behind patella (anterior to medial epicondyle)
    - Ascends anteromedial thigh
  - Drains: into femoral vein at the saphenous opening
  - Tributaries:
    - At the ankle branches from sole of foot through the medial marginal vein
    - In the lower leg the anterior and posterior tibial veins and many cutaneous veins
    - In the thigh numerous tributaries; those from the medial and posterior parts of the thigh frequently unite to form a large *accessory saphenous vein*
    - Near the saphenous opening the superficial epigastric, superficial iliac circumflex, and superficial external pudendal veins

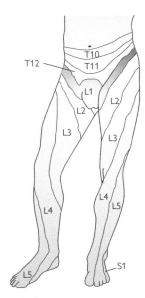

Figure A.2.1 Dermatomes of lower limb

2.1.4 Lymph nodes/vessels

- The lymph nodes of the groin are arranged into *superficial* and *deep* groups.
- Superficial:
  - Located: in the superficial fascia and arranged in 2 chains
  - Longitudinal:
    - Lie along the terminal portion of the saphenous vein
    - Receive lymph from the majority of the superficial tissues of the lower limb
  - Horizontal:
    - Lie parallel to the inguinal ligament
    - Receive lymph from the superficial tissues of the lower trunk (below umbilicus), buttock, external genitalia, and lower half of anal canal
- Deep:
  - Located: medial to the femoral vein (usually 3 of them)
  - Drain:
    - All of the tissues deep to the fascia lata of the lower limb
    - Skin and superficial tissues of the heel and lateral aspect of the foot

2.1.5 Muscles

Figure A.2.2 shows the muscles of the front of the lower limb.

- Sartorius:
  - Actions:
    - Flexion of the hip
    - Abduction of the hip
    - Lateral rotation of the hip
    - Flexion of the knee
    - ('Tailor's position' of sitting cross-legged)
  - Innervation: L2–L3 = femoral nerve

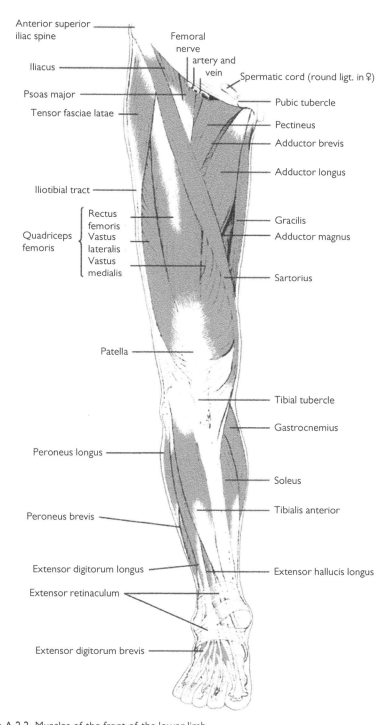

Figure A.2.2 Muscles of the front of the lower limb

Reproduced with permission from MacKinnon P, Morris J. (2005). *Oxford Textbook of Functional Anatomy*, Vol. 1.
Oxford: Oxford University Press, © 2005.

- Iliacus:
  - Actions: flexion of the hip
  - Innervation: L2 = femoral nerve
- Psoas major:
  - Actions:
    - Flexion of the hip
    - Postural muscle controlling deviation of the trunk when standing
  - Innervation: L1–L3 = femoral nerve
- Pectineus:
  - Actions:
    - Adduction of the hip
    - Flexion of the hip
  - Innervation: L2–L3 = femoral nerve, obturator nerve
- Quadriceps femoris (rectus femoris, vastus lateralis, vastus medialis, vastus intermedialis):
  - Actions:
    - Extension of the knee
    - Stabilization of the knee
    - Flexion of hip (only rectus and weak)
  - Innervation: L2–4 = femoral nerve

2.1.6 Movements

- Hip flexion:
  - 0–120°
  - Iliacus
  - Psoas major
  - Rectus femoris
  - Sartorius
  - Pectineus
- Knee extension:
  - Quadriceps femoris

2.1.7 Femoral sheath

- The *femoral sheath* is an inferior prolongation of the extraperitoneal fascia from the abdomen. It is a funnel-shaped tube emerging from behind the inguinal ligament and ending 4cm inferior to this. It contains the femoral artery and femoral vein, *not* the femoral nerve.
- The *femoral canal* is the short, conical medial compartment of the femoral sheath that lies between the medial edge of the femoral sheath and the femoral vein. This space allows the femoral vein to expand with increased venous return from the lower limb.
- The *femoral ring* is the small (1cm) superior end (abdominal opening) of the femoral canal. Its boundaries are:
  - Laterally—femoral vein
  - Posteriorly—superior ramus of pubis
  - Medially—lacunar ligament and conjoint tendon
  - Anteriorly—medial part of inguinal ligament
- The *femoral artery* is a continuation of the external iliac artery. It commences at the mid-inguinal point behind the inguinal ligament.
- The *femoral vein* lies immediately medial to the femoral artery in the groin. This is clinically significant in that it allows simple palpation to identify the site for central line insertion.

- The *femoral nerve* is derived from the posterior divisions of L2–L4 (see Figure A.2.3). It passes under the inguinal ligament immediately lateral to the femoral artery. 5cm distal to the inguinal ligament it divides into:
  - Superficial:
    - *Medial* and *intermediate cutaneous branches* supplying skin over the anterior and medial thigh
    - 2 muscular branches (*pectineus* and *sartorius*)
  - Deep:
    - 4 muscular branches (*quadriceps femoris*)
    - *Saphenous nerve* descending beyond the knee supplying skin over medial aspect of leg and foot

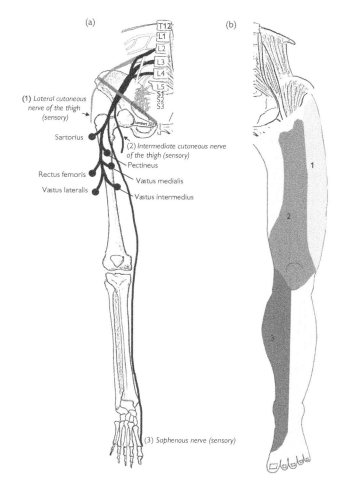

Figure A.2.3 (a) Femoral nerve: supply to muscles. (b) Femoral nerve: supply to skin; 1 = lateral cutaneous nerve of the thigh (L2–3), 2 = anterior (intermediate) cutaneous femoral nerve (L2–3), 3 = saphenous nerve (L3–4)

2.1.8 Patellar region

- The 4 parts of the quadriceps unite with their tendons to form the quadriceps tendon, which attaches to the patella.
- The *patellar ligament* is a continuation of this, and attaches the apex of the patella (inferiorly) and the tibial tuberosity.
- This is therefore the true insertion of the quadriceps and the patella is thus a sesamoid bone.
- The patella site in the femoral groove: the *medial patellar ligament* and the *vastus medialis* muscle are important structures in preventing the patella from dislocating or subluxing laterally.

2.2 Medial thigh

2.2.1 Muscles and movements

- Adductor longus:
  - Actions: adduction of the hip
  - Innervation: L2–L4 = obturator nerve
- Adductor brevis:
  - Actions: adduction of the hip
  - Innervation: L2–L4 = obturator nerve
- Adductor magnus:
  - Actions:
    - Adduction of the hip
    - Extension of the hip
  - Innervation:
    - L2–L4 = obturator nerve (adduction)
    - L4 = sciatic nerve (extension)
- These 2 muscles also have a role in medial femoral rotation (but to a lesser extent than *gluteus medius* and *gluteus minimis*).
- Obturator externus:
  - Actions: lateral rotation of the hip
  - Innervation: L3 + L4 = obturator nerve
- To test adduction strength the examiner slips their active hand under the medial aspect of the patient's knee and applies increasing resistance as the patient adducts their thigh toward the midline.

2.2.2 Arteries and nerves

- The *profunda femoris artery* is the chief artery to the thigh and is the largest branch of the femoral artery.
- The *obturator artery* arises from the internal iliac artery and assists the profunda femoris artery in supplying the adductor muscles of the thigh.
- The *obturator nerve* supplies:
  - Muscular:
    - Adductor longus
    - Adductor brevis
    - Adductor magnus
    - Gracilis
    - Obturator externus
    - Pectineus
  - Cutaneous: skin of medial aspect of thigh

2.3 Hip joint and gluteal region

2.3.1 Cutaneous innervation

- Cutaneous supply is via both the posterior and anterior rami of the lumbosacral nerves (see Figure A.2.4).

2.3.2 Muscles and movements

Figure A.2.5 shows the muscles at the back of the lower limb.

- Gluteus maximus:
  - Actions:
    - Extension of the hip
    - Lateral rotation of the hip
  - Innervation: L5–S2 = Inferior gluteal nerve
- Gluteus medius:
  - Actions:
    - Abduction of the hip
    - Medial rotation of the hip
    - Prevents pelvis tilting to unsupported side when walking
  - Innervation: L5 + S1 = superior gluteal nerve
- Gluteus minimus:
  - Actions:
    - Abduction of the hip
    - Medial rotation of the hip
    - Prevents pelvis tilting to unsupported side when walking
  - Innervation: L5 + S1 = superior gluteal nerve

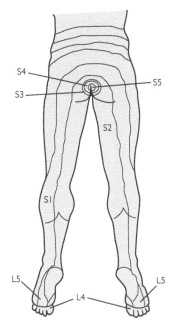

Figure A.2.4 Dermatomes of lower limb

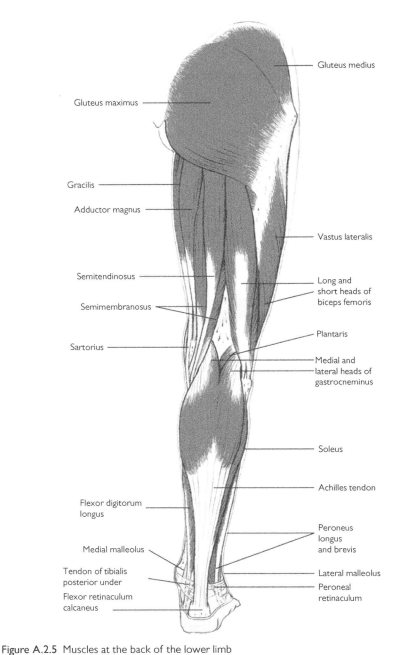

Figure A.2.5 Muscles at the back of the lower limb

Reproduced with permission from MacKinnon P, Morris J. (2005). *Oxford Textbook of Functional Anatomy*, Vol. 1. Oxford: Oxford University Press, © 2005.

- Piriformis:
  - Action: lateral rotation of the hip
  - Innervation: branches of ventral rami of S1 + S2 from sacral plexus
- Piriformis, obturator internus, and quadratus femoris act together synergistically to laterally rotate the extended hip, abduct the flexed hip, and steady the femoral head in the acetabulum.

2.3.3 Sciatic nerve

- The sciatic nerve originates from the anterior primary rami of the sacral plexus (L4–S3).
- It leaves the pelvis through the greater sciatic foramen (inferior to piriformis) and descends in the midline deep to gluteus maximus.
- It divides into its terminal branches in the mid-thigh (tibial nerve and common peroneal nerve).

2.3.4 Clinical relevance for IM injections

- With respect to the sciatic nerve, the buttock has a side of safety (lateral) and a side of danger (medial).
- Injections in the medial side may injure the sciatic nerve and its branches to the hamstrings.
- Injections can be made safely only into the superolateral part of the buttock (see Figure A.2.6).

2.3.5 Hip joint

- The bony acetabulum consists of:
  - Ileum (superior)
  - Ischium (postero-inferior)
  - Pubis (anterior)
- The inferior margin is completed by the *transverse acetabular ligament*.
- From the floor of the acetabulum, the weak *ligamentum teres* attaches to the femoral head.
- The main stability of the joint is provided by 3 ligaments—the *iliofemoral ligament*, the *pubofemoral ligament* and the *ischiofemoral ligament*.
- The capsule of the hip joint is attached proximally to the acetabulum and the transverse acetabular ligament. It attaches distally to the intertrochanteric line and to the bases of the trochanters. This capsule carries some fibres forming *retinacula*, which contain blood vessels derived from branches of the *circumflex femoral arteries*.
- The nerve supply is from branches of the femoral, sciatic, and obturator nerve.

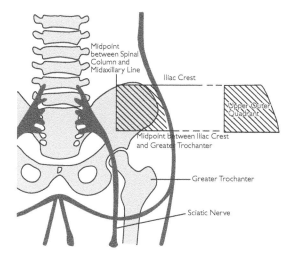

Figure A.2.6 Safe area of buttock

2.3.6 Movements

- Flexion:
  - 0–120°
  - Iliacus
  - Psoas major
  - (Rectus femoris)
  - (Sartorius)
  - (Pectineus)
- Extension:
  - 0–20°
  - Gluteus maximus
  - Hamstrings:
    - Biceps femoris
    - Semimembranosus
    - Semitendinosus
- Adduction:
  - 0–30°
  - Adductor magnus
  - Adductor longus
  - Adductor brevis
  - (Gracilis)
  - (Pectineus)
- Abduction:
  - 0–45°
  - Gluteus medius
  - Gluteus minimis
  - Tensor fascia latae
- External rotation:
  - 0–45°
  - Piriformis
  - Obturator internus
  - Obturator externus
  - Gemellus inferior
  - Gemellus superior
  - Quadratus femoris
  - Gluteus maximus
- Internal rotation:
  - 0–45°
  - Tensor fascia latae
  - Gluteus medius
  - Gluteus minimis

2.4 Posterior thigh compartment

2.4.1 Muscles and movements

- Biceps femoris:
  - Actions:
    - Extension of the hip
    - Flexion of the knee
  - Innervation: L5–S2 = sciatic nerve

- Semitendinosus:
  - Actions:
    - Extension of the hip
    - Flexion of the knee
  - Innervation: L5–S2 = sciatic nerve
- Semimembranosus:
  - Actions:
    - Extension of the hip
    - Flexion of the knee
  - Innervation: L5–S2 = sciatic nerve
- To test the integrity of the hamstrings, position the patient so they are flexed at the waist with their torso lying on the bed and they are standing on the floor. Then ask them to flex their knees and lift their legs off the floor. This demonstrates at least grade III power.

2.4.2 Sciatic nerve

- The sciatic nerve has a curved course through the gluteal region but descends into the thigh in the midline posteriorly.
- It divides into its terminal branches (tibial and common peroneal nerve) at a point roughly a hand's-breadth above the popliteal crease.
- It supplies:
  - Nerve to quadratus femoris
  - Nerve to obturator internus
  - Muscular branches to hamstrings

2.5 Popliteal fossa and knee

2.5.1 Boundaries and composition of the popliteal fossa

- The popliteal fossa is rhomboidal in shape (see Figure A.2.7).

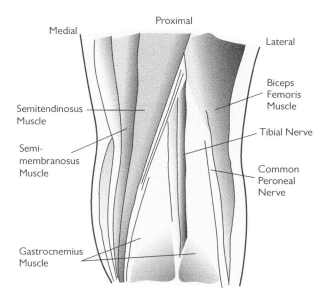

Figure A.2.7 Popliteal fossa

- Its boundaries are:
  - Biceps tendon (superolateral)
  - Semimembranosus (superomedial)
  - Semitendinosus (superomedial)
  - Medial head gastrocnemius (inferomedial)
  - Lateral head gastrocnemius (inferolateral)
  - Skin and fascia (roof)
  - Femur (floor)
  - Popliteus (floor)
- The contents of the fossa are (deep to superficial): the *popliteal artery*, the *popliteal vein*, and the *tibial nerve*. The *common peroneal nerve* runs along the medial border of biceps tendon and then out of the fossa.
- Because the popliteal artery is deep, it is very difficult to feel the popliteal pulse. If it is easily palpable then a popliteal aneurysm should be considered. Palpation of the pulse is performed by placing the patient prone with the leg flexed to relax the popliteal fascia and hamstrings.

2.5.2 Muscles and movements

- Popliteus:
  - Actions:
    - Initiation of flexion of the knee
    - Lateral rotation of the femur on the tibia (thus 'unlocking' the extended knee joint)
    - Posterior draw of lateral meniscus in knee flexion
  - Innervation: L4–S1 = tibial nerve

2.5.3 Knee joint

- The knee joint is a synovial hinge joint that also allows a small degree of rotation.
- The femoral and tibial condyles articulate medially and laterally, and the patella articulates with the femur between them. The condyles are anatomically adapted to allow the 'screw-home' movement of knee locking in extension.
- The *articular capsule* is strong and fibrous. It attaches to the femur superiorly (proximal to condyles) and to the articular margin of the tibia inferiorly. There are 2 openings— on the lateral condyle for popliteus, and anteriorly to communicate with the *suprapatellar bursa*.
- Ligaments:
  - Medial collateral: resists valgus deformity
  - Lateral collateral: resists varus deformity
  - Oblique popliteal: strengthens the capsule posteriorly
  - Anterior cruciate: prevents posterior displacement of the femur on the tibia
  - Posterior cruciate: prevents anterior displacement of the femur on the tibia
- The menisci are crescentic fibrocartilage that act as 'shock-absorbers' and facilitate lubrication of the knee joint.
- Bursae (see Figure A.2.8):
  - Suprapatellar: communicates with knee joint
  - Semimembranosus
  - Popliteus: communicates with knee joint
  - Anserine: communicates with knee joint
  - Gastrocnemius: communicates with knee joint
  - Subcutaneous prepatellar
  - Subcutaneous infrapatellar
  - Deep infrapatellar

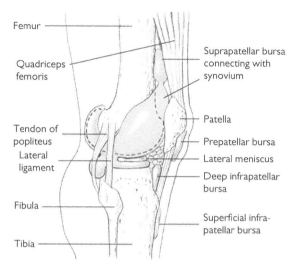

Figure A.2.8 Synovial membrane and bursae of knee

Reproduced with permission from MacKinnon P, Morris J. (2005). *Oxford Textbook of Functional Anatomy*, Vol. 1. Oxford: Oxford University Press, © 2005.

2.5.4 Movements

- Extension:
  - Quadriceps femoris
- Flexion:
  - Hamstrings
  - Gracilis
  - Gastrocnemius
  - Sartorius
- Internal rotation of tibia (unlocking):
  - Popliteus
- The knee is a major weightbearing joint, and its stability depends almost entirely on its associated ligaments and muscles. The collateral ligaments prevent disruption of the sides of the knee joint. The anteroposterior relationship of the femur and the tibia is maintained by the cruciate ligaments and the tibial spine.

2.6 Anterior leg

2.6.1 Muscles

- Tibialis anterior:
  - Actions:
    - Dorsiflexion of the ankle
    - Inversion of the foot
  - Innervation: L4–L5 = deep peroneal nerve
- Extensor hallucis longus:
  - Actions:
    - Extension of the big toe
    - Dorsiflexion of the ankle
  - Innervation: L5–S1 = deep peroneal nerve

- Extensor digitorum longus:
  - Actions:
    - Extension of lateral four digits
    - Dorsiflexion of the ankle
  - Innervation: L5–S1 = deep peroneal nerve
- Peroneus tertius:
  - Actions:
    - Dorsiflexion of the ankle
    - (Eversion of the foot)
  - Innervation: L5–S1 = deep peroneal nerve
- Gracilis:
  - Actions:
    - Adduction of the hip
    - Flexion of the hip
    - (Medial rotation of the hip)
  - Innervation: L2–L3 = obturator nerve
- The tendons of the 4 parts of the quadriceps femoris unite to form the *quadriceps tendon*. This broad band attaches to the patella. The *patellar ligament* attaches the patella to the tibial tuberosity and is the continuation of the quadriceps tendon.
- There are 4 main bursae around the patella:
  - Suprapatellar—between femur and quadriceps tendon
  - Subcutaneous prepatellar—between skin and patella
  - Subcutaneous infrapatellar—between skin and tibial tuberosity
  - Deep intrapatellar—between patellar ligament and tibia

2.7 Dorsum of the foot

2.7.1 Innervation
See Figures A.2.9–A.2.11.

2.7.2 Vessels
- The *dorsalis pedis artery* is a direct continuation of the *anterior tibial artery* distal to the front of the ankle joint midway between the malleoli.
- It is flanked on either side by *tibialis anterior* and *extensor digitorum longus*.
- The artery travels anteromedially down the dorsum of the foot to the base of the metatarsals before passing towards the sole at the first interosseous space.

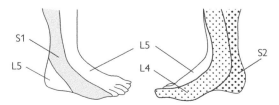

Figure A.2.9 Dermatomes of foot

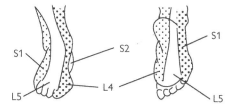

Figure A.2.10 Dermatomes of sole

2.8 Lateral leg

2.8.1 Muscles

- Peroneus longus:
  - Actions:
    - Eversion of the foot
    - (Plantarflexion of the ankle)
  - Innervation: L5–S2 = superficial peroneal nerve
  - Insertion: base of 1st metatarsal + medial cuneiform
- Peroneus brevis:
  - Actions:
    - Eversion of the foot
    - (Plantarflexion of the ankle)
  - Innervation: L5–S2 = superficial peroneal nerve
  - Insertion: base of 5th metatarsal
- The tendons of both peroneus longus and brevis pass posteriorly to the lateral malleolus and are held in place underneath the *peroneus retinaculum*. As such these tendons are commonly injured (strained) with ankle inversion injuries.

2.9 Posterior leg (calf)

- The deep veins form an extensive network within the posterior compartment of the calf (around soleus) from which blood is assisted upwards against gravitational

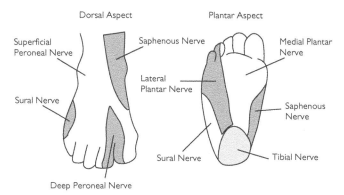

Figure A.2.11 Innervation of the foot

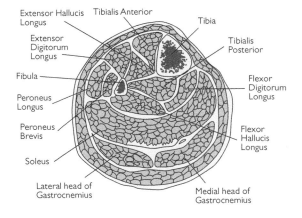

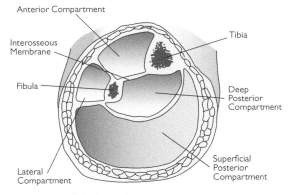

Figure A.2.12 Compartments of the lower leg

forces by muscular contraction during exercise. Failure of this 'muscle pump' to work efficiently (e.g. during long flights) may cause *deep vein thrombosis* (DVT).

- Fascial septa and the interosseous membrane of the lower leg divide the leg into 4 compartments (see Figure A.2.12). Following fractures of the leg, oedema within one or more compartments can lead to obstruction of blood flow with consequent infarction of tissue—'*compartment syndrome*'.
- The calf muscles can be divided into 2 groups—superficial and deep:
  - The superficial group comprises 3 muscles:
    - Gastrocnemius
    - Soleus
    - Plantaris
  - The deep group comprises:
    - Popliteus
    - Flexor hallucis longus
    - Flexor digitorum longus
    - Tibialis posterior

2.9.1 Muscles and movements

Figure A.2.13 shows the deep muscles of the calf.

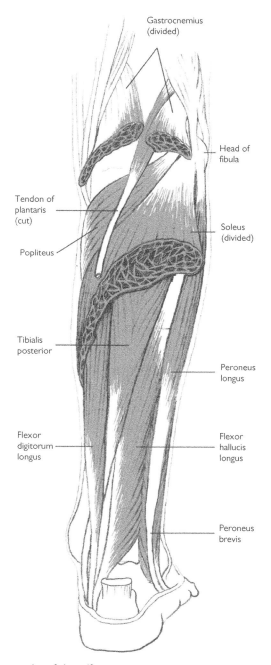

Gastrocnemius
(divided)

Head of
fibula

Tendon of
plantaris
(cut)

Popliteus

Soleus
(divided)

Tibialis
posterior

Peroneus
longus

Flexor
digitorum
longus

Flexor
hallucis
longus

Peroneus
brevis

Figure A.2.13 Deep muscles of the calf

Reproduced with permission from MacKinnon P, Morris J. (2005). *Oxford Textbook of Functional Anatomy*, Vol. 1. Oxford: Oxford University Press, © 2005.

- Gastrocnemius:
  - Actions:
    - Plantar flexion of the foot
    - (Flexion of the knee)
  - Innervation: S1 + S2 = tibial nerve
- Soleus:
  - Actions:
    - Plantar flexion of the foot
    - ('Muscle pump')
  - Innervation: S1 + S2 = tibial nerve
- Flexor digitorum longus:
  - Actions:
    - Flexion of the lateral 4 toes
    - (Plantar flexion of the foot)
  - Innervation: S2 + S3 = tibial nerve
- Flexor hallucis longus:
  - Actions:
    - Flexion of the great toe
    - (Plantar flexion of the foot)
  - Innervation: S2 + S3 = tibial nerve
- Tibialis posterior:
  - Actions:
    - Plantar flexion of the foot
    - Inversion of the foot
  - Innervation: L4 + L5 = tibial nerve
  - Insertions: tuberosity of navicular, medial, and lateral cuneiforms, and cuboid and bases of 2nd, 3rd, and 4th metatarsals

2.9.2 Vessels

- The *posterior tibial artery* provides the main blood supply to the foot. It is the largest terminal branch of the *popliteal artery*.
- At the ankle the posterior tibial artery runs posterior to the medial malleolus from which it is separated by the tendons of the tibialis posterior and flexor digitorum longus.

2.9.3 Nerves

- The *tibial nerve* crosses the popliteal fossa and descends in the median plane of the calf, deep to soleus.
- Together with the posterior tibial artery it passes behind the medial malleolus.
- It supplies all the muscles of the posterior (flexor) compartment of the lower leg.

2.10 Sole of the foot

- The sole is described as consisting of an aponeurosis and 4 muscle layers.
- The plantar arteries and nerves lie between the 1st and 2nd muscle layers.
- This has implications for the structures likely to be compromised when the sole is injured.

2.10.1 The four muscle layers

- 1st layer (not required).
- 2nd layer:
  - Tendon of flexor digitorum longus
  - Tendon of flexor hallucis longus

- 3rd layer (not required).
- 4th layer:
  - Tendon of tibialis posterior
  - Tendon of peroneus longus

2.11 Ankle and foot joints; joint dynamics

2.11.1 Ankle joint

- The ankle joint is a synovial hinge joint. The inferior ends of the tibia and fibula form a deep socket (*mortise*) into which the talus fits, allowing weightbearing through the joint from talus to tibia. The lateral and medial malleoli act as stabilizers by gripping the talus as it moves anteriorly and posteriorly.
- The ankle joint is reinforced medially by the strong *deltoid ligament* that attaches proximally to the medial malleolus and distally to the talus/calcaneus/navicular.
- The ankle is reinforced laterally by the '*lateral*' ligament, which consists of three bands:
  - The anterior talofibular ligament from the lateral malleolus to the neck of the talus
  - The posterior talofibular ligament from the malleolar fossa to the lateral tubercle of the talus
  - The calcaneofibular ligament from the tip of the lateral malleolus to the lateral surface of the calcaneus

2.11.2 Ankle movements

- The movements of the ankle are dorsiflexion and plantarflexion. As such, the axis of rotation of the ankle is usually stated to be horizontal (or transverse).
- The superior articulating surface of the talus is wedge shaped from front to back. The ankle is very stable during dorsiflexion because in this position the trochlea of the talus fills the mortise formed by the malleoli. The ankle joint is relatively unstable during plantarflexion because the trochlea of the talus is narrower posteriorly and therefore does not fill the mortise. As a result inversion, eversion, abduction, and adduction occur only in plantarflexion.

2.11.3 Tarsal joints

- All the foot bones are united by interosseous dorsal and plantar ligaments. The plantar ligaments are important in maintaining the arches of the foot.
- The *plantar calcaneonavicular ligament* or 'spring ligament' runs from the sustentaculum tali of the calcaneus to the postero-inferior surface of the navicular (medial). It supports the head of the talus and thus supports the arch of the foot. If it yields the patient becomes 'flat-footed'. It contains elastic fibres, giving elasticity to the arch and spring to the foot.

2.11.4 Foot movements

- Inversion and eversion of the foot involve the midtarsal and subtalar joints.
- The subtalar joint involves the talus, calcaneus, and navicular bones (the *talocalcaneal* joint and the *talocalcaneonavicular* joint).
- The midtarsal joint comprises the calcaneus, cuboid, talus, and navicular bones (the *calcaneocuboid* joint and the *talonavicular* joint). See Figure A.2.14.
- Tibialis anterior and tibialis posterior invert the foot. Peroneus longus and peroneus brevis evert the foot.

2.11.5 Supporting mechanisms of the foot

- When standing normally the calcaneus and the metatarsal heads rest on the floor. Between these weightbearing points are arches of the foot.

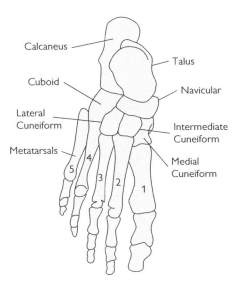

Figure A.2.14 Bones of the foot

- The medial longitudinal arch comprises calcaneus, talus (apex), navicular, the 3 cuneiforms, and 3 medial metatarsals. The arch is bound together by the spring ligament and the deltoid ligament. It is also supported by the tendon of tibialis anterior and posterior and peroneus longus. Without these the ligaments cannot maintain the medial arch and would become permanently stretched.
- The lateral longitudinal arch comprises calcaneus, cuboid, and the 2 lateral metatarsals. Its stability is enhanced by 2 strong plantar ligaments together with the tendons of peroneus longus and peroneus brevis.

2.12 Lower limb innervation

- Clinical effects of damage to the following nerves:
  - Femoral nerve:
    - Instability of the knee ('buckling') on climbing stairs
    - Numbness of the medial side of thigh and calf
    - Quadriceps muscle weakness and wasting; loss of knee jerk
  - Lateral cutaneous femoral nerve:
    - Anterolateral thigh burning, tingling, or numbness
    - Symptoms worse on standing, walking, or hip extension
  - Obturator nerve:
    - Exercise-related groin pain
    - If severe, loss of adduction and internal rotation
    - Gait with externally rotated foot
  - Sciatic nerve:
    - Weakness of knee flexion, and foot plantarflexion
    - Weak or absent ankle jerk
    - 'Sciatica' pain down back of thigh and calf and sole of foot
    - If severe, loss of sensation

- Common peroneal nerve:
  - Foot drop
  - High stepping gait (loss of dorsiflexion of foot)
  - Decreased sensation to top of foot

2.13 Lower limb osteology

- You should be familiar with the normal X-ray appearances of all the bones and joints of the lower limb.
- You should also be aware of the typical radiological appearances of fractures of the femur, tibia, fibula, ankle malleoli, and foot.

CHAPTER A3

Thorax

CONTENTS

3.1 Thoracic body wall

3.1.1 Dermatomes

See Figure A.3.1.

3.1.2 Osteology of the body wall

- Thoracic part of the vertebral column:
  - Concave forwards
  - 12 vertebrae
  - Intervertebral discs
- Typical thoracic vertebrae:
  - Body is medium sized
  - Body is heart shaped
  - Spines are long and angled down
  - Costal facets for articulation of heads of rib
  - Facets on transverse processes for articulation of tubercles of rib
  - See Figure A.3.2
- Sternum:
  - 3 parts:
    - Manubrium
    - Body
    - Xiphoid process
  - See Figure A.3.3
- Ribs:
  - 12 pairs of thoracic ribs:
    - Rib 1 is atypical
    - Ribs 2–7 are true ribs
    - Ribs 8–12 are false ribs

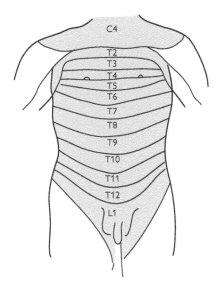

Figure A.3.1 Dermatomes of thorax and abdomen

3.1.3 Joints between ribs and vertebrae

- 1st rib:
  - Head articulates via a single synovial joint with the vertebral body of T1 vertebrae only—it *does not* articulate with C7 vertebrae
  - Articular part of rib tubercle articulates with its own transverse process via a synovial joint (i.e. with T1 vertebrae)
  - Anterior end of 1st rib attached to sternum via its costal cartilage
- True ribs (2–7):
  - The demifacets of the head of the rib articulate with the demifacets of its own vertebrae and the vertebrae above (i.e. 5th rib with 5th and 4th vertebrae). These are synovial joints
  - Articular part of rib tubercle articulates with its own transverse process (i.e. 5th rib with T5 vertebrae) via synovial joint
  - Anterior end of true ribs attached to sternum via its costal cartilage

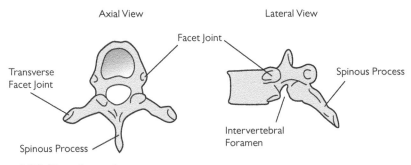

Figure A.3.2 Thoracic vertebrae

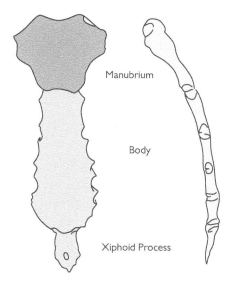

Manubrium

Body

Xiphoid Process

Figure A.3.3 Sternum

- False ribs (8–12):
  - Ribs 8 and 9 articulate with the vertebrae in the same way as the typical ribs
  - The heads of ribs 10–12 articulate with their corresponding vertebrae *only* via synovial joints (i.e. 10th rib with T10 vertebrae)
  - The tubercle of the 10th rib articulates with the transverse process of the T10 vertebrae
  - The tubercle is absent in the 11th and 12th ribs

3.1.4 Costochondral joints

- Costal cartilages are hyaline cartilage.
- 1st costal cartilages:
  - Articulate with the manubrium
  - No movement is possible at these joints
- 2nd costal cartilages:
  - Articulate with the manubrium and the body of the sternum
  - These joints are mobile synovial joints
- 3rd–7th costal cartilages:
  - Articulate with the body of the sternum via mobile synovial joints
- 6th–10th costal cartilages:
  - Articulate with each other via synovial joints
- 11th and 12th costal cartilages:
  - Embedded in the muscles of the abdominal wall and do not articulate with the other cartilages or the sternum

3.1.5 Muscles

- Arranged in three layers:
  - External intercostal muscle:
    - From: inferior border of rib
    - To: superior border of rib below
    - Direction of fibres: downwards and forwards
    - Nerve supply: intercostal nerves

- Internal intercostal muscle:
  - From: inferior border of rib
  - To: superior border of rib below
  - Direction of fibres: downwards and backwards
  - Nerve supply: intercostal nerves
- Transversus thoracis (innermost intercostals):
  - From: adjacent ribs
  - To: adjacent ribs
  - Direction of fibres: incomplete layer
  - Nerve supply: intercostal nerves

3.1.6 Thoracic movements in respiration

- The chest wall and muscles play a vital role in respiration.
- Respiration has both thoracic and abdominal components.
- It consists of 2 phases: inspiration and expiration.
- Inspiration:
  - The ribs are elevated during inspiration
  - The anterior aspect of each rib is usually below the level of the posterior ends
  - Muscle contraction causes the anterior aspect of each rib to rise above the posterior end. This is the *pump-handle* action of breathing. All of the ribs are drawn together and raised towards the fixed 1st rib
  - At the same time the lateral aspect of each rib is raised so that they swing upwards in a *bucket-handle* action, which increases the transverse diameter of the chest
  - The false ribs open out anteriorly, like the opening of a book or set of callipers
  - In quiet respiration these movements are carried out by the external intercostals muscles, assisted by the scalene muscles
  - In forced inspiration these muscles are supported by other muscles attached to the ribs, including the pectoral muscle, sternocleidomastoid, serratus anterior, and latissimus dorsi
  - Abdominal breathing is facilitated by contraction of the diaphragm, which descends as it contracts, increasing the vertical diameter of the thorax
- Expiration:
  - This is largely a passive process that occurs as the muscles described above relax and the elastic lungs recoil. Forced expiration is predominately assisted by contraction of the abdominal musculature
  - When multiple ribs are fractured in multiple places a *flail segment* is produced. The process of respiration is disturbed as this section is discontinuous from the rest of the thoracic cage. This results in uncoordinated movement of the chest wall, with the flail segment moving paradoxically, and can lead to respiratory distress and hypoventilation

3.1.7 Intercostal structures

- Muscle layers:
  - External intercostals
  - Internal intercostals
  - Transverses thoracis
- Fascia:
  - Endothoracic fascia—lined internally by parietal pleura
- Contents:
  - Intercostal vein
  - Intercostal artery
  - Intercostal nerve
- Neurovascular bundle lies between internal intercostals and innermost intercostals/ transverses thoracis. See Figure A.3.4.

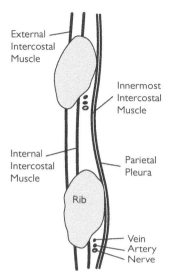

External Intercostal Muscle

Innermost Intercostal Muscle

Internal Intercostal Muscle

Parietal Pleura

Rib

Vein
Artery
Nerve

Figure A.3.4 Intercostal bundle

3.1.8 Pleural aspiration/chest drain insertion

- When performing needle aspiration of the chest cavity or inserting a chest drain, knowledge of the anatomy of the intercostal space is essential.
- These procedures should be performed in the triangle of safety in the 5th intercostal space, just anterior to the midaxillary line. It is important to pass the needle or tube over the lower rib to avoid the intercostal neurovascular bundle, which sits under the intercostal groove of the upper rib, as shown in Figure A.3.4.

3.2 The diaphragm

- Diaphragm:
  - From:
    - Xiphoid process
    - Lower 6 costal cartilages
    - 1st 3 lumbar vertebrae
  - To: central tendon
  - Nerve supply: phrenic nerve (C3, C4, C5)
  - Action:
    - Most important muscle of respiration
    - Pulls central tendon downwards
    - Increases vertical diameter of thorax
    - Assists in raising lower ribs
    - Used in abdominal straining
- The diaphragm has a right and left dome. The right dome is higher than the left due to the position of the liver.
- It is composed of striated muscle.
- Injury to the right or left phrenic nerve in the neck can cause paralysis of the corresponding dome of the diaphragm.

3.2.1 Surface markings of the diaphragm

- During mid-respiration the surface markings are:
  - Central tendon: directly behind xiphisternal joint
  - Right dome: at level of upper border of 5th rib in midclavicular line
  - Left dome: at level of lower border of 5th rib in midclavicular line

3.2.2 Openings of the diaphragm

- There are three main openings.
- Aortic opening:
  - Vertebral level: T12 (between crura)
  - Structures transmitted:
    - Aorta
    - Azygous vein
    - Thoracic duct
- Oesophageal opening:
  - Vertebral level: T10 (right crus)
  - Structures transmitted:
    - Oesophagus
    - Right and left vagus nerves
    - Oesophageal branches of left gastric vessels
    - Lymphatics (from lower third of oesophagus)
- Vena caval opening:
  - Vertebral level: T8 (central tendon)
  - Structures transmitted:
    - Inferior vena cava
    - Branches of right phrenic nerve

3.2.3 Diaphragmatic hernias

- Congenital:
  - Bochdalek's hernia: hernia through the pleuriperitoneal canal, more common on left side (as this closes last)
  - Absence of diaphragm
  - Absence of central tendon
  - These hernias are associated with respiratory distress and lung hypoplasia and must be treated surgically, after resuscitation of the baby. Up to 50% of babies born with these congenital hernias will not survive
  - Morgagni hernias: small defects in the anterior diaphragm close to the sternum. Rarely cause lung hypoplasia, but require surgical repair
- Acquired:
  - Hiatus hernia: part of the stomach herniates through the oesophageal opening in the diaphragm. There are two types:
    - Sliding: most common. Associated with raised intra-abdominal pressure and obesity. Stomach 'slides' through oesophageal opening. Reflux occurs
    - Rolling: fundus of stomach passes alongside the oesophagus into the chest. Reflux does not occur, but the fundus may become incarcerated and subsequent strangulation/perforation may occur

3.2.4 Surgical approach to the thorax

- Emergency thoracotomy can be performed to gain access to the heart and contents of the thorax. This is particularly useful in penetrating chest trauma:
  - Whilst standing on the left side of the patient, abduct the left arm
  - Begin your incision at the medial end of the left 5th intercostal space

- Make the incision laterally, along the upper border of the 6th rib, into the axilla
- The incision can be extended medially
- Rib retractors are used to gain access to the chest
- Strong scissors can be used to cut through the sternum, into the right 5th intercostal space
- The heart can then be identified and the pericardium opened
- Myocardial defects can then be closed directly
- Cardiac massage can also be performed

3.3 Thoracic inlet

- Boundaries:
  - Posterior: T1 vertebra
  - Lateral: medial borders of 1st ribs and their costal cartilages
  - Anterior: superior border of manubrium
- Contents:
  - Figure A.3.5 demonstrates the anatomy of the thoracic inlet.

3.4 Trachea

- The trachea is 10–12cm in length. It is a tube-like structure and is approximately 2.5cm in diameter.
- Origin: below the cricoid cartilage of the larynx in the neck, at the level of the C6 vertebrae.
- Termination: at the level of the sternal angle in the thorax at the level of the T4 vertebra, where it divides into the right and left main bronchi.
- Structure: fibroelastic wall, with embedded U-shaped rings of hyaline cartilage. These rings are deficient posteriorly, so as not to interfere with transmission of food in the oesophagus, which lies directly behind.
- Lining: pseudostratified ciliated columnar epithelium. Cilia move small particles upwards. Larger particles are removed by coughing.
- Innervation: branches of vagus and recurrent laryngeal nerves.

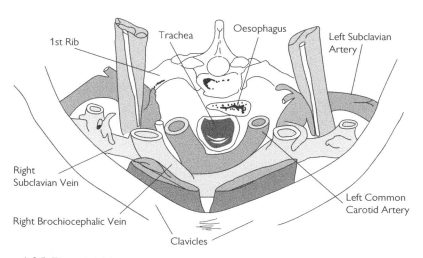

Figure A.3.5 Thoracic inlet

3.4.1 Relations of the trachea in the neck

- Posterior:
  - Oesophagus
  - Recurrent laryngeal nerves (in groove between the trachea and the oesophagus)
- Lateral:
  - Thyroid isthmus at 2nd–4th tracheal rings
  - Carotid sheath
  - Anterior jugular veins

3.4.2 Mediastinal relations of the trachea

- Anterior:
  - Sternum
  - Thymus
  - Left brachiocephalic vein
  - Origin of brachiocephalic artery
  - Origin of left common carotid artery
  - Arch of aorta
- Posterior:
  - Oesophagus
  - Recurrent laryngeal nerves (in groove between trachea and oesophagus)
- Right side:
  - Azygous vein
  - Right vagus nerve
  - Pleura
- Left side:
  - Arch of aorta
  - Left common carotid artery
  - Left subclavian artery
  - Left vagus nerve
  - Left phrenic nerve
  - Pleura

3.5 Thymus

- Lymphatic tissue moulded around great vessels and trachea.
- Lies in anterior mediastinum between manubrium and pericardium.
- Relatively largest at birth. Increases in size until puberty and then involutes.
- Blood supply from inferior thyroid and internal thoracic arteries.

3.6 Pericardium and heart

3.6.1 Pericardium

- This is a fibroserous sac enclosing the heart and the roots of the great vessels.
- It is located posterior to the body of the sternum and the 2nd–6th costal cartilages.
- Pain sensation is via the phrenic nerves—thus the diaphragmatic pain of acute pericarditis.
- Fibrous pericardium:
  - Strong outer layer

- Attachments:
  - Inferior: central tendon of diaphragm
  - Anterior: via sternopericardial ligaments to sternum
- Fuses with the outer layer of great vessels that pass through it:
  - Aorta
  - Pulmonary trunk
  - Superior vena cava
  - Inferior vena cava
  - Pulmonary veins
- Serous pericardium:
  - Has both parietal and visceral layers
  - Parietal layer:
    - Lines the fibrous pericardium
    - Reflects around roots of great vessels
    - Becomes continuous with the visceral layer
  - Visceral layer:
    - Closely applied to the heart
    - Space between parietal and visceral layers is the pericardial cavity
    - Cavity contains small amount of pericardial fluid
    - This lubricates the movement of the heart

3.6.2 Heart

- The heart lies within the pericardium and is a pyramid shape, with the base lying opposite the apex.
- Surfaces of the heart:
  - Sternocostal:
    - Right atrium
    - Right ventricle
  - Diaphragmatic:
    - Right ventricle
    - Left ventricle
  - Posterior (base):
    - Left atrium
  - Apex:
    - Left ventricle
- Borders of the heart:
  - Right:
    - Right atrium
  - Left:
    - Left atrium
    - Left ventricle
  - Superior:
    - Roots of great vessels
  - Inferior:
    - Right ventricle
    - Apex of left ventricle

3.6.3 Surface markings of the heart

- Apex: left 5th intercostal space 9cm from midline.
- Superior border: extends from 2nd left costal cartilage 1.5cm from edge of sternum to 3rd right costal cartilage 1.5cm from the sternum.

- Right border: extends from 3rd right costal cartilage 1.5cm from the sternum to the 6th right costal cartilage 1.5cm from the sternum.
- Left border: extends from 2nd left costal cartilage 1.5cm from the edge of the sternum to apex of heart as previously described.
- Inferior border: extends from 6th right costal cartilage 1.5cm from the edge of the sternum to apex of heart as previously described.

3.6.4 The heart valves

- There are 4 heart valves:
    - Tricuspid valve: between right atrium and right ventricle
    - Mitral valve: between left atrium and left ventricle
    - Pulmonary valve: guards pulmonary orifice
    - Aortic valve: guards aortic orifice
- Surface markings of heart valves:
    - Tricuspid valve: behind right half of sternum opposite 4th intercostal space
    - Mitral valve: behind left half of sternum opposite 4th costal cartilage
    - Pulmonary valve: behind medial end of 3rd left costal cartilage and sternum
    - Aortic valve: behind left half of sternum opposite 3rd intercostal space
- Auscultation points for the heart valves:
    - Tricuspid valve: right sternal edge, 5th intercostal space
    - Mitral valve: at apex beat (left 5th intercostal space 9cm from midline)
    - Pulmonary valve: left sternal edge, 3rd costal cartilage
    - Aortic valve: right sternal edge, 2nd intercostal space

3.6.5 Origin of great vessels

- Ascending aorta:
    - Commences at base of left ventricle
    - Runs upwards and forwards to lie behind right half of sternum; at the level of the sternal angle here it becomes the arch of the aorta
- Pulmonary trunk:
    - Commences at the upper part of right ventricle
    - Runs upwards, backwards, and to the left
    - Terminates at the concavity of the aortic arch by dividing into the right and left pulmonary arteries
- The ascending aorta and pulmonary trunk are enclosed together in a layer of serous pericardium and lie within the fibrous pericardium.

3.6.6 Conducting system of the heart

- Cardiac muscle contraction is controlled by groups of specialized cardiac muscle cells, which are organized in the following way.
- Sinoatrial (SA) node:
    - Pacemaker for the heart; sets the rate of impulse conduction
    - Located in the wall of the right atrium
- Atrioventricular (AV) node:
    - Electrical impulses from the SA node are conducted through the atria to the AV node
    - Located in the wall of the interatrial septum
- Bundle of His:
    - Conducts electrical impulses to the ventricles
    - Divided into right and left branches and transmits impulses to Purkinje fibres
    - Located in the interventricular septum

- Purkinje fibres:
  - Conduct impulses to the right and left ventricles
  - These fibres are in the subendocardial tissue

3.6.7 Cardiac blood supply

- The blood supply for the heart comes from the right and left coronary arteries and their branches. (See Figure A.3.6.)
- Right coronary artery:
  - Origin: arises from the aortic root
  - Supplies:
    - Right ventricle
    - SA node (via SA nodal artery) in 60% of individuals
    - Varying portions of the atria
    - Part of interventricular septum AV node
  - Branches:
    - Right marginal branch (supplies right ventricle)
    - SA nodal artery (supplies SA node in 60% of people)
    - Posterior interventricular branch (gives supply to both ventricles)
    - AV nodal artery (supplies AV node)
- Left coronary artery:
  - Origin: arises from aortic root

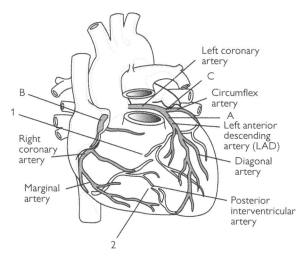

Figure A.3.6 Location of two typical intercoronary anastomoses and three sites of predilection for coronary occlusion. Anastomosis 1 depicts the communication in the posterior part of the coronary sulcus between the right coronary artery (RCA) and the circumflex branch of the left coronary artery (LCA). Anastomosis 2 shows the communication in the posterior interventricular sulcus between the posterior and anterior interventricular branches of the RCA and LCA. Notice the three most common locations of coronary occlusion. They are, in descending order of frequency, the anterior interventricular branch of the LCA (site A), the RCA (site B), and the circumflex branch of the LCA (site C)

Lachman's Case Studies in Anatomy by Seidon and Corbett (2013) Fig. 21.2. By permission of Oxford University Press, USA.

- Supplies:
  - Left ventricle
  - SA node (via SA nodal artery) in 40% of individuals
  - Varying portions of the atria
  - Part of interventricular septum
- Branches:
  - Left anterior descending artery (supplies right and left ventricles and the interventricular septum)
  - Circumflex branch (supplies left atrium and left ventricle)
  - SA nodal artery (supplies SA node in 40% of people)

3.6.8 Emergency pericardiocentesis

- Haemorrhage into the pericardial sac following trauma may inhibit cardiac output. This is known as cardiac tamponade.
- In order to drain the blood from the pericardium, pericardiocentesis is performed:
  - An 18G needle is connected to a syringe and a three-way-tap
  - The needle is inserted just below the xiphisternum
  - The needle is directed superiorly and posteriorly, aiming towards the tip of the right scapula
  - Aspirate as the needle is advanced, until blood is aspirated
  - By removing even 20–50mL of blood, cardiac function can be improved until definitive surgery or thoracotomy
  - (In most people a standard cannula will not be long enough to get into the pericardial space and a special pericardiocentesis needle will be needed)

3.7 Oesophagus

- The oesophagus is a muscular tube extending from C6 (at the level of the cricoid cartilage) to T10. It is approximately 25cm long.
- It has 2 layers of muscle, an inner circular layer and an outer longitudinal layer. It is lined with stratified squamous epithelium.
- It can be divided into cervical, thoracic, and abdominal sections. See Table A.3.1.

3.8 Pleura and lungs

3.8.1 Pleura

- Each pleural cavity is composed of a thin serous membrane, invaginated by the lung.
- The visceral pleura is closely related to the lung and is continuous with the parietal pleura, which is applied to the inner aspect of the thoracic wall.
- Lungs conform to the shape of the pleura, but don't take up the full capacity. This allows expansion during respiration.

3.8.2 Surface markings of pleura

- Pleura extends above the level of the clavicles.
- Follows a curved line from sternoclavicular joint to junction of inner third and outer two-thirds of the clavicle, with the pleural apex 2.5cm above the clavicle.
- Pleural line on each side passes from behind the sternoclavicular joint; meet in the midline at the level of the 2nd costal cartilage.
- On the right side the pleura passes inferiorly down to the 6th costal cartilage, then crosses the 8th rib in the midclavicular line, the 10th rib in the midaxillary line, and the 12th rib at the border of erector spinae.

Table A.3.1 Oesophageal sections

	Cervical	Thoracic	Abdominal
Relations: Posterior	C6 and C7	T1–T10 Thoracic duct Azygous vein Descending aorta	Pierces diaphragm at T10 (*as described in Section 3.2.2*) Left crus of diaphragm
Anterior	Trachea Recurrent laryngeal nerve	Trachea Left recurrent laryngeal nerve Left main bronchus Pericardium	Left lobe of liver
Right lateral	Thyroid	Mediastinal pleura Azygous vein	
Left lateral	Thyroid	Arch of aorta Thoracic duct Mediastinal pleura Thoracic duct Left subclavian artery	
Points of constriction	Where pharynx joins upper end, 6cm from incisor teeth	Where left bronchus and aortic arch cross, 25cm from incisor teeth	Where oesophagus passes through diaphragm, 41cm from incisor teeth
Nerve supply	Recurrent laryngeal Sympathetic fibres from middle cervical ganglion	Vagus nerve Sympathetic trunk Greater splanchnic nerve	Vagus plexuses Oesophageal plexus

- On the left side the pleura reaches the 4th costal cartilage and then indents laterally, separated from the chest wall by the pericardium. This means the left 4th and 5th intercostal spaces are not covered with pleura at their medial ends. Aspiration at this point would enter the pericardium without piercing the pleura. Otherwise the pleura continues to follow the same route as described for the right.
- The pleura extends above the clavicle into the neck, and below the 12th ribs, and so is vulnerable to stab wounds and incisions at these points.

3.8.3 Nerve supply of pleura
- Visceral pleura receives autonomic nerve supply from the pulmonary plexus. It is sensitive to stretch, but insensitive to pain.
- Parietal pleura receives nerve supply from the intercostal nerves and the phrenic nerves. It is sensitive to pain and pressure.

3.8.4 Lungs
- Lungs are soft, spongy, and elastic.
- Right lung divided into 3 lobes:
  - Upper lobe
  - Middle lobe
  - Lower lobe
- Right lung has 2 fissures:
  - Upper and middle lobes separated by transverse fissure
  - Lower lobe separated from upper and middle lobes by oblique fissure (see Figure A.3.7)

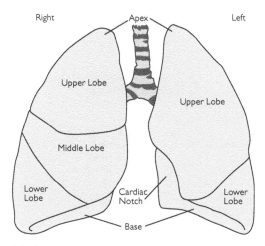

Figure A.3.7 Lobes of the lungs

- Left lung divided into 2 lobes:
  - Upper lobe
  - Lower lobe
  - Lingula is equivalent of middle lobe and lies between cardiac notch and oblique fissure
- Left lung has 1 fissure:
  - Oblique fissure
- Bronchi:
  - The trachea terminates at the level of the sternal angle and divides into left and right main bronchi
  - The right main bronchus is wider, shorter (2.5cm), and more vertical than the left. It is therefore more likely for a foreign body to be lodged here than in the left main bronchus. It divides into bronchi to the middle and lower lobes
  - The left main bronchus is approximately 5cm long and divides into bronchi to the upper and lower lobes
- Blood supply:
  - Pulmonary trunk arises from the right ventricle of the heart. Beneath the aortic arch it divides into the right and left pulmonary arteries
  - Alveoli receive deoxygenated blood from the pulmonary arteries. Oxygenated blood is then drained through the alveolar capillaries to the tributaries of the pulmonary veins, and finally into the pulmonary veins themselves
- Lung roots:
  - Formed by the structures that are entering or leaving the lung—the bronchi, pulmonary artery and veins, lymph vessels, bronchial vessels, and nerves. See Figure A.3.8
  - They connect the lung roots to the mediastinum
  - They are surrounded by a tubular sheath of pleura, which connects the mediastinal parietal pleura to the visceral pleura covering the lungs

3.8.5 Surface anatomy of the lungs

- Follows a curved line from sternoclavicular joint to junction of inner third and outer two-thirds of the clavicle, with the lung apex 2.5cm above the clavicle.

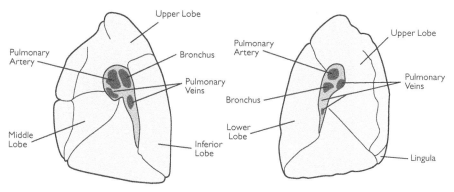

Figure A.3.8 Lung roots

- Anterior border of the right lung runs from behind the sternoclavicular joint downwards to the level of the sternal angle, almost reaching the midline. It then continues downwards to the xiphisternal joint.
- Anterior border of the left lung has a similar course, but at the level of the 4th costal cartilage it deviates laterally beyond the lateral level of the sternum, to form the cardiac notch. It then continues downwards to the xiphisternal joint.
- In mid-inspiration the lower border of the lung follows a curving line, crossing the 6th rib at the midclavicular line, the 8th rib in the midclavicular line, and the 10th rib adjacent to the vertebral column posteriorly.
- The posterior border of the lung extends from the spinous process of C7 downwards to the level of T10, about 4cm from the midline.
- The oblique fissure lies on the line from the root of the spine of the scapula obliquely down, anterior, and lateral, along the course of the 6th rib to the 6th costochondral junction.
- On the right side the horizontal fissure lies on the line along the 4th costal cartilage, to meet the oblique fissure in the midaxillary line.

3.8.6 Lymph drainage

- The lymph drainage of the lung is carried out by lymph vessels originating in superficial and deep plexuses within the lung.
- Superficial drainage occurs over the surface of the lung, then via the bronchopulmonary nodes in the hilum of the lung.
- Deep drainage occurs via the deep plexus along the course of the bronchi and pulmonary vessels to the bronchopulmonary nodes on the hilum of the lung.
- All the lymph from the superficial and deep plexuses then leaves the hilum via the tracheobronchial nodes and then into the bronchomediastinal trunks.

3.8.7 Nerve supply of the lungs

- At each lung root is a pulmonary plexus composed of efferent and afferent autonomic nerve fibres from the sympathetic trunk, and parasympathetic fibres of the vagus nerve.
- Sympathetic efferent fibres cause bronchodilatation and vasoconstriction.
- Parasympathetic efferent fibres cause bronchoconstriction and vasodilatation.
- Afferent impulses pass to the CNS via both sympathetic and parasympathetic nerves.

CHAPTER A4

Abdomen

CONTENTS

4.1 Abdominal wall

4.1.1 Regions of the abdominal wall

The abdominal wall is subdivided into regions as seen in Figure A.4.1.

4.1.2 Muscles of the anterior abdominal wall

Figure A.4.2 shows the muscles of the anterior abdominal wall.

- External oblique:
  - Origin: lower 8 ribs
  - Insertion:
    - Xiphoid process
    - Linea alba
    - Pubic crest
    - Pubic tubercle
    - Iliac crest
    - (Is the origin of the inguinal ligament)
  - Innervation:
    - Lower 6 thoracic nerves
    - Iliohypogastric nerve
    - Ilioinguinal nerve
  - Action:
    - Supports abdominal contents
    - Assists in trunk flexion and rotation
    - Compresses abdominal contents
    - Assists in forced expiration, defecation, parturition, micturition, vomiting

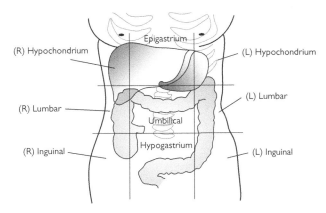

Figure A.4.1 Regions of the abdominal wall

- Internal oblique:
  - Origin:
    - Lumbar fascia
    - Iliac crest
    - Lateral two-thirds of inguinal ligament
  - Insertion:
    - Lower 3 ribs and costal cartilages
    - Xiphoid process
    - Linea alba
    - Symphysis pubis
  - Innervation:
    - Lower 6 thoracic nerves
    - Iliohypogastric nerve
    - Ilioinguinal nerve
  - Action: same range of actions as external oblique
- Transversus:
  - Origin:
    - Lower 6 costal cartilages
    - Lumbar fascia
    - Iliac crest
    - Lateral third of inguinal ligament
  - Insertion:
    - Xiphoid process
    - Linea alba
    - Symphysis pubis
  - Innervation:
    - Lower 6 thoracic nerves
    - Ilioinguinal nerve
    - Iliohypogastric nerve
  - Action: compresses abdominal contents
- Rectus abdominis:
  - Origin:
    - Symphysis pubis
    - Pubic crest

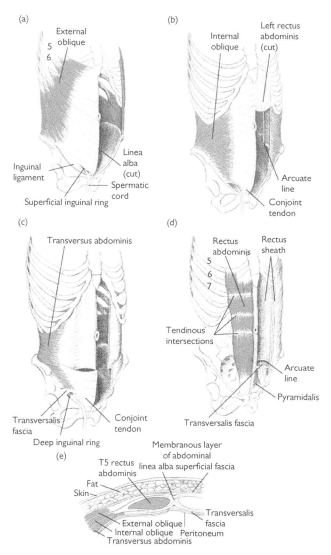

(a)

External oblique
5
6

Inguinal ligament

Superficial inguinal ring

Linea alba (cut)

Spermatic cord

(b)

Internal oblique

Left rectus abdominis (cut)

Arcuate line

Conjoint tendon

(c)

Transversus abdominis

Transversalis fascia

Deep inguinal ring

Conjoint tendon

(d)

Rectus abdominis
5
6
7

Rectus sheath

Tendinous intersections

Transversalis fascia

Arcuate line

Pyramidalis

(e)

T5 rectus abdominis

Fat

Skin

Membranous layer of abdominal superficial fascia

linea alba

External oblique
Internal oblique
Transversus abdominis

Transversalis fascia

Peritoneum

Figure A.4.2 Muscles of the anterior abdominal wall: (a) external oblique; (b) internal oblique; (c) transversus abdominis; (d) rectus abdominis; (e) section through anterior abdominal wall. The aponeuroses of the abdominal wall muscles which form the rectus sheath interdigitate to form the midline linea alba

Reproduced with permission from MacKinnon P, Morris J. (2005). *Oxford Textbook of Functional Anatomy*, Vol. 2. Oxford: Oxford University Press, © 2005.

- ■ Insertion:
  - ● 5th–7th costal cartilages
  - ● Xiphoid process
- ■ Innervation: lower 6 thoracic nerves

- Action:
  - Compresses abdominal contents
  - Flexes vertebral column
  - Assists expiration

4.1.3 Rectus sheath

- The rectus sheath is a fibrous sheath enclosing the rectus abdominis muscle.
- It is formed mainly by the aponeurosis of the 3 main abdominal muscles described previously (external oblique, internal oblique, and transversus). See Figure A.4.3.
- It is best considered in 3 sections:
  - Above the level of the costal margin:
    - The anterior rectus sheath is formed by the external oblique aponeurosis only
    - There is no aponeurosis from internal oblique or transversus at this level
    - There is no posterior rectus sheath
    - Rectus femoris lies directly on 5th–7th costal cartilages
  - From the costal margin to the anterior superior iliac spine (ASIS) and arcuate line:
    - The anterior rectus sheath is formed by the external oblique aponeurosis and the anterior part of the split internal oblique aponeurosis
    - The posterior rectus sheath is formed by the posterior part of the split internal oblique aponeurosis and the transversus abdominis aponeurosis
  - From the ASIS and arcuate line to the pubis:
    - The anterior rectus sheath is formed by the combined aponeuroses of external oblique, internal oblique, and transversus
    - The posterior rectus sheath is absent and the rectus abdominis lies on transversalis fascia (which is thickened here to form the iliopubic tract)

4.1.4 Contents of the rectus sheath

- The rectus sheath contains:
  - Pyramidalis muscle (if present)
  - Superior epigastric vessels
  - Inferior epigastric vessels

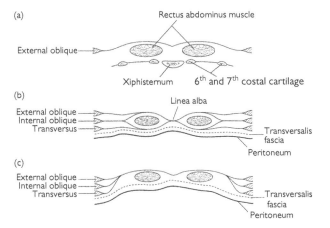

Figure A.4.3 The formation of the rectus sheath: a) above the costal margin; b) above the arcuate line; c) below the arcuate line

- Nerves and vessels from T7 to T12
- Posterior intercostal nerves

4.2 Inguinal region

4.2.1 The inguinal canal

- This is an oblique passage through the lower part of the abdominal wall. It allows passage of structures from the testis to the abdomen in males and the passage of the round ligament of the uterus from the uterus to the labium majus in females.
- It is around 6cm long in the adult and lies parallel and above the inguinal ligament, from the deep inguinal ring to the superficial inguinal ring.

4.2.2 Boundaries of the inguinal canal

- Roof:
  - The arching lower fibres of internal oblique and transversus muscles
- Anterior wall:
  - Aponeurosis of external oblique along entire length
  - Reinforced by internal oblique in lateral third
- Posterior wall:
  - Fascia transversalis along entire length
  - Reinforced by conjoint tendon in medial third (this is the common tendon of insertion of internal oblique and transversus at the pubic crest)
- Floor:
  - The inguinal ligament (rolled under inferior edge of the aponeurosis of external oblique)
  - At the medial end the lacunar ligament contributes to the floor

4.2.3 Openings of the inguinal canal

- Superficial inguinal ring:
  - Triangular-shaped defect in the external oblique aponeurosis
  - Lies above and medial to the pubic tubercle
  - Margins of the superficial ring give rise to the external spermatic fascia
- Deep inguinal ring:
  - Oval opening in the transversalis fascia
  - Lies 1.3cm above the inguinal ligament, midway between ASIS and symphysis pubis
  - Margins of the deep ring give rise to the internal spermatic fascia

4.2.4 Contents of the inguinal canal (and spermatic cord)

- Vas deferens.
- Arterial structures:
  - Testicular artery
  - Artery to the vas deferens
  - Cremasteric artery
- Venous structures:
  - Pampiniform plexus
- Lymphatic vessels.
- Nerves:
  - Genital branch of the genitofemoral nerve
  - Sympathetic nerves (accompany arteries)
  - Ilioinguinal nerve
- Processus vaginalis.

4.3 Testis, epididymis, and spermatic cord

4.3.1 Spermatic cord

- The covering of the spermatic cord consists of 3 concentric layers, acquired as the processus vaginalis descends through the layers of the abdominal wall:
  - Internal spermatic fascia: from transversalis fascia
  - Cremasteric fascia: from internal oblique and transversus
  - External spermatic fascia: from external oblique

4.3.2 The testes

- Lie within the scrotum, with the left testis usually slightly higher than the right. See Figure A.4.4.
- The testis is surrounded by a tough, fibrous capsule called the tunica albuginea.
- Blood supply is from the testicular artery, which arises from the abdominal aorta and runs in the spermatic cord.
- The testis is suspended in the scrotum on the spermatic cord. Twisting or torsion of the testis therefore leads to occlusion of the testicular artery and, if not treated, possible necrosis of the testis.
- Lymph drainage of the testis is via the para-aortic lymph nodes. The coverings of the testis drain to the external iliac nodes. The scrotum drains to the superficial inguinal lymph nodes.
- Innervation is via sympathetic fibres derived from T6–T10 and afferent fibres that accompany them. Testicular pain is therefore often referred to the abdomen.

4.3.3 Descent of the testes

- The testes begin development in the abdomen from the mesodermal cells of the gonadal ridge covering the embryonic kidney, the mesonephros.
- Each is embedded in the upper end of the gubernaculum, a thick gelatinous cord of mesenchyme.
- The gubernaculum extends downwards through the region that will become the inguinal canal and on to the genital swelling that will become the scrotum or labium majus.
- The gubernaculum swells and draws the testis down towards the developing scrotum, along with a diverticulum of peritoneum called the processus vaginalis.
- The testis drags behind it the vas deferens, which develops from the mesonephric duct, along with its accompanying blood vessels and lymphatics.

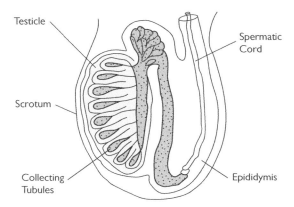

Figure A.4.4 Outline diagram of testis

- The coverings of the cord form around these structures, resulting in the 3 concentric layers of fascia described previously.
- The gubernaculum ends up as a remnant in the scrotum and the vas passes down through the inguinal canal.
- In the female, the ovary only descends to the pelvis, so the inguinal canal contains only the remnants of the gubernaculum.
- The processus vaginalis pinches off, forming the tunica vaginalis of the testis.
- This embryological pathway explains the structure and content of the inguinal canal and spermatic cord.

4.3.4 Vas deferens

- The vas deferens is a thick-walled tube, approximately 18cm long.
- It allows the transport of mature sperm from the epididymis to the ejaculatory duct and urethra.
- It arises from the tail of the epididymis and runs upwards through the inguinal canal. It leaves via the deep inguinal ring and passes around the inferior epigastric artery. It then passes along the lateral wall of the pelvis, downwards and backwards, and crosses the ureter at the level of the ischial spine.
- It continues medially and downwards along the posterior surface of the bladder and opens out to form an ampulla, which then joins the duct of the seminal vesicle, forming the ejaculatory duct.
- The ejaculatory ducts pierce the posterior surface of the prostate and open into the prostatic portion of the urethra, where the seminal fluid and sperm are drained.

4.4 Topography of the abdominal cavity

- Structures within the abdomen can be divided up into intraperitoneal and retroperitoneal structures.
- Retroperitoneal structures lie behind the peritoneum, whilst intraperitoneal structures lie within the peritoneum.
- Intraperitoneal structures are suspended within the peritoneal cavity by 3 different types of tissues.
- A mesentery is a 2-layered fold of peritoneum that connects parts of the intestine to the posterior abdominal wall. An example is the mesentery of the small intestine.
- Omenta are 2-layered folds of peritoneum that connect the stomach to other viscera, for example, the lesser omentum connects the lesser curvature of the stomach to the liver.
- Peritoneal ligaments are 2-layered folds of peritoneum connecting solid viscera to the abdominal walls, for example, the falciform ligament connects the liver to the diaphragm and anterior abdominal wall.
- The position of an organ within the abdomen, whether it is retroperitoneal or intraperitoneal, whether it is suspended, and whether it is a solid or hollow viscus, all have an impact on that organ's susceptibility to different types of injury.
- Compressive forces from direct blows or from external compression against a fixed object (e.g. seatbelt pressing against the spinal column) commonly cause tears and bleeding of solid organs. These forces may also cause deformity of hollow organs, resulting in raised intraluminal pressure and rupture of the viscus.
- Deceleration forces cause stretching and linear shearing between relatively fixed and free objects. These longitudinal shearing forces tend to rupture supporting structures at the junction between free and fixed segments.
- Common injuries resulting from this mechanism include liver injuries, where the liver is attached by the ligamentum teres, and bowel injuries at their mesenteric attachments.

- Intraperitoneal organs:
  - Stomach
  - Liver
  - Gallbladder
  - Spleen
  - Jejunum
  - Ileum
  - Transverse colon
  - Sigmoid colon
  - Uterus
  - Ovaries
- Retroperitoneal organs:
  - Kidneys
  - Adrenal glands
  - Aorta
  - Inferior vena cava
  - Urinary bladder
  - Prostate
  - Vagina
  - Rectum
  - Pancreas (except for tail)
  - Duodenum (2nd and 3rd portions)
  - Ascending colon
  - Descending colon

4.5 Peritoneum

- The peritoneum is a thin, serous membrane lining the pelvic and abdominal cavities and covering the viscera of the abdomen and pelvis.
- It has 2 layers:
  - Parietal peritoneum:
    - Lines walls of abdominal and pelvic cavities
    - Sensitive to pain, temperature, touch, and pressure
    - Abdominal section supplied by lower 6 thoracic and 1st lumbar nerves
    - Diaphragmatic section supplied by phrenic nerves and lower 6 thoracic nerves
    - Pelvic section supplied by obturator nerve
  - Visceral peritoneum:
    - Covers the organs
    - Sensitive only to stretch and tearing
    - Supplied by autonomic afferent nerves that supply viscera or travel in mesentery
  - Peritoneal fluid:
    - Between layers of peritoneum
    - Lubricates and facilitates free movement

4.5.1 Functions of the peritoneum

- Allows free movement of the viscera.
- Suspends the viscera within the abdominal cavity.
- Transmits nerves, blood vessel, and lymphatics to viscera.
- Leucocytes in peritoneal fluid absorb contaminants.

- Seals areas of infection.
- Stores fat.

4.5.2 Peritoneal compartments

- The peritoneum is divided into 3 sections:
  - Supracolic
  - Infracolic
  - Pelvic
- The division between the supracolic and infracolic compartments is the transverse mesocolon. This attaches along the posterior abdominal wall from the lower border of the pancreas and extends to the right over the duodenum to the right kidney at the right colic (hepatic) flexure. On the left the attachment is over the lower part of the left kidney, at the left colic (splenic) flexure.
- Infracolic compartment:
  - The infracolic compartment is further divided into right and left infracolic compartments by the root of the mesentery, which begins on the left at the duodenojejunal junction and runs down and to the right at a 45° angle to the right iliac fossa
  - The infracolic compartment contains small intestine and the ascending and descending colon
- The sigmoid mesocolon:
  - An inverted V-shaped fold of peritoneum
  - It begins on the medial side of the left psoas major and runs upwards and backwards to its apex, overlying the bifurcation of the left common iliac vessels and left ureter
  - It then bends downwards to end at the level of the 3rd sacral vertebra in the median plane
- Supracolic compartment:
  - This compartment contains the stomach, liver, and spleen
- Greater omentum:
  - Connects the greater curvature of the stomach to the transverse colon
  - It hangs down in front of the coils of small intestine, like an apron, and then folds back on itself to attach to the transverse colon

4.6 Gastrointestinal tract

4.6.1 Abdominal oesophagus

See Table A.4.1 for details relating to the oesophagus.

4.6.2 Prevention of reflux

- There is no anatomical sphincter at the lower end of the oesophagus. There is, however, a circular layer of muscle that acts as a physiological sphincter. Contraction of this sphincter under vagal control prevents regurgitation of stomach contents. Contraction is augmented by hormonal control by secretin, glucagons, and cholecystokinin.
- Fibres of right crus of diaphragm help prevent reflux.
- Muscularis mucosa has mucosal flaps that help to prevent reflux.

4.6.3 Stomach

- The stomach is almost J-shaped with an anterior and posterior surface and a greater and lesser curvature.
- The lesser curvature is attached to the lesser omentum.
- The greater curvature is attached to the greater omentum (to the left this is continuous with the gastrosplenic ligament).
- It has 2 openings, the cardiac and pyloric openings.

Table A.4.1 Oesophageal relations

Relations:	
Posterior	Pierces diaphragm at T10
	Left crus of diaphragm
	Right vagus nerve
	Left lobe of liver
Anterior	Covered with peritoneum
	Left vagus nerve
Points of constriction	Where oesophagus passes through diaphragm, 41cm from incisor teeth
Nerve supply	Vagus plexuses
	Oesophageal plexus
Blood supply	Branches from left gastric artery
Venous drainage	Left gastric vein (tributary of portal vein)

4.6.4 Structure of the stomach

See Figure A.4.5.

- Cardia:
  - Lies to the left of the midline, at approximately T10
  - Cardiac opening between oesophagus and cardia
  - Most fixed portion of stomach
- Fundus:
  - Dome shaped
  - Projects above the cardia and is in contact with the diaphragm
  - Usually full of gas
- Body:
  - Largest section of stomach
  - Extends from cardiac orifice to the incisura angularis, a constant notch at the lower end of the lesser curvature
  - In the erect position may reach the level of the umbilicus at T10
- Pylorus:
  - Tubular-like portion of the stomach
  - Pyloric antrum links pylorus and the body

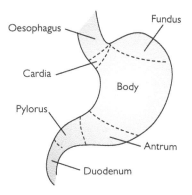

Figure A.4.5 Structure of the stomach

- Thick muscular wall called the pyloric sphincter—this is a true anatomical sphincter, unlike the cardiac sphincter
- The pyloric opening lies to right of midline at level of L1 when in recumbent position
- Pyloric sphincter controls rate of passage of stomach contents into duodenum

4.6.5 Relations of the stomach (from left to right)

- Anterior:
  - Diaphragm
  - Anterior abdominal wall
  - Left lobe of the liver
- Posterior:
  - Lesser sac
  - Diaphragm
  - Aorta
  - Pancreas
  - Spleen
  - Left kidney
  - Left adrenal gland
  - Transverse mesocolon
  - Transverse colon

4.6.6 Blood supply of the stomach

Figure A.4.6 shows the arterial supply to the stomach.

- Left gastric artery:
  - Derived from the coeliac axis
  - Runs along lesser curvature
  - Anastomoses with right gastric artery
- Right gastric artery:
  - Derived from hepatic artery
- Right gastroepiploic artery:
  - Arises from gastroduodenal branch of hepatic artery
  - Runs along greater curvature
  - Anastomoses with left gastroepiploic artery
- Left gastroepiploic artery:
  - Arises from splenic artery
  - Runs along greater curvature
  - Anastomoses with right gastroepiploic artery
- Short gastric arteries:
  - Arise from splenic artery
  - Supply fundus
- Venous drainage:
  - Veins are named in reflection of the arteries and drain into portal system
- Lymphatics:
  - Area supplied by splenic artery drains to lymph nodes at hilum of spleen, then to those along the pancreas, and finally to the coeliac nodes
  - Cardia drains along left gastric artery to coeliac nodes
  - Remainder drains to coeliac nodes via hepatic artery and gastroepiploic vessels
  - Retrograde spread may occur into hepatic nodes at porta hepatis

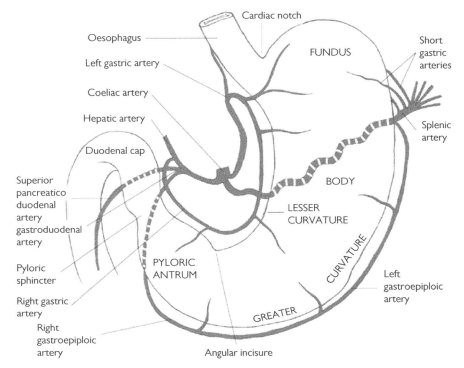

Figure A.4.6 Arterial supply to the stomach

Reproduced with permission from MacKinnon P, Morris J. (2005). *Oxford Textbook of Functional Anatomy*, Vol. 2. Oxford: Oxford University Press, © 2005.

4.6.7 Nerve supply

- Vagus nerves supply the stomach.
- Anterior and posterior vagi enter abdomen via oesophageal opening in diaphragm and supply parasympathetic fibres.
- Anterior nerve (from left vagus) lies in contact with anterior oesophagus, is close to the wall of the stomach, and supplies the anterior aspect.
- Branches:
  - Gastric branches
  - Hepatic branches
  - Branches to pyloric antrum
- Posterior nerve (from right vagus) is further away in loose connective tissue and supplies the posterior aspect.
- Branches:
  - Coeliac branch
  - Numerous branches to posterior stomach
- Sympathetic nerve supply is via coeliac plexus.

4.6.8 Duodenum

- The duodenum is the first part of the small intestine. It runs from the pylorus of the stomach to the jejunum.
- It is situated in epigastric and umbilical region of the abdomen and divided into 4 parts.

- It is a C-shaped tube, approximately 25cm long, and receives openings of bile ducts and pancreatic ducts. It is largely retroperitoneal.

4.6.9 First part of duodenum

- First 5cm is intraperitoneal, the remainder is retroperitoneal
- Begins at pylorus
- Runs upwards and backwards on the right side of L1
- Lies on transpyloric plane
- Relations:
  - Anterior:
    - Right lobe of liver
    - Gallbladder
  - Posterior:
    - Lesser sac
    - Gastroduodenal artery
    - Bile duct
    - Portal vein
    - IVC
  - Superior:
    - Entrance to lesser sac
  - Inferior:
    - Head of pancreas

4.6.10 Second part of duodenum

- 8cm long.
- Runs vertically downwards anterior to right kidney.
- Lies to right of L2 and L3.
- Halfway down medial border bile ducts and pancreatic ducts enter medial wall where they unite to form major duodenal papilla.
- Relations:
  - Anterior:
    - Fundus of gallbladder
    - Right lobe of liver
    - Transverse colon
    - Small intestine
  - Posterior:
    - Hilum of right kidney
    - Right ureter
  - Laterally:
    - Ascending colon
    - Right colic flexure
    - Right lobe of liver
  - Medially:
    - Head of pancreas
    - Bile duct
    - Main pancreatic ducts

4.6.11 Third part of duodenum

- 8cm long.
- Runs horizontally to left.
- Crosses L3 and follows lower margin of head of pancreas.

- Relations:
  - Anterior:
    - Root of mesentery of small intestine
    - Coils of jejunum
  - Posterior:
    - Right ureter
    - Right psoas
    - IVC
    - Aorta
  - Superior:
    - Head of pancreas
  - Inferior:
    - Coils of jejunum

4.6.12 Fourth part of duodenum

- 5cm long.
- Runs upwards and left to the duodenal flexure (held in place by ligament of Treitz).
- Attached to right crus of diaphragm.
- Relations:
  - Anterior:
    - Beginning of root of mesentery
    - Coils of jejunum
  - Posterior:
    - Left margin of aorta
    - Medial border of left psoas

4.6.13 Blood supply of duodenum

- Upper half supplied by superior pancreaticoduodenal artery (from gastroduodenal).
- Lower half supplied by inferior pancreaticoduodenal artery (from superior mesenteric artery).

4.6.14 Jejunum and ileum

- Together measure approximately 6 metres in length.
- Gradual change from one to the other.
- Jejunum begins at duodenojejunal flexure.
- Ileum ends at ileocaecal junction.
- Blood supply:
  - Supplied by branches from the superior mesenteric artery, which run in the mesentery to supply the gut
  - Anastomose to form a series of arcades
  - Lowest part of ileum supplied by ileocolic artery
- Nerve supply:
  - Supplied by vagal sympathetic and parasympathetic nerves from the superior mesenteric plexus
  - Pain fibres pass to the spinal cord via the splanchnic nerves and pain from this region is referred to the dermatomes supplied by T9–T11. Pain is therefore felt in the umbilical region first and only later localizes to the inguinal region (as seen when a coil of small intestine incarcerates within a hernia and only localizes once it becomes inflamed)

4.6.15 Traumatic injury to jejunum and ileum

- Jejunum and ileum are susceptible to trauma due to their being freely mobile but attached to the posterior abdominal wall by the mesentery of the small intestine.

- They can also be compressed against the vertebral column and the sacral margin, again making them susceptible to blunt trauma.

4.6.16 Meckel's diverticulum

- A diverticulum can occur in the ileum, which can be clinically significant. Classically said to occur in 2% of the population, 2 feet (60cm) from the caecum, and 2 inches (5cm) long.
- True diverticulum and contains all 3 layers of intestinal wall. Most common congenital abnormality of small bowel.
- May be attached to umbilicus by a fibrous cord, or be adherent to it. May contain ectopic gastric or pancreatic mucosa.
- Can present clinically in a number of ways:
  - Haemorrhage or perforation (due to gastric mucosa)
  - Volvulus leading to obstruction
  - Intussusception with Meckel's as apex
  - Meckel's diverticulitis (mimics appendicitis)

4.6.17 Caecum

- Part of large intestine in right iliac fossa.
- It is guarded by ileocaecal valve to prevent reflux of material into ileum.
- It is a blind-ended pouch, 6cm in length.
- The appendix is attached to caecum.
- Relations:
  - Anterior:
    - Coils of small intestine
    - Part of greater omentum
    - Anterior abdominal wall of RIF
  - Posterior:
    - Psoas and iliacus muscles
    - Lateral cutaneous nerve of thigh
    - (Due to these posterior relations localized infection may cause pain when psoas is stretched or on movement of the hip)

4.6.18 Appendix

- The position of the appendix varies. Common sites are:
  - Retrocaecal:
    - 62% of population
    - Poorly localizing signs
    - Proximity to ureter—white cells in urine
    - May lie between caecum and psoas (pain on psoas stretch)
  - Pelvic:
    - 34% of population
    - Increased nausea and vomiting
    - May cause pain on hip rotation
  - Pre-ileal:
    - 1%
  - Post-ileal:
    - 0.5%
    - Poorly localized pain
  - Rare sites:
    - RUQ appendix
    - Situs inversus LIF appendix
    - Long appendix—tip can be anywhere!

- Classically pain of appendicitis felt at McBurney's point: point one-third of the way from ASIS to the umbilicus.

4.6.19 Colon

- Ascending colon:
  - Lies in right lower quadrant and is approximately 15cm long
  - Extends upwards from caecum to inferior surface of right lobe of liver
  - Here it turns to the left, forming the right colic flexure (hepatic flexure), and becomes continuous with the transverse colon
  - Rarely has a mesentery
  - Usually retroperitoneal
- Relations:
  - Anterior:
    - Coils of small intestine
    - Greater omentum
    - Anterior abdominal wall
  - Posterior:
    - Iliacus
    - Iliac crest
    - Quadratus lumborum
    - Origin of transversus abdominis
    - Lower pole of right kidney
    - Iliohypogastric and ilioinguinal nerves
- Transverse colon:
  - Extends across the abdomen in the umbilical region and is approximately 38cm long
  - Intraperitoneal
  - Begins at right colic flexure and hangs downwards, supported by transverse mesocolon, before ascending to the left colic flexure (splenic flexure)
  - Attached to pancreas via mesocolon
  - Left colic flexure is higher than the right and suspended from diaphragm by the phrenicocolic ligament
  - Position of the transverse colon is variable due to the length of the mesocolon
  - Mesentery attached to superior border, greater omentum attached to inferior border
- Relations:
  - Anterior:
    - Greater omentum
    - Anterior abdominal wall
  - Posterior:
    - 2nd part of duodenum
    - Head of pancreas
    - Coils of small intestine
- Descending colon:
  - Approximately 25cm long, lies in left upper and lower quadrants
  - Extends from left colic flexure (splenic flexure) to pelvic brim, where it becomes continuous with the sigmoid colon
  - Rarely has a mesentery
  - Usually retroperitoneal
- Relations:
  - Anterior:
    - Coils of small intestine

- Greater omentum
- Anterior abdominal wall
  - ■ Posterior:
    - Lateral border of left kidney
    - Origin of transversus abdominis muscle
    - Quadratus lumborum
    - Iliac crest
    - Iliacus
    - Left psoas
    - Iliohypogastric nerve
    - Ilioinguinal nerve
    - Lateral cutaneous nerve of the thigh
    - Femoral nerve
- Sigmoid colon:
  - ■ 25–40cm long, continuation of descending colon
  - ■ Becomes continuous with rectum in front of S3
  - ■ Attached to posterior abdominal wall by sigmoid mesocolon
  - ■ Sigmoid mesocolon hangs down from an inverted V-shaped root overlying the bifurcation of the common iliac artery
- Relations:
  - ■ Anterior:
    - In male: urinary bladder
    - In female: posterior surface uterus; upper part of vagina
  - ■ Posterior:
    - Rectum
    - Sacrum

4.6.20 Blood supply of the large bowel

Figure A.4.7 shows the anatomy and blood supply of the large bowel.

- Superior mesenteric artery supplies:
  - ■ Via ileocolic branch:
    - 1st part of ascending colon
    - Caecum
    - Appendix
  - ■ Via right colic branch: ascending colon
  - ■ Via middle colic branch: transverse colon
- Inferior mesenteric artery supplies:
  - ■ Via left colic branch: descending colon
  - ■ Via sigmoid branches: sigmoid colon
  - ■ Via superior rectal branch: rectum

- Branches of superior and inferior mesenteric arteries anastomose with their neighbours above and below, forming a continuous chain of anastomoses known as the marginal artery (of Drummond).
- Mesenteric arteries may be occluded by disease of the aorta.
- Inferior mesenteric artery susceptible to atherosclerotic disease and can result in infarction of the bowel.
- Marginal artery provides anastomosis between superior and inferior mesenteric arteries, but is not always well developed and is often deficient just proximal to the splenic flexure where the 2 main artery territories meet.
- Interruption of arterial supply can result in ischaemic colitis.

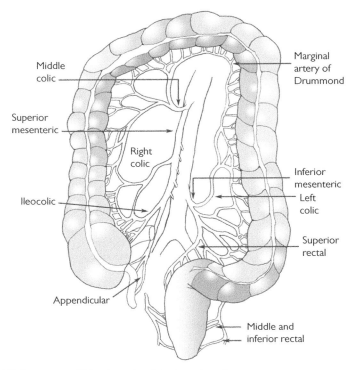

Figure A.4.7 Anatomy and blood supply of the large bowel

Reproduced with permission from MacKay GJ, Dorrance HR, Molloy RG, et al. (2010). *Oxford Specialist Handbook of Colorectal Surgery*. Oxford: Oxford University Press, © 2010.

4.6.21 Nerve supply of the large bowel

- Pain receptors transmit signals via sympathetic fibres that pass along arteries to the aortic plexus (T10–L2).
- Main motor fibres for proximal colon, as far as distal transverse colon, come from vagus nerve.
- Distal large bowel receives motor innervation from sacral nerves.
- Intramural plexuses in the bowel wall connect with extrinsic nerves.

4.7 Liver and biliary tract

4.7.1 Surface markings of liver

- Lies under the cover of the lower ribs on the right side.
- Convex upper surface is moulded to shape of diaphragm and lies below it, rising to the approximate level of the xiphisternal joint.
- Lower border roughly corresponds to the right costal margin (although at the midline it crosses the epigastrium below the margin).
- In infants, the liver may extend 1 or 2 finger-breadths below the costal margin.
- In adults, a hard, enlarged liver edge may be palpated below the costal margin, most easily on deep inspiration when the diaphragm pushes the liver down.

4.7.2 Lobes of the liver

- 4 lobes:
  - Right lobe
  - Left lobe
  - Caudate lobe
  - Quadrate lobe
- The liver is wedge shaped and has an upper diaphragmatic surface and a lower postero-inferior or visceral surface. (See Figure A.4.8)
- Diaphragmatic surface:
  - Convex and lies under diaphragm

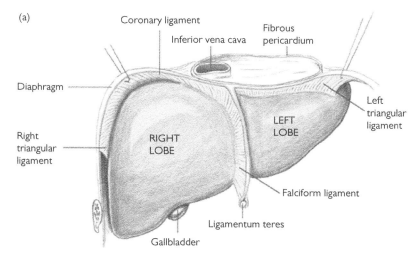

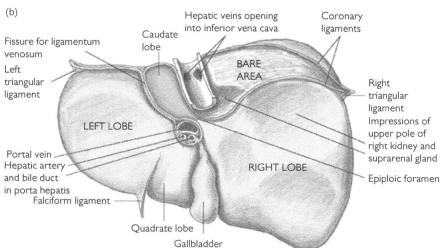

Figure A.4.8 (a) Anterior and (b) posterior views of the liver and its peritoneal reflections

- Has superior, posterior, anterior, and right surfaces
- Covered by peritoneum, which attaches it to the diaphragm
- Postero-inferior surface:
  - Moulded to shape of adjacent viscera
  - Irregular
  - In contact with:
    - Abdominal oesophagus
    - Stomach
    - Duodenum
    - Right colic flexure
    - Right kidney
    - Right adrenal gland
    - Gallbladder
    - IVC
- Anterior relations:
  - Diaphragm
  - Right and left costal margins
  - Right and left pleura and inferior lung margins
  - Xiphoid process
  - Anterior abdominal wall

4.7.3 Liver lobules

- The liver is constructed from smaller building blocks, called liver lobules, and the liver as a whole is surrounded by a fibrous capsule.
- These lobules each have a central vein (a tributary of the hepatic veins) and between the lobules are spaces called the portal canals.
- These spaces contain branches of the hepatic artery and portal vein and a bile duct tributary. Together these 3 vessels are known as the *portal triad*.
- Arterial and venous supply passes between the liver cells by means of sinusoids and then drains into the central vein.

4.7.4 Ligaments of the liver

- The main stability of the liver comes from support by the attachment of the hepatic veins to the IVC.
- The liver ligaments provide additional stability for the liver:
- Falciform ligament:
  - Double fold of peritoneum
  - Ascends from umbilicus to liver
  - Contains the ligamentum teres in its free margin (remains of umbilical vein)
  - Divides into:
    - Coronary ligament: formed by right layer
    - Left triangular ligament: formed by left layer
    - Right triangular ligament: extremity of coronary ligament
    - (Fibres of coronary ligament are widely spaced leaving a bare area on the liver, devoid of peritoneum)
- Ligamentum teres:
  - Contains remains of umbilical vein
  - Passes into fissure on visceral surface of liver
  - Joins left branch of portal vein in porta hepatis
- Ligamentum venosum:
  - Remains of ductus venosus

- Attached to left branch of portal vein
- Situated on visceral surface of liver

4.7.5 Blood supply of liver

- The liver is highly vascular and receives approximately 1.5L of blood per minute. 30% of this blood comes from the hepatic artery, a branch of the coeliac artery (oxygenated blood). 70% comes from the portal vein (deoxygenated blood, rich in products of digestion).
- This blood travels to the central vein of each liver lobule, as described above.
- Central veins drain into right and left hepatic veins, which open directly into the IVC. Right lobe of liver receives blood mainly from intestine. Left, caudate, and quadrate lobes receive blood mainly from stomach and spleen.
- This distribution may explain the pattern of metastasis to the liver.

4.7.6 Lymph drainage

- Liver produces around one-third of body lymph.
- Lymph vessels leave liver via the porta hepatis.
- Coeliac and posterior mediastinal lymph nodes are responsible for drainage.

4.7.7 Gallbladder

- Pear-shaped sac on undersurface of liver.
- Function is to store bile, and concentrate this by absorbing water.
- Divided into a fundus, body, and neck.
- Fundus:
  - Rounded and projects below the liver
- Body:
  - In contact with visceral surface of liver
  - Directed upwards, backwards, and to the left
- Neck:
  - Becomes continuous with cystic duct
- Hartmann's pouch:
  - A dilated area of the gallbladder neck just before the point where it joins the cystic duct
  - Gallstones commonly lodge at this site
- Relations:
  - Anterior:
    - Anterior abdominal wall
    - Inferior surface of liver
  - Posterior:
    - Transverse colon
    - 1st and 2nd parts of duodenum
- The posterior relationship of the gallbladder to the duodenum and transverse colon means that gallstones can sometimes erode through into these structures, and may then lead to gallstone ileus.
- Surface markings: fundus of gallbladder lies opposite tip of right 9th costal cartilage, where lateral edge of right rectus abdominis crosses costal margin.

4.7.8 Biliary ducts

- Bile is secreted by the liver, concentrated and stored in the gallbladder, and delivered into the duodenum to assist digestion.
- Right and left hepatic ducts arise from the right and left lobes of the liver respectively, in the porta hepatis.

- The right and left hepatic ducts run a short course and then unite to form the common hepatic duct.
- Common hepatic duct then unites with the cystic duct from the gallbladder to form the common bile duct.
- Common bile duct is approx 8cm long and is divided into 3 parts:
  - 1st part: lies in the free margin of the lesser omentum, in front of the portal vein and to the right of the hepatic artery
  - 2nd part: lies behind the 1st part of the duodenum, to the right of the gastroduodenal artery
  - 3rd part: lies in a groove on the posterior surface of the head of the pancreas, and comes into contact with main pancreatic duct
- Common bile duct ends by piercing the medial wall of the 2nd part of the duodenum, approximately halfway down its length.
- Usually it is joined by the main pancreatic duct, and together they open into the duodenal wall at the ampulla of Vater.
- The ampulla of Vater opens into the duodenal lumen via the major duodenal papilla and both these structures are surrounded by the sphincter of Oddi.
- There are normal variants of this arrangement where the pancreatic and common bile ducts pierce the duodenum separately.

4.7.9 Nerve supply of bile ducts

- Supply is sympathetic and parasympathetic vagal fibres from the coeliac plexus.
- Biliary colic occurs when the smooth muscle of the gallbladder spasms to try and dislodge a gallstone. Afferent fibres ascend through the coeliac plexus and greater splanchnic nerves to the thoracic nerves, and referred pain is felt in the right upper quadrant or epigastrium (T7, T8, T9).

4.7.10 Portal vein

- Porta hepatis is the hilum of the liver.
- Contains:
  - Left and right hepatic duct, forming the common hepatic duct
  - Hepatic artery
  - Portal vein
- Portal vein:
  - Formed by superior mesenteric and splenic veins
  - Normal portal pressure 5–10mmHg above IVC pressure
  - Portal hypertension can occur in cirrhotic and other disease processes of the liver, which cause obstruction in the portal tree
- Portal hypertension causes:
  - Development of collateral portosystemic circulation
  - Splenomegaly
  - Hepatic failure
  - Ascites
- There are 4 main areas of portosystemic anastomosis developed in portal obstruction:
  - Between left gastric vein and the oesophageal veins—leads to oesophageal varices
  - Between the obliterated umbilical vein and superior and inferior epigastric veins—leads to caput medusae
  - Between the superior and inferior rectal veins—leads to haemorrhoids
  - Retroperitoneal and diaphragmatic anastomoses—leads to potential intraoperative problems

4.8 Pancreas

- The pancreas is a gland with both exocrine and endocrine functions.
- Exocrine—pancreatic juice excreted into the duodenum, containing:
  - Enzymes:
    - Amylase
    - Lipase
    - Trypsinogen and chymotrypsinogen
    - Peptidases
  - Bicarbonate ions
  - Sodium ions
  - Water
- Endocrine:
  - Insulin from ß-cells in islets of Langerhans
  - Glucagon from α-cells in islets of Langerhans
  - Somatostatin from δ-cells in islets of Langerhans
  - Pancreatic polypeptide from F cells
- Anatomically the pancreas is divided into a head, neck, body, and tail:
  - Head:
    - Disc shaped
    - Lies in C-shaped concavity of duodenum
    - Has an uncinate process, which lies behind the superior mesenteric vessels
  - Neck:
    - Constricted section of pancreas
    - Lies in front of portal vein and origin of superior mesenteric artery
  - Body:
    - Passes left and upwards across the midline, forming part of stomach bed
  - Tail:
    - Lies within the lienorenal ligament and is in contact with the hilum of the spleen

4.8.1 Relations of the pancreas

- Anterior (from R to L):
  - Transverse colon
  - Transverse mesocolon
  - Lesser sac
  - Stomach
- Posterior (from R to L):
  - Bile duct
  - Portal vein
  - Splenic vein
  - IVC
  - Aorta
  - Superior mesenteric artery
  - Left psoas muscle
  - Left adrenal gland
  - Hilum of spleen

4.8.2 Surface marking of pancreas

- Lies across the transpyloric plane, with the head below and to the right, the neck on the plane, and the body and tail above and to the left.

- Transpyloric plane:
  - Horizontal plane through the tips of the 9th costal cartilages, at the point where the lateral margin of rectus abdominis crosses the costal margin
  - Lies at level of L1
  - Passes through:
    - Neck of pancreas
    - Pylorus of stomach
    - Duodenojejunal junction
    - Hila of kidneys

4.8.3 Blood supply of pancreas

- Supply from the splenic and pancreaticoduodenal arteries.
- Corresponding veins drain to the portal system.

4.8.4 Lymph drainage

- Lymph drains to nodes situated along the arteries and then to coeliac and superior mesenteric lymph nodes.

4.8.5 Innervation

- Innervation is from sympathetic and parasympathetic vagal nerve fibres.
- Pain is referred to T6–T10 dermatomes.

4.9 Spleen

- Largest lymphoid organ.
- Various functions:
  - Filtering blood—macrophages remove cellular and non-cellular material (e.g. bacteria, defective red cells, and platelets)
  - Haemopoiesis—in foetus and if demand exceeds marrow capacity
  - Immune—antigen recognition
  - Opsonization—antibody synthesis
  - Protection from infection—splenectomy leaves patients more prone to infection (from capsulated organisms)
  - Iron reutilization

4.9.1 Surface markings of the spleen

- Situated in left upper quadrant, lying under cover of 9th–11th ribs.
- Long axis corresponds to the 10th rib.
- Does not normally project forwards in front of midaxillary line.
- Lower pole may be palpated in children.
- Splenic enlargement:
  - A pathologically enlarged spleen extends downwards and medially
  - As it projects below the left costal margin its anterior border can be palpated through the anterior abdominal wall

4.10 Posterior abdominal wall

4.10.1 Muscles of the posterior abdominal wall

- Psoas:
  - Origin: transverse processes, bodies, and intervertebral discs of T12, L1–L5
  - Insertion: lesser trochanter of femur

- ■ Innervation: lumbar plexus
- ■ Action:
  - ● Flexes thigh on trunk
  - ● If thigh is fixed, flexes trunk on thigh (e.g. sitting up)
- ● Quadratus lumborum:
  - ■ Origin:
    - ● Iliolumbar ligament
    - ● Iliac crest
    - ● Transverse processes of lower lumbar vertebrae
  - ■ Insertion: 12th rib
  - ■ Innervation: lumbar plexus
  - ■ Action:
    - ● Fixes 12th rib during inspiration
    - ● Depresses 12th rib during forced expiration
    - ● Laterally flexes vertebral column (same side)
- ● Iliacus:
  - ■ Origin: iliac fossa
  - ■ Insertion: lesser trochanter of femur
  - ■ Innervation: femoral nerve
  - ■ Action:
    - ● Flexes thigh on trunk
    - ● If thigh is fixed, flexes trunk on thigh (e.g. sitting up)
- ● NB Iliacus and psoas are often grouped together and referred to as iliopsoas.
- ● Each of the 3 muscles is covered with a layer of thick fascia, derived from the lumbar fascia.

4.10.2 Vessels of posterior abdominal wall

- ● Aorta:
  - ■ Surface markings:
    - ● Lies in the midline of the abdomen and bifurcates into the right and left common iliac arteries at the level of L4
    - ● Runs behind peritoneum on anterior surfaces of lumbar vertebrae
    - ● Enters abdomen through aortic opening in diaphragm at T12
  - ■ Branches:
    - ● 3 anterior visceral branches: coeliac; superior mesenteric; inferior mesenteric
    - ● 3 lateral branches: suprarenal; renal; testicular/ovarian
    - ● 5 lateral abdominal wall branches: inferior phrenic; 4 lumbar
    - ● 3 terminal branches: 2 common iliac; median sacral
- ● IVC:
  - ■ Surface markings:
    - ● Lies on the right side of the aorta, formed by the union of the common iliac veins behind the right common iliac artery at L5
    - ● Pierces central tendon of diaphragm at T8
  - ■ Tributaries:
    - ● 2 anterior visceral tributaries: hepatic veins
    - ● 3 lateral visceral tributaries: right suprarenal vein; renal vein; right testicular/ovarian vein
    - ● 5 lateral abdominal wall tributaries: inferior phrenic vein; 4 lumbar veins
    - ● 3 veins of origin: 2 common iliacs; 1 median sacral

4.10.3 Lumbar plexus

See Table A.4.2 and Figure A.4.9.

Table A.4.2 Nerves of the lumbar plexus

Branch	Nerve roots	Structures supplied
Iliohypogastric nerve	L1	External oblique Internal oblique Transversus abdominis Skin of lower anterior abdominal wall and buttock
Ilioinguinal nerve	L1	External oblique Internal oblique Transversus abdominis Skin of upper medial aspect of thigh Root of penis/scrotum Mons pubis/labia majorum
Lateral cutaneous nerve of the thigh	L2/L3	Skin of anterior and lateral thigh
Genitofemoral nerve	L1/L2	Cremaster muscle Cremasteric reflex Skin of anterior surface of thigh
Femoral nerve	L2/L3/L4	Iliacus Pectineus Sartorius Quadriceps femoris Skin of anterior surface of thigh Skin of medial side of leg and foot Branches to hip and knee joints
Obturator nerve	L2/L3/L4	Gracilis Adductor brevis Adductor longus Obturator externus Pectineus Adductor portion of adductor magnus Skin of medial surface of thigh Branches to hip and knee joints
Segmental branches		Quadratus lumborum and psoas

4.10.4 Lumbar sympathetic trunk

- Continuous with thoracic and pelvic sympathetic trunks.
- Runs down along medial border of psoas on bodies of lumbar vertebrae.
- Enters abdomen behind medial arcuate ligament and runs down to pelvis by passing behind common iliac vessels.
- Right trunk lies behind right border of IVC.
- Left trunk lies close to left border of aorta.
- Possesses 4/5 segmentally arranged ganglia, with the first 2 often fused together.

4.10.5 Lymph vessels of the posterior abdominal wall

- Lymph nodes are closely related to the aorta.
- Preaortic lymph nodes:
  - Coeliac nodes

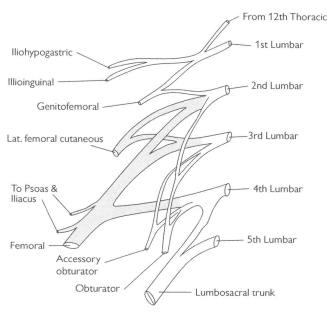

Figure A.4.9 The lumbar plexus

    ■ Superior mesenteric nodes
    ■ Inferior mesenteric nodes
- Drain lymph from:
    ■ The GI tract from lower third of oesophagus to halfway down anal canal
    ■ Spleen
    ■ Pancreas
    ■ Gallbladder
    ■ Greater part of liver
- Para-aortic lymph nodes:
    ■ Drain lymph from:
        ● Kidneys
        ● Adrenals
        ● Testes/ovaries
        ● Uterine tubes
        ● Fundus of uterus
        ● Deep lymph of abdominal wall
        ● Common iliac nodes

4.11 Kidneys, ureters, and bladder

- Each kidney is approximately 11cm long, 6cm wide, and 3cm thick.
- Each has:
    ■ An anterior and posterior surface
    ■ An upper and lower pole
    ■ A hilum (situated at the middle of the medial border)

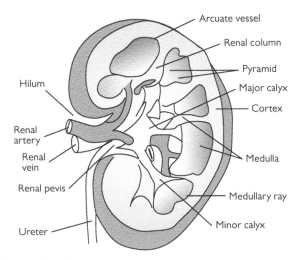

Figure A.4.10 Outline of a kidney

- The renal vein, renal artery, and renal pelvis enter and leave at the level of the hilum in that order, moving anterior to posterior (although the exact anatomy of the contents of the hilum is variable). See Figure A.4.10.
- The kidneys are retroperitoneal and lie (from medial to lateral) on psoas, quadratus lumborum, and the origin of transversus abdominis.
- The upper border of the kidney lies directly on the diaphragm. They are largely under the cover of the costal margin. The right kidney is slightly lower than the left, due to the large right lobe of the liver. With contraction of the diaphragm during normal respiration the kidneys move downwards in vertical direction by around 2.5cm.
- In an individual with poorly developed abdominal musculature, the right kidney may be palpated in the right lumbar region at the end of deep inspiration. The left kidney is not normally palpable.
- On the anterior abdominal wall the hilum of the kidney lies on the transpyloric plane (see Chapter A4, Section 4.8.2) approximately 3 finger-breadths from the midline.
- On the back the kidneys extend from the spine of T12 to the spine of L3 and the hila are at L1.

4.11.1 Relations of the right kidney

- Anterior:
  - Adrenal gland
  - Liver
  - 2nd part of duodenum
  - Right colic flexure
- Posterior:
  - Diaphragm
  - Costodiaphragmatic recess of pleura
  - 12th rib
  - Psoas, quadratus lumborum, and transversus abdominis
  - Subcostal, iliohypogastric, and ilioinguinal nerves

4.11.2 Relations of the left kidney

- Anterior:
  - Adrenal gland
  - Spleen
  - Stomach
  - Pancreas
  - Left colic flexure
  - Coils of jejunum
- Posterior:
  - Diaphragm
  - Costodiaphragmatic recess of the pleura
  - 11th and 12th ribs
  - Psoas, quadratus lumborum, and transversus abdominis
  - Subcostal, iliohypogastric, and ilioinguinal nerves

4.11.3 Coverings of the kidney

- Kidneys have 4 layers of coverings (from deep to superficial):
  - Fibrous capsule
  - Perirenal fat
  - Renal fascia
  - Pararenal fat
- Renal fascia:
  - Tough areolar membrane that splits to enclose the kidney and perinephric fat
  - Condensation of connective tissue, encloses kidneys and adrenals
  - Continuous laterally with transversalis fascia
  - Rupture of an abscess in the kidney into the perinephric tissue results in pus being trapped within the renal fascia
  - This perinephric abscess is contained within the fascia, and points posteriorly above the iliac crest. A large mass may form, with tenderness over the affected kidney. Onset is slow due to the containment of pus within the renal fascia.

4.11.4 Blood supply of kidney

- The renal arteries arise from the aorta at the level of L2. Main arteries divide into posterior and anterior branches. May be a separate upper pole vessel in some patients.
- Each renal artery divides into approximately 5 segmental arteries that enter the kidney at the hilum, which then supply different sections of the kidney.
- These segmental arteries subdivide into lobar arteries and then divide again into interlobar arteries. The interlobar arteries then give off arcuate arteries, which are arranged like umbrella spokes between the cortex and the medulla.
- Renal arteries are end arteries and occlusion results in infarction of the kidney.

4.11.5 Lymphatic drainage

- The lymph vessels follow the renal artery and drain into the para-aortic and lumbar lymph nodes.

4.11.6 Renal colic

- The nerve supply to the kidney is via coeliac plexus, sympathetic trunk, and spinal nerves.
- The pain from renal calculi is colicky in nature and typically radiates from the 'loin to groin'. The renal pelvis and ureter have afferent nerves that run to T11–L2.

- The severe colicky pain occurs when strong peristaltic waves try to push the calculi along the ureter and the pain is referred to the areas supplied by T11–L2: the loin, groin, and flank. If the stone passes into the lower ureter, the pain may be felt in the scrotum or testis in the male, or in the labium majora in the female.
- In addition, pain can sometimes be felt in the front of the thigh, as pain can be referred along the femoral branch of the genitofemoral nerve.

4.11.7 Structure of the kidney

- The kidney is divided into the dark brown outer cortex and a lighter brown inner medulla.
- The medulla is made up of approximately 12 renal pyramids, with the base facing the cortex and the apex (renal papilla) facing medially.
- The pyramids indent approximately 12 minor calyces, which unite to form 2 or 3 major calyces, and in turn these join to form the renal pelvis.
- The renal pelvis may be intra- or extrarenal and is continuous with the upper ureter, which usually lies behind the renal artery in the hilum.

4.11.8 The nephron

- The glomerulus is formed by a group of capillaries, supplied by an afferent arteriole, which invaginates into the Bowman's capsule. It is drained by the efferent arteriole. See Figure A.4.11.
- The glomerular membrane allows passage of small neutral substances into the Bowman's capsule.
- The loop of Henle allows water, sodium, and chloride to be reabsorbed in the descending limb, whilst the ascending limb is impermeable to water but allows re-absorption of sodium and chloride ions.
- This acts as a counter-current multiplier, with the cortex being isotonic and the medulla hypotonic, which allows the formation of dilute urine.

4.11.9 Ureters

- The ureters are muscular tubes extending from the kidneys to the bladder. Urine is propelled along the ureters by peristaltic action.
- The ureter emerges from the hilum of the kidney and runs retroperitoneally downwards on the psoas muscle, along the route of the tips of the transverse processes of the lumbar vertebrae:

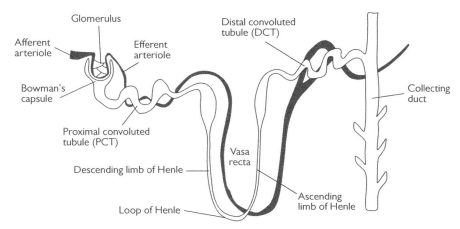

Figure A.4.11 The nephron

- Enters pelvis by crossing the bifurcation of the common iliac artery, in front of the sacroiliac joint
- Then runs down lateral wall of the pelvis to the level of the ischial spine, where it turns medially to enter the bladder at its lateral angle
- This path can be traced on X-rays, and calculi are sometimes visible along the route of the ureter in plain films. Contrast examination (e.g. IVU) can also be used to visualize the ureters.
- Due to the proximity of the right ureter to the appendix, it can be involved in adhesions from a perforated appendix and is at risk during surgery for appendicitis.

4.11.10 Urinary bladder

- The urinary bladder stores urine. It has a capacity of around 500mL in adults.
- In adults it lies behind the symphysis pubis and is entirely within the pelvis when empty.
- When full, its superior border rises up to the hypogastric region, and in children the superior aspect also lies intrabdominally. This makes the bladder more prone to injury from abdominal trauma.
- The empty bladder is pyramidal in shape. See Figure A.4.12.
- Apex:
  - Points anteriorly and lies behind the upper margin of the symphysis pubis
  - Attached to the umbilicus via the urachus (median umbilical ligament)
- Base:
  - Posterior surface
  - Faces posteriorly and is triangular in shape
  - Superolateral angles are joined by ureters and the inferior angle gives rise to the urethra
  - Upper part is covered with peritoneum, forming rectovesical pouch
- Superior surface:
  - Completely covered with peritoneum
  - As bladder fills the superior surface becomes ovoid and bulges into abdomen
- Inferolateral surface:
  - Lies behind the pubic bones

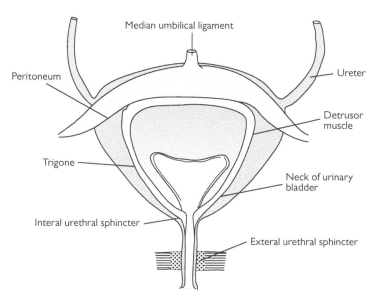

Figure A.4.12 The bladder

- Neck:
  - Neck of the bladder lies inferiorly
- Trigone:
  - The trigone of the bladder is an area of mucous membrane covering the internal surface of the base of the bladder
  - It lies between the two ureteral orifices superiorly and the urethral orifice inferiorly
- Posterior relations of the bladder:
  - Male:
    - Seminal vesicles
    - Vas deferens
    - Ureters
    - Rectum
  - Female:
    - Uterus
    - Vagina

4.11.11 Nerve supply to bladder

- From the hypogastric plexus.
- Sympathetic postganglionic neurons (L1, L2) are vasomotor to the vessels of the bladder and motor to the trigone region and smooth muscle of the urethra at the internal urethral orifice.
- Parasympathetic fibres arise as splanchnic nerves from S2–S4 and pass through hypogastric plexus to reach the bladder wall.
- Afferent sensory fibres reach the CNS via the splanchnic nerves, though some travel via the hypogastric plexus with the sympathetics to L1, L2.
- Sympathetic nerves inhibit contraction of the detrusor muscle and stimulate contraction of the bladder sphincter.
- Parasympathetic nerves stimulate contraction of the detrusor muscle and inhibit the action of the bladder sphincter.

4.11.12 Control of micturition

- Reflex action—also under control of higher centres of brain (once toilet-trained).
- Reflex initiated when stretch receptors detect bladder volume >300mL.
- Afferent impulses pass up pelvic splanchnic nerves to S2–4 and also via hypogastric plexus to L1, L2—conscious desire to micturate.
- Efferent parasympathetic impulses leave cord at S2–4 and travel via pelvic splanchnic nerves and hypogastric plexuses to the bladder wall.
- Smooth muscle of the bladder wall (detrusor) is made to contract and the bladder sphincter is made to relax.
- The urethral sphincter also receives efferent impulses from S2–4 via the pudendal nerve and also relaxes.
- Once urine enters the urethra, additional afferent impulses reinforce this reflex action, and contraction of abdominal muscles assists micturition.
- In continent individuals this reflex is inhibited by the cerebral cortex until it is appropriate to micturate.
- Inhibitory pathways in the corticospinal tracts pass to S2–4 and cause contraction of urinary sphincters, to allow voluntary control of micturition.

4.11.13 Spinal injury and bladder control

- Initial 'spinal shock phase':
  - Atonic bladder:
    - Bladder wall relaxed
    - Bladder sphincter contracted

- Urethral sphincter relaxed
- Bladder becomes distended, then overflows
- Lasts a few days to weeks
- Cord lesion above S2–4:
  - Automatic reflex:
    - Bladder fills and empties as a reflex activity every 1–4 hours
- Cord lesion destroying S2–4:
  - Autonomous:
    - No reflex control
    - Bladder fills to capacity and overflows
    - Constant dribbling

4.12 Pelvis

4.12.1 The pelvic cavity

- The pelvis is made from a pair of inominate bones, forming the lateral and anterior walls, and the sacrum and coccyx, forming the posterior wall. See Figure A.4.13.
- Inominate bones formed from 3 fused bones:
  - Ilium
  - Ischium
  - Pubis
- Sacroiliac joints are part synovial, part fibrocartilaginous and are reinforced by the ligaments of the pelvis:
  - Sacrotuberous ligament:
    - Extends from lateral part of sacrum and coccyx and posterior inferior iliac spine to the ischial tuberosity
    - Strong
  - Sacrospinous ligament:
    - Triangular in shape
    - Base attached to lateral part of sacrum and coccyx

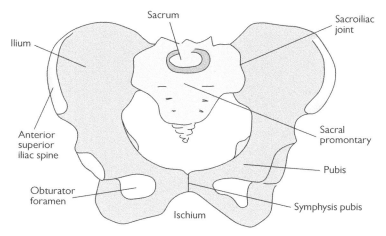

Figure A.4.13 The bones of the pelvis

- Apex attached to ischial spine
- Strong
  - Iliolumbar ligament:
    - Connects tip of L5 transverse process to the iliac crest
  - Posterior sacroiliac ligaments:
    - Suspend sacrum between the iliac bones
    - Very strong
  - Anterior sacroiliac ligaments:
    - Situated on anterior of joint
    - Thin structure
  - Sacrococcygeal joint:
    - Cartilaginous joint between sacrum and coccyx, supported by ligaments
    - Mobile joint
- The symphysis pubis is a cartilaginous joint, with a fibrocartilaginous disc interposed between cartilaginous articular surfaces.
- Pelvis is lined with muscles and fascia, to support the pelvic organs. The pelvic floor is a layer of muscle that divides the pelvis into the main pelvic cavity (above the pelvic floor) and the perineum below.

4.12.2 Rectum and anus

- The rectum is approximately 13cm long and begins anterior to S3, where the transverse mesocolon ends. It is a continuation of the sigmoid colon without structural differentiation.
- The peritoneum covers the upper third of the rectum at the front and sides.
- The peritoneum covers the middle third of the rectum at the front only.
- It passes downwards in front of the sacrum and coccyx and ends by piercing the pelvic diaphragm to become the anus.
- Puborectalis portion of the levator ani muscles forms a sling at the junction of the rectum and anus, and pulls this part of the bowel forwards, forming the anorectal angle.
- The anal canal has 2 layers of circular muscle making up the wall, an internal anal sphincter of smooth muscle and an external anal sphincter of skeletal muscle. The puborectalis muscle is continuous with the external anal sphincter at this level.

4.12.3 Relations of the rectum and anus

Figure A.4.14 shows the sagittal section of the female pelvis.

- Posterior relations (both sexes):
  - Sacrum
  - Coccyx
  - Levatores ani
  - Sacral plexus
  - Sympathetic trunks
- Anterior relations (male):
  - Sigmoid colon
  - Posterior surface of bladder
  - Termination of vas deferens
  - Termination of seminal vesicles
  - Prostate
- Anterior relations (female):
  - Rectouterine pouch
  - Posterior surface of vagina
  - Cervix

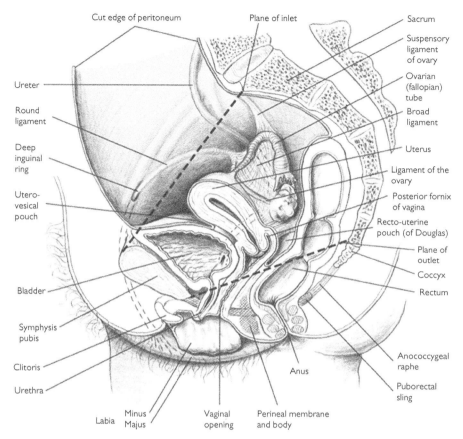

Figure A.4.14 Sagittal section of female pelvis

Reproduced with permission from MacKinnon P, Morris J. (2005). *Oxford Textbook of Functional Anatomy*, Vol. 2. Oxford: Oxford University Press, © 2005.

- (On PR examination, only the prostate/cervix and the coccyx can be palpated in a 'normal' examination.)
- The prostate and rectum are separated by the strong rectovesical fascia (of Denonvilliers), which helps prevent local spread of rectal carcinoma to the prostate and vice versa.

4.12.4 Innervation of rectum and anus

- The sympathetic nerve supply is from branches from the hypogastric and coeliac plexuses.
- The parasympathetic supply is from S2–4 via the pelvic splanchnic nerves.

4.12.5 Blood supply of the rectum and anus

- Superior rectal artery: terminal branch of inferior mesenteric artery.
- Median sacral artery: from internal iliac artery.
- Middle rectal artery: from internal iliac artery.
- Inferior rectal arteries: from internal pudendal branch of internal iliac artery.

4.12.6 Lymph drainage of rectum and anus

- The lymph drainage of the rectum and anus is to the pararectal nodes and then along the branches of the arteries.
- Lymph from the upper and middle sections accompanies the superior rectal artery to the inferior mesenteric nodes. Lymph from the lower part of the rectum and anus is drained accompanying the middle rectal artery to the internal iliac nodes.

4.12.7 Defecation

- The rectum is empty until there is an increase in activity in the left side of the colon (e.g. after eating a meal). As faeces enter the rectum, the person has the sensation of needing to pass stool. Sitting or crouching straightens the anorectal angle, and stool can enter the anal canal.
- The person is able to distinguish gas from solids. Anal sphincter is under voluntary control.
- The normal pressure of the anal sphincter (45–90mmHg) can be doubled by squeeze pressure. Diaphragm, levator ani, and abdominal wall muscles all contract to aid defecation. The rectum can accommodate up to 400mL of faeces.

4.12.8 Anal region in spinal pathology

- Examination of the anus and rectum is important when patients present with spinal pathology. The skin around the anus is supplied by S5, S4, S3 in concentric circles and loss of sensation here can suggest spinal injury or cauda equine.
- Loss of anal tone is also suggestive of serious spinal pathology as the anal sphincter is supplied by S2–4.

4.13 Prostate

- The prostate is a glandular organ with a fibrous capsule, lying inferior to the bladder.
- It surrounds the prostatic urethra and is approximately 3cm long.
- The normal prostate weighs approximately 20g.

4.13.1 Relations

- Superiorly: neck of bladder
- Inferiorly: urogenital diaphragm
- Anteriorly: symphysis pubis (connected by puboprostatic ligaments)
- Posteriorly: rectum (separated by rectovesical fascia (of Denonvilliers))
- The base of the prostate lies against the bladder neck and is pierced by the urethra at its centre.
- The apex of the prostate lies against the urogenital diaphragm, and the urethra leaves the prostate just above the apex on the posterior surface.
- The prostate is anatomically divided into 5 lobes:
  - Anterior
  - Middle
  - Posterior
  - Right lateral
  - Left lateral
- The middle lobe contains a large amount of glandular tissue and so is often principally affected in benign prostatic hypertrophy (BPH).
- This middle lobe enlarges upwards and encroaches on the bladder sphincter, causing the urinary symptoms associated with BPH (enlargement of lateral lobes contributes to this, often leading to urinary retention).

- In BPH the enlarged prostate usually has a regular contour when palpated per rectum.
- Malignant enlargement of the prostate tends to occur in the periphery of the prostate, and is limited by the prostatic capsule.
- In malignant enlargement the prostate often feels hard and irregular when palpated per rectum.
- Blood supply: internal pudendal, inferior vesical, and middle rectal arteries.
- Venous drainage: peri-prostatic plexus.
- Lymph drainage: drains into the internal/external iliac, sacral, and vesical lymph nodes.

4.14 Female reproductive system

4.14.1 Uterus

- Hollow pear-shaped organ with thick, muscular walls. See Figure A.4.9.
- In a nulliparous adult it measures:
  - 8cm long
  - 5cm wide
  - 2.5cm thick
- It is divided into the fundus, body, and cervix, as shown in Figure A.4.15.
- The relations of the uterus are:
  - Anteriorly:
    - Superior surface of bladder
    - Uterovesical pouch
    - Anterior fornix of vagina (cervix)
  - Posteriorly: rectouterine pouch (of Douglas)
  - Laterally:
    - Broad ligament/uterine vessels
    - Ureter
    - Lateral fornix of vagina
    - Round ligaments
    - Uterine (Fallopian) tubes

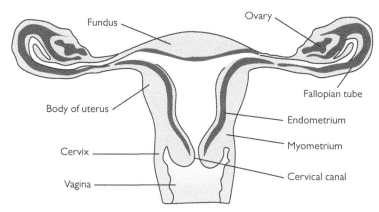

Figure A.4.15 The normal uterus

4.14.2 Uterine (Fallopian) tubes

- The uterine tubes are 10–12cm long and run from the superolateral sides of the body of the uterus to the pelvic wall. Each uterine tube is contained within the broad ligament, a sheet of peritoneum draped over the tubes.
- Each tube is divided into:
  - Indundibulum: trumpet-shaped opening into the peritoneal cavity, positioned over the ovary
  - Ampulla: wide, thin-walled, and tortuous
  - Isthmus: narrow, straight, and thick-walled
  - Intramural part: pierces uterine wall
- Ectopic pregnancy occurs when a fertilized ovum implants outside the uterine cavity. The commonest site for implantation is the uterine tube (97%). Of these tubal pregnancies, 75% occur in the ampulla and 25% in the isthmus. The remaining 3% of ectopics occur intra-abdominally, in the ovary or the cervix.

4.14.3 Blood supply of the uterus and ovary

- The uterus is supplied by the uterine artery (a branch of the internal iliac artery). It runs in the base of the broad ligament, and 2cm lateral to the cervix it passes anterior and superior to the ureter ('water under the bridge') to reach the uterus at the level of the internal os.
- The artery ascends tortuously up the lateral side of the body of the uterus and then turns laterally and inferiorly, where it terminates by anastomosing with the terminal branches of the ovarian artery.
- The uterine tubes receive blood supply from both the uterine and ovarian arteries. Erosion of the tube by an ectopic pregnancy results in effusion of a large quantity of blood into the peritoneal cavity, leading to peritonitis.
- Innervation of uterus and uterine tubes—from the inferior hypogastric plexus.

4.14.4 Ovary

- The ovary is an almond-shaped organ, measuring approximately 4cm × 2cm, lying against the lateral wall of the pelvis in the ovarian fossa.
- It is attached to the posterior aspect of the broad ligament by the mesovarium. The suspensory ligament of the ovary is a fold of peritoneum, which merges with the peritoneum over psoas. The round ligament of the ovary is the remnant of the gubernaculum and links the medial edge of the ovary with the lateral wall of the uterus.
- Blood supply of the ovary—via the ovarian artery, a direct branch of the aorta.
- Lymph drainage of the ovary follows the ovarian artery to the para-aortic nodes.
- Innervation of the ovary is derived from the aortic plexus, and from T10, T11. There may also be fibres from the inferior hypogastric plexus, and ovarian pain may be felt paraumbilically or in the thigh, as in appendicitis.
- The pathological ovary can cause local pressure on the lateral cutaneous nerve of the thigh, which will again lead to pain in the thigh.

4.14.5 Vagina

- The vagina surrounds the cervix of the uterus and then passes forwards and downwards through the pelvic floor to open into the vestibule.
- The vestibule is the area enclosed by the labia minora and contains the urethral orifice, which lies immediately behind the clitoris.
- In the adult the vagina is usually 7–8cm long.
- Its relations are:
  - Anterior:
    - Base of bladder
    - Urethra

- Posterior:
  - Rectouterine pouch (of Douglas)
  - Anterior wall of rectum
  - Perineal body
  - Anal canal
- Superior: ureter
- Lateral:
  - Levator ani muscles
  - Pelvic fascia
- Structures palpable on digital vaginal examination:
  - Cervix
  - Uterus (bimanual palpation)
  - Adnexae (bimanual palpation)
  - Vaginal walls

4.15 Male urogenital region

4.15.1 Male urethra

- The male urethra is approximately 20cm in length. It extends from the neck of the bladder to the external meatus on the glans penis.
- It is divided into 3 parts:
  - Prostatic urethra:
    - Approximately 3cm long
    - Passes through prostate
    - Widest and most dilatable portion of urethra
  - Membranous urethra:
    - Approximately 1.5cm long
    - Lies within the urogenital diaphragm surrounded by the urethral sphincter muscle
    - Least dilatable part of the urethra
  - Penile urethra:
    - Approximately 15.5cm long
    - Enclosed in the bulb and corpus spongiosum of penis
    - External meatus is the narrowest part of the whole urethra
    - Urethra within the glans penis is dilated to form the fossa terminalis (navicular fossa)
    - Bulbourethral glands open into penile urethra below urogenital diaphragm

4.15.2 Scrotum

- The scrotum is an out-pouching of the anterior abdominal wall and contains the testes, epididymis, and lower ends of the spermatic cords.
- The innervation of the scrotal skin is from L1, S2, S3.
- The anterior surface is supplied by the ilioinguinal nerves, and the genital branch of the genitofemoral nerves.
- The posterior surface is supplied by branches of the peroneal nerves and the posterior cutaneous nerves of the thigh.
- The lymph drainage of the scrotum is via the medial group of superficial inguinal lymph nodes.

4.15.3 Penis

- The penis has a fixed root and a body, which is free.

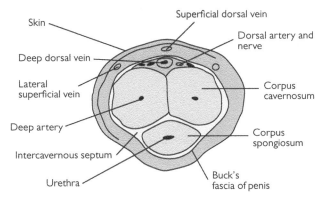

Figure A.4.16 Cross-section of the penis

- The root of the penis is made up of 3 bodies of erectile tissue:
  - Bulb of penis
  - Right crus
  - Left crus
- The bulb is situated in the midline and is attached to the undersurface of the urogenital diaphragm.
- The bulb is traversed by the urethra and is covered by the bulbospongiosus muscles.
- Each crus is attached to the side of the pubic arch and is covered by the ischiocavernosus muscle.
- The bulb continues forward and becomes the corpus spongiosum.
- The crura continue forward and merge, forming the corpora cavernosa.
- The body of the penis is made up of 3 cylinders of erectile tissue, enclosed in a tubular sheath of fascia (Buck's fascia).
- A cross-section through the body of the penis is shown in Figure A.4.16, demonstrating each of the different layers.
- The penis is innervated by the pudendal nerves and the pelvic plexuses (S2–4).

Head and neck

CONTENTS

5.1 Fascial layers of the neck

- Superficial fascia:
  - Thin layer enclosing the platysma muscle
  - Embedded in it are superficial vessels and lymph nodes along with cutaneous nerves
- Deep cervical fascia:
  - Areolar tissue supporting the structures of the neck
  - It condenses to form 4 well-defined fibrous sheets:
    - Investing fascia: completely encircles the neck
    - Prevertebral fascia: lies in front of the prevertebral muscles
    - Pretracheal fascia: allows movement of trachea during swallowing
    - Carotid sheath: surrounds internal jugular vein, common carotid artery, and vagus nerve

5.2 Tissue spaces of the neck

- These are potential spaces within the neck, and are important as infections originating in the mouth, pharynx, teeth, and oesophagus can spread throughout them.
- There are 4 main clinically important fascial spaces in the neck (see Figure A.5.1):
  - *Prevertebral space*: space between the vertebral bodies and the prevertebral fascia
  - *Retropharyngeal space*: space between the middle layer of deep cervical fascia anteriorly and the deep layer of the deep cervical fascia posteriorly. It extends from the skull base to T4
  - *Parapharyngeal space*: the parapharyngeal space is the shape of an inverted pyramid with its base attaching to the skull base and the apex at the level of the hyoid bone. It is bordered by the nasopharynx and oropharynx and by the retropharyngeal space

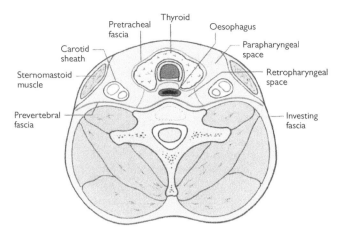

Figure A.5.1 Fascial layers and spaces of the neck

Reproduced with permission from Corbridge, Steventon. (2009). *Oxford Handbook of ENT and Head and Neck Surgery* (2 ed). Oxford: Oxford University Press, © 2009.

- *Submandibular space*: below the mandible and mylohyoid muscle, bordered medially by the anterior belly of the digastric muscle, posteriorly by the posterior border of the submandibular gland, it reaches inferiorly to the level of the hyoid bone
- Infection in the tissue spaces: organisms from the pharynx, teeth, mouth, and oesophagus can enter the fascial spaces and can then spread from one to the other along fascial planes. Dental infections may spread from the mandible into the submandibular space and then spread throughout the spaces. It is possible for blood, pus, or air in the retropharyngeal space to spread downwards into the superior mediastinum.
- *Ludwig's angina*: acute infection of the submandibular space, usually secondary to dental infection. Pus can fill the space, pushing the tongue forward and upward, and downwards spread may lead to vocal cord oedema and airway obstruction.

5.3 Triangles of the neck

5.3.1 Muscles of the neck

- Platysma:
  - Origin: deep fascia over pectoralis major and deltoid
  - Insertion: body of mandible and angle of mouth
  - Innervation: facial nerve (cervical branch)
  - Action: depresses mandible and angle of mouth
- Sternocleidomastoid:
  - Origin: manubrium and middle third of clavicle
  - Insertion: mastoid process
  - Innervation: spinal part of accessory nerve, C2, C3
  - Actions:
    - Two muscles together extend head and flex neck
    - One muscle alone rotates head to opposite side

- Suprahyoid muscles: act as effectors of swallowing
  - Digastric
  - Stylohyoid
  - Geniohyoid
  - Mylohyoid
- Infrahyoid muscles: act as laryngeal depressors
  - Sternothyroid
  - Sternohyoid
  - Thyrohyoid
  - Omohyoid

5.3.2 Boundaries of the anterior triangle

- Medial: the midline.
- Lateral: anterior border of sternocleidomastoid.
- Superior: lower border of the mandible.
- Roof: investing fascia.
- Floor: prevertebral fascia.

5.3.3 Boundaries of the posterior triangle

- Anterior: sternocleidomastoid.
- Posterior: trapezius.
- Base: middle third of clavicle.
- Roof: investing fascia.
- Floor: pevertebral fascia.

5.4 Thyroid

- Consists of right and left lobes connected by a narrow isthmus. Very vascular organ, contained within a sheath derived from the pretracheal deep fascia.
- Each lobe is pear shaped and lies with its apex on the lamina of the thyroid cartilage and its base at the level of the 4th or 5th tracheal ring. The isthmus lies across the midline at the level of the 2nd, 3rd, and 4th tracheal rings. Sometimes a pyramidal lobe is present and projects upwards from the isthmus.

5.4.1 Relations of the lobes

- Lateral:
  - Sternothyroid
  - Sternohyoid
  - Sternocleidomastoid
  - Omohyoid
- Medial:
  - Larynx
  - Pharynx
  - Trachea
  - Oesophagus
  - External laryngeal nerve
  - Recurrent laryngeal nerve (in groove between trachea and oesophagus)
- Posterior:
  - Parathyroids
  - Carotid sheath and its contents

- Inferior thyroid artery
- Thoracic duct (left lobe only)

5.4.2 Relations of the isthmus

- Anterior:
  - Sternothyroids
  - Sternohyoids
  - Anterior jugular veins
  - Fascia
  - Skin
- Posterior:
  - 2nd, 3rd, 4th tracheal rings

5.4.3 Blood supply of thyroid

- Superior thyroid artery (from the external carotid).
- Inferior thyroid artery (from the thyrocervical trunk of the subclavian).
- Thyroidea ima artery (present in 3% of individuals, from brachiocephalic or aortic arch).
- Lymphatic drainage:
  - Upper section: anterior-superior group of deep cervical nodes
  - Lower section: posterior-inferior group of deep cervical lymph nodes
  - (Some nodes descend to paratracheal nodes)

5.5 Trachea

- The trachea is a mobile tube.
- It commences at the lower border of the cricoid cartilage of the larynx at C6. Extends downwards in the midline of the neck.
- Divides into 2 main bronchi at the level of the intervertebral disc between T4 and T5.
- C-shaped rings of hyaline cartilage keep the lumen patent.

5.5.1 Relations of the trachea in the neck

- Anteriorly:
  - Skin
  - Fascia
  - Isthmus of thyroid
  - Anterior jugular venous arch
  - Thyroidea ima artery (in 3%)
  - Inferior thyroid veins
- Posteriorly:
  - Recurrent laryngeal nerves
  - Oesophagus
  - Vertebral column
- Laterally:
  - Lobes of thyroid (as far as 5th/6th ring)
  - Carotid sheath

5.5.2 Emergency tracheotomy/cricothyroidotomy

- The thyroid and cricoid cartilages are palpated and identified.
- A tube is then inserted through the cricothyroid membrane, either by needle cricothyroidotomy, or by making an incision and passing a tube into the trachea.

5.6 Oesophagus

- The oesophagus extends from the pharynx to the stomach.
- Its relations in the neck are:
  - Anterior:
    - Trachea
    - Recurrent laryngeal nerves (in groove between trachea and oesophagus)
  - Posterior:
    - Prevertebral layer of deep cervical fascia
    - Vertebral column
    - Longus colli muscle
  - Lateral:
    - Lobes of thyroid
    - Carotid sheath
    - Thoracic duct (left side)

5.7 Cervical sympathetic trunk

- The cervical section of the sympathetic trunk is divided into 3 ganglia.

5.7.1 Superior cervical ganglion

- Large and immediately below the skull.
- Branches:
  - Internal carotid nerve: forms internal carotid plexus
  - Gray rami communicantes: to anterior rami of C1–4
  - Arterial branches: to common and external carotid arteries
  - Cranial nerve branches: join 9th, 10th, and 12th cranial nerves
  - Pharyngeal branches: join glossopharyngeal and vagus nerve pharyngeal branches and form pharyngeal plexus
  - Superior cardiac branch: descends to cardiac plexus

5.7.2 Middle cervical ganglion

- Small and lies at level of cricoid cartilage.
- Branches:
  - Gray rami communicantes: to anterior rami C5–6
  - Thyroid branches: pass along inferior thyroid artery
  - Middle cardiac branch: descends to cardiac plexus

5.7.3 Inferior cervical ganglion

- Fuses with 1st thoracic ganglion to form stellate ganglion.
- Branches:
  - Gray rami communicantes: to anterior rami of C7–8
  - Arterial branches: to subclavian and vertebral arteries
  - Inferior cardiac branch: descends to cardiac plexus

5.7.4 Horner's syndrome

- The cervical sympathetic trunk gives supply to the head and neck via the stellate ganglion, and this includes fibres that supply the orbit. When this nerve supply is interrupted it leads to Horner's syndrome.

- This is characterized by:
  - Constriction of the pupil
  - Ptosis
  - Enophthalmos
- Causes of Horner's syndrome include:
  - Traumatic injury
  - Malignancy (Pancoast's tumour of lung)
  - Cervical rib

5.8 Root of the neck

- Scalenus anterior:
  - Origin: transverse processes of C3–6
  - Insertion: 1st rib
  - Innervation: C4–6
  - Action:
    - Elevates 1st rib
    - Laterally flexes and rotates cervical section of vertebral column

5.8.1 Phrenic nerve in the root of the neck

- Phrenic nerve arises from C3, 4, 5 of the cervical plexus.
- The roots of the phrenic nerve unite at the lateral border of scalenus anterior at the level of the cricoid cartilage.
- The nerve runs down, vertically across the front of scalenus anterior, behind the prevertebral layer of deep fascia.
- The nerve crosses scalenus anterior from its lateral to its medial border and enters the thorax by crossing in front of the subclavian artery and behind the origin of the brachiocephalic vein.
- Relations of phrenic nerve in neck:
  - Anteriorly:
    - Prevertebral deep fascia
    - Internal jugular vein
    - Superficial cervical artery
    - Suprascapular artery
    - Thoracic duct (left side)
    - Origin of brachiocephalic vein
  - Posteriorly:
    - Scalenus anterior
    - Subclavian artery
    - Cervical dome of pleura

5.8.2 Recurrent laryngeal nerves

- Both recurrent laryngeal nerves arise from the vagi.
- Left nerve hooks around arch of aorta.
- Right nerve passes beneath subclavian artery.
- Recurrent laryngeals ascend in the groove between the trachea and oesophagus. Pass behind pretracheal fascia and lie next to medial surface of the thyroid lobes.

5.8.3 Deep cervical lymphatics

- Deep cervical lymph nodes form a chain along the course of the internal jugular vein.

- 2 major lymph nodes:
  - Jugulodogastric node:
    - Below and behind angle of mouth
    - Drains tonsil and tongue
  - Jugulo-omohyoid node:
    - Related to intermediate tendon of omohyoid
    - Drains the tongue

5.8.4 Subclavian vein

- The axillary vein continues as the subclavian vein as it crosses the junction of the 1st rib, behind the clavicle.
- The subclavian vein ends behind the sternoclavicular joint, where it joins the internal jugular vein to form the brachiocephalic vein.
- The subclavian vein is below and in front of the subclavian artery and above and in front of the cervical dome of the pleura.
- On the left side the thoracic duct enters the subclavian vein, and so central venous cannulation is safer on the right side:
  - It is safest to approach from below the clavicle
  - The patient is positioned supine, arms by their side, and with their head turned to the opposite side
  - The skin is prepared and local anaesthetic instilled
  - The Seldinger technique is used, and the needle is inserted directly below the clavicle, at the junction of the proximal third and medial third of the clavicle
  - The needle tip is slowly advanced towards the suprasternal notch, along the under-surface of the clavicle
  - Gentle aspiration allows the operator to know when the vein is entered
  - The guidewire can now be sited and then the catheter placed over this and sutured in place
- The anatomy of the region can lead to the following complications:
  - Pneumothorax/haemothorax (proximity of pleura)
  - Arteriovenous fistula (puncture of subclavian artery)
  - Thoracic duct injury (if inserted on left)
  - Catheterization of neck or axillary veins
  - Brachial plexus injury
  - Cardiac arrhythmias/rupture of right atrium

5.8.5 Subclavian artery

- The subclavian artery is divided into 3 parts by the scalenus anterior muscle:
  - The 1st part extends from its origin (on the left from the arch of the aorta and on the right from the brachiocephalic artery) to the medial border of scalenus anterior
  - The 2nd part lies posterior to scalenus anterior
  - The 3rd part extends from the lateral border of scalenus anterior to the outer border of the 1st rib
- Subclavian artery can be palpated by pressing down, backwards, and medially on the clavicular head of sternocleidomastoid (its transverse cervical branch can be palpated 1 finger-breadth above and parallel to the clavicle).

5.9 The face

See Table A.5.1 for facial muscles.

5.9.1 The modiolus

- The modiolus is a chiasma of facial muscles held together by fibrous tissue.

Table A.5.1 Muscles of the facial region

Muscle		Origin	Insertion	Innervation	Action
Obicularis occuli	Palpebral part	Medial palpebral ligament	Lateral palpebral raphe	Facial nerve	Closes eyelids Dilates lacrimal sac
	Orbital part	Medial palpebral ligament and adjoining bone	Loops return to origin	Facial nerve	Folds skin around orbit (to protect eye)
Levator palpebrae superioris		Lesser wing of sphenoid	Anterior surface and upper border of superior tarsal plate	Occulomotor (voluntary) Sympathetics (involuntary)	Raises upper eyelid
Occipito-frontalis	Occipital belly	Occipital bone	Epicranial aponeurosis	Facial nerve	Moves scalp on skull and raises eyebrows
	Frontal belly	Skin and superficial fascia of eyebrows	Epicranial aponeurosis	Facial nerve	Moves scalp on skull and raises eyebrows
Obicularis oris		Maxilla, mandible, and skin	Encircles oral orifice	Facial nerve	Compresses lips together
Buccinator		Maxilla, mandible, and pterygo-mandibular ligament	Maxilla, mandible and pterygo-mandibular ligament	Facial nerve	Compresses cheeks and lips against teeth
Temporalis		Floor of temporal fossa	Coronoid process of mandible	Mandibular division of trigeminal	Elevates mandible Posterior fibres retract mandible
Masseter		Zygomatic arch	Lateral surface of ramus of mandible	Mandibular division of trigeminal	Elevates mandible (occludes teeth)
Lateral pterygoid (2 heads)		Greater wing of sphenoid and lateral pterygoid plate	Neck of mandible and articular disc	Mandibular division of trigeminal	Pulls neck of mandible forwards
Medial pterygoid		Tuberosity of maxilla and lateral pterygoid plate	Medial surface of angle of mandible	Mandibular division of trigeminal	Elevates mandible

- It is located lateral and slightly superior to each angle of the mouth.
- It is important in moving the mouth and in facial expression.
- Innervated by the facial nerve.
- Blood supply from labial branches of the facial artery.
- It is contributed to by the following muscles:
    - Orbicularis oris
    - Buccinator

- Levator anguli oris
- Depressor anguli oris
- Zygomaticus major
- Risorius quadratus labii superioris
- Quadratus labii inferioris

5.9.2 The facial nerve

- The motor part of the facial nerve (CN VII) emerges from the stylomastoid foramen (as shown in Figure A.5.2).
- It gives off 2 branches immediately before it enters the parotid gland:
  - 1. Muscular branch to posterior belly of digastric and stylohyoid
  - 2. Posterior auricular nerve
- The nerve then enters the parotid gland and divides into its 5 terminal branches, which emerge from the parotid:
  - 1. Temporal branch:
    - Emerges from upper border of gland
    - Supplies: anterior auricular muscle; superior auricular muscle; frontal belly of occipitofrontalis; orbicularis oculi; corrugator supercilii
  - 2. Zygomatic branch:
    - Emerges from anterior border of gland
    - Supplies: orbicularis oculi
  - 3. Buccal branch:
    - Emerges from anterior border of gland
    - Supplies: buccinator; muscles of upper lip and nostril
  - 4. Mandibular branch:
    - Emerges from anterior border of gland
    - Supplies: muscles of lower lip
  - 5. Cervical branch:
    - Emerges from lower border of gland
    - Supplies: platysma; depressor anguli oris muscle

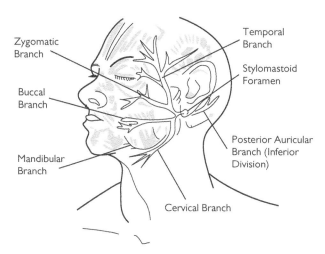

Figure A.5.2 The facial nerve

5.9.3 Sensory nerve supply of the face

- The sensory supply of the face is from the trigeminal nerve.
- The trigeminal nerve is subdivided into 3 divisions, each of which contains several branches. These supply sensation to the face as shown in Figure A.5.3.
  - 1. Ophthalmic division, 5 branches:
    - Lacrimal
    - Supraorbital
    - Supratrochlear
    - Infratrochlear
    - External nasal
  - 2. Maxillary division, 3 branches:
    - Zygomaticotemporal
    - Zygomaticofacial
    - Infra-orbital
  - 3. Mandibular division, 3 branches:
    - Auriculotemporal
    - Buccal
    - Mental
- The areas of Figure A.5.3 show the dermatomes of the head and neck and which nerves supply them.
- This dermatomal distribution is important clinically as trigeminal neuralgia and shingles from herpes zoster infection create pain in a dermatomal distribution. The vesicles of shingles also appear in a dermatomal distribution.
- Sturge–Weber syndrome affects the trigeminal nerve, and the associated port-wine birth mark is due to an abundance of capillaries around the ophthalmic branch of the trigeminal nerve.

5.9.4 Facial artery

- The facial artery is a branch of the external carotid artery.
- It leaves the external carotid near the lingual artery and reaches the border of the mandible, just anterior to the masseter muscle.

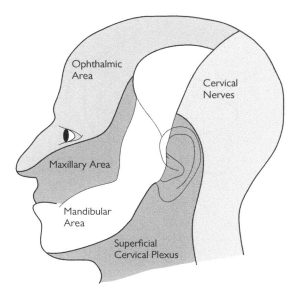

Figure A.5.3 Dermatomes of the face

- From here it runs a tortuous course past the angle of the mouth and along the side of the nose.
- From the side of the nose the artery is sometimes renamed the angular artery and runs upwards to reach the medial angle of the eye, where it anastomoses with orbital vessels.
- The torturosity of the artery allows it to stretch when the mouth is opened wide (e.g. when yawning).
- 4 branches of the facial artery:
  - Submental artery
  - Inferior labial artery
  - Superior labial artery
  - Lateral nasal artery

5.9.5 Superficial temporal artery

- The superficial temporal artery is a terminal branch of the external carotid artery.
- Deep to the mandible, within the substance of the parotid gland, the external carotid divides into its 2 terminal branches, the maxillary artery and the superficial temporal artery.
- The superficial temporal branch curls behind the neck of the mandible and runs upwards to supply the superficial tissues of the temple and scalp.
- It crosses the root of the zygomatic arch, in front of the auriculotemporal nerve and the auricle. Its pulsation can be felt at this point.
- The artery ascends into the scalp and divides into anterior and posterior divisions.
- There are 8 branches of the external carotid artery, each shown on Figure A.5.4.

5.9.6 Venous drainage of the face

- Facial vein forms at the medial angle of the eye from the supraorbital and supratrochlear veins.
- As the supraorbital vein is connected to the superior ophthalmic vein, and this in turn communicates with the cavernous sinus, there is a pathway from the facial vein into the cavernous sinus.
- This is clinically important as infection in the face can spread to the cavernous sinus, resulting in cavernous sinus thrombosis, which can be fatal.

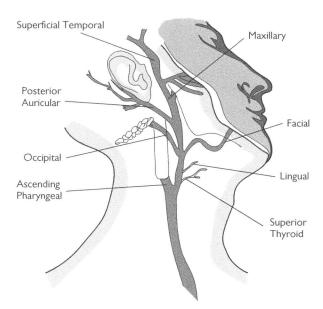

Figure A.5.4 Branches of external carotid artery

- The facial vein descends behind the facial artery to the inferior margin of the body of the mandible.
- It then passes superficially to the submandibular gland and drains into the internal jugular vein.

5.9.7 Lymph drainage of the face

- Drainage is via 3 groups of nodes:
  - Submandibular lymph nodes drain:
    - Forehead
    - Anterior portion of the face
  - Preauricular lymph nodes drain:
    - Lateral portion of face
  - Submental lymph nodes drain:
    - Lower lip
    - Chin

5.10 The scalp

- The scalp is made up of 5 layers, which can be remembered by each letter of the word *SCALP*:
  - *S*kin
  - *C*onnective tissue
  - *A*poneurosis
  - *L*oose areolar tissue
  - *P*eriosteum

5.10.1 Arterial supply of scalp

- The scalp has a rich anastomosing network of arteries to supply nourishment to the hair follicles, as shown in Figure A.5.5.
- These arteries come from branches of both the external and internal carotid arteries:
  - Supratrochlear arteries
  - Supraorbital arteries
  - Superficial temporal arteries
  - Posterior auricular arteries
  - Occipital arteries
- This rich arterial supply means that scalp wounds may demonstrate profuse bleeding, as the arteries have deep dermal attachments.

5.10.2 Venous drainage of the scalp

- Veins draining the scalp accompany the arteries:
  - Supratrochlear veins
  - Supraorbital veins
  - Superficial temporal veins
  - Posterior auricular veins
  - Occipital veins
- The veins communicate freely with each other and in addition are connected to the diploic veins of the skull bones and, via emissary vessels, to the intercranial venous sinuses.
- This means that scalp infections can lead to osteomyelitis of the skull bones, and venous sinus thrombosis. Pus can also spread throughout the potential space below the aponeurosis.

5.10.3 Innervation of the scalp

- Figure A.5.5 shows the sensory innervation of the scalp and compares this with the arterial supply.

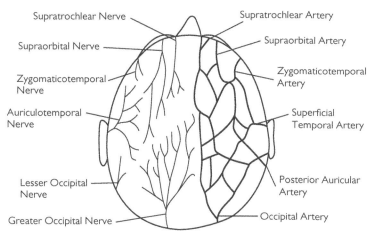

Figure A.5.5 Innervation and arterial supply of the scalp

5.10.4 Temporal fossa

- The boundaries of the temporal fossa:
  - Superior: superior temporal line on the side of the skull
  - Anterior: frontal process of zygomatic bone
  - Inferior: zygomatic arch (formed by the zygomatic process of the temporal bone and the temporal process of the zygomatic bone)
- Contents of temporal fossa:
  - Temporalis (see Table A.5.1)
  - Temporal fascia
  - Deep temporal nerves
  - Auriculotemporal nerve
  - Superficial temporal artery
  - Deep temporal arteries
- These structures are at risk if there is a fracture or injury in this region.

5.10.5 Parotid gland

- The parotid is the largest of the salivary glands.
- It is situated below the external auditory meatus, in a deep hollow bounded by the ramus of the mandible, the mastoid process, and the styloid process. It lies in front of the sternocleidomastoid.
- It is surrounded by the parotid sheath, a strong layer of investing fascia, which limits the swelling of the gland and causes the pain associated with parotid inflammation (e.g. in mumps).
- Structures within the parotid gland:
  - Facial nerve and branches (see Chapter A5, Section 5.9.2 on facial nerve)
  - Retromandibular vein
  - External carotid artery
  - Parotid lymph nodes
- The parotid duct emerges from the gland and passes forwards over the lateral surface of the masseter muscle. At the anterior border of masseter, it turns medially and pierces buccinator, then passes forwards to open into the mouth, opposite the 2nd upper molar tooth.
- Innervation of parotid:
  - Secretomotor function supplied by parasympathetics from CN IX

- Sensory supply from the auriculotemporal nerve
- Sympathetic supply from the external carotid artery nerve plexus

5.10.6 Infratemporal fossa

- This region is situated beneath the skull base, between the ramus of the mandible and pharynx.
- Contents:
  - Lateral pterygoid (see Table A.5.1)
  - Medial pterygoid (see Table A.5.1)
  - Mandibular division of trigeminal nerve
  - Otic ganglion
  - Chorda tympani (branch of CN VII)
  - Maxillary artery
  - Pterygoid venous plexus
  - Maxillary vein

5.10.7 Maxillary artery

- This is a terminal branch of the external carotid artery.
- It gives off several branches in the infratemporal fossa:
  - Inferior alveolar artery (follows alveolar nerve)
  - Middle meningeal artery (important supply to meninges of skull)
  - Branches to external auditory meatus and tympanic membrane
  - Branches to the muscles of mastication
  - Branches to nose and palate

5.10.8 Pterygoid venous plexus

- Venous plexus related to the pterygoid muscles, which drains into the maxillary vein, and then to the retromandibular vein in the parotid.
- Communicates with the facial vein via the deep facial vein.
- Consequently infection in this region can spread to the ophthalmic veins and the cavernous sinus, causing cavernous sinus thrombosis as described previously.
- The pterygoid venous plexus is susceptible to injury when a dentist inserts a mandibular nerve block, as the needle is inserted lateral to the pterygomandibular ligament to access the inferior alveolar nerve.

5.10.9 Mandibular nerve

- This division of the trigeminal nerve traverses the middle cranial fossa and emerges through the foramen ovale in the greater wing of the sphenoid bone.
- The mandibular nerve then descends until it reaches the border of the lateral pterygoid, where it divides into a small anterior and a large posterior division.
- Branches from anterior division:
  - Masseteric nerve
  - Deep temporal nerves
  - Nerve to lateral pterygoid
  - Buccal nerve (does not supply buccinator, which is supplied by facial nerve)
- Branches from posterior division:
  - Auriculotemporal nerve (supplies sensation to skin of auricle, external auditory meatus, tympanic membrane, parotid gland, TMJ, branches to scalp)
  - Conveys parasympathetic fibres to the parotid
  - Lingual nerve (supplies sensation to the tongue, gives no branches in infratemporal fossa, joined by chorda tympani at lower border of lateral pterygoid, frequently receives a branch from inferior alveolar nerve)
  - Inferior alveolar nerve (supplies sensation to teeth of lower jaw and skin of face, gives a branch which supplies mylohyoid and anterior belly of digastric)

5.10.10 Chorda tympani

- This is a branch of the facial nerve, which enters the infratemporal fossa through the petrotympanic fissure.
- The nerve carries secretomotor parasympathetic fibres to the submandibular and sublingual salivary glands.
- It joins the lingual nerve and carries taste fibres from the anterior two-thirds of the tongue.

5.10.11 Glossopharyngeal nerve (cranial nerve IX)

- Leaves the skull through the jugular foramen.
- Contributes to the pharyngeal plexus.
- Supplies motor innervation to stylopharangeus.
- Supplies parasympathetic fibres to the parotid via the otic ganglion.
- Receives sensory fibres from the tonsils, posterior third of tongue, and the middle ear.
- Receives sensory fibres from the oropharynx and is involved in the gag reflex.
- Receives visceral sensory fibres from the carotid bodies and carotid sinus.

5.10.12 Vagus nerve (cranial nerve X)

- Leaves the skull through the jugular foramen.
- Supplies motor fibres to:
  - Constrictor muscles of pharynx
  - Intrinsic muscles of larynx
  - Involuntary muscle of heart, bronchi, and trachea
  - Involuntary muscle of alimentary tract
  - Liver
  - Pancreas
- Receives sensory fibres from:
  - Epiglottis and vallecula
  - Afferent fibres from the structures it supplies with motor fibres
- Nucleus ambiguus: situated posterior to the inferior oliviary nucleus in the upper medulla, this nucleus gives rise to the efferent motor fibres of the vagus and glossopharyngeal nerves, and parasympathetic fibres to the heart. The cranial portion of the accessory nerve also receives contributions from this nucleus.

5.10.13 Accessory nerve (cranial nerve XI)

- Leaves the skull through the jugular foramen.
- Cranial portion gives motor supply to:
  - Muscles of soft palate
  - Muscles of pharynx and larynx
- Spinal portion gives motor supply to:
  - Sternocleidomastoid
  - Trapezius

5.10.14 Hypoglossal nerve (cranial nerve XII)

- Leaves skull through the hypoglossal canal.
- Gives motor supply to:
  - Muscles of the tongue (except palatoglossus)

5.10.15 Maxillary division of trigeminal nerve (cranial nerve V)

- Leaves skull through foramen rotundum.
- Receives sensory fibres from:
  - Skin over maxilla
  - Upper lip

- Teeth of upper jaw
- Mucous membranes of nose
- Maxillary air sinus
- Palate

5.10.16 Pterygopalatine fossa

- Small space behind and below the orbital fossa.
- Communicates:
  - Laterally with the infratemporal fossa (through the pterygomaxillary fissure)
  - Medially with the nasal cavity, through the spenopalatine foramen
  - Superiorly with the skull through the foramen rotundum
  - Anteriorly with the orbit through the inferior orbital fissure
- Contains the pterygopalatine ganglion, which provides sensory, secretomotor, and sympathetic innervation of the nasal cavity, lacrimal glands, paranasal sinuses, pharynx, and gingiva.
- Injury from facial trauma that involves the pterygopalatine ganglia can cause a decrease in tear production and dry nasal mucosa, along with decreased sensation in the region supplied by the ganglion.

5.11 Nose and paranasal region

- The nose is made up of the external nose and the nasal cavity.

5.11.1 External nose

- Framework of external nose made up of:
  - Nasal bones
  - Frontal process of maxilla
  - Nasal part of frontal bone
  - Upper nasal cartilage
  - Lower nasal cartilage
  - Septal cartilage
- Cutaneous innervation is via the ophthalmic and maxillary branches of the trigeminal nerve (see Chapter A5, Section 5.9.3).
- Blood supply is from branches of the facial artery and ophthalmic artery.

5.11.2 Nasal cavity

- The nasal cavity extends from the nares to the posterior nasal aperture (choanae).
- It is divided into right and left halves by the nasal septum.
- Each half has a floor, a roof, and a medial and lateral wall.
- Floor:
  - Palatine process of maxilla
  - Horizontal plate of the palatine bone (upper surface of hard palate)
- Roof:
  - Body of sphenoid bone
  - Cribriform plate of ethmoid bone
  - Frontal bone
  - Nasal bone
  - Nasal cartilages
- Medial wall:
  - Nasal septum

- Lateral wall:
  - The lateral wall has 3 projections:
    - Superior nasal concha
    - Middle nasal concha
    - Inferior nasal concha
- Below each of the nasal conchae is an area known as a meatus (e.g. superior meatus lies below superior concha):
  - Superior meatus: receives openings of posterior ethmoidal sinuses
  - Middle meatus: receives openings of middle ethmoidal sinuses, maxillary sinus, and the frontal and anterior ethmoidal sinuses
  - Inferior meatus: receives opening of the nasolacrimal duct (which carries tears from the lacrimal sac into the nasal cavity)
- The sphenoethmoidal recess lies above the superior concha and receives the opening of the sphenoidal sinuses.

5.11.3 Innervation of nasal cavity

- Specialized olfactory cells ascend through the cribriform plate to the olfactory bulbs, where they are supplied by the olfactory nerve.
- Sensory nerves are derived from the ophthalmic and maxillary divisions of the trigeminal nerve:
  - Anterior nasal cavity: anterior ethmoidal nerve
  - Posterior nasal cavity: nasal, nasopalatine, and palatine branches of pterygopalatine ganglion

5.11.4 Blood supply of nasal cavity

- Arterial supply is derived mainly from branches of the maxillary artery.
- On the nasal septum there is a region called Little's area, where 4 arteries anastomose:
  - Anterior ethmoid artery (branch of ophthalmic artery)
  - Great palatine artery (branch of maxillary artery)
  - Sphenopalatine artery (branch of maxillary artery)
  - Superior labial artery (branch of facial artery)
- This area is commonly the source of epistaxis.

5.11.5 Paranasal sinuses

- The paranasal sinuses are arranged in pairs as shown in Figures A.5.6 and A.5.7. They are filled with air and lined with mucoperiosteum.
- They act as resonators of sound and reduce the weight of the skull.
- The mucus produced drains into the nose and is removed from the body.
- When the sinuses become blocked the patient's voice changes.
- At birth the maxillary and sphenoidal sinuses are present only in rudimentary form.
- They enlarge after the age of 8 years and are fully formed by adolescence.

5.12 Mouth and hard palate

- The mucous membrane of the mouth receives its sensory innervation mainly from branches of the trigeminal nerve:
  - Roof of mouth:
    - Greater palatine nerve
    - Nasopalatine nerve
  - Floor of mouth:
    - Lingual nerve
    - Taste fibres in chorda tympani
  - Cheek:
    - Buccal nerve

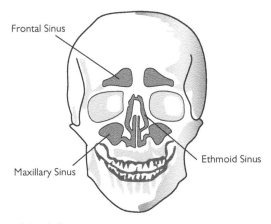

Figure A.5.6 Sinuses of the skull

5.12.1 Permanent teeth

- 32 permanent teeth
- In each jaw there are:
  - 2 canines
  - 4 premolars
  - 6 molars
- Approximate ages of eruption are:
  - 1st molars: 6 years
  - Central incisors: 7 years
  - Lateral incisors: 8 years
  - 1st premolars: 9 years
  - 2nd premolars: 10 years
  - Canines: 11 years
  - 2nd molars: 12 years
  - 3rd molars (wisdom teeth): 17–30 years

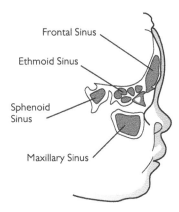

Figure A.5.7 Lateral view of the skull sinuses

5.12.2 Innervation

- The teeth of the upper jaw are innervated by the maxillary division of the trigeminal via the anterior superior alveolar nerve and posterior superior alveolar nerves.
- The teeth of the lower jaw are innervated by the mandibular division of the trigeminal via the inferior alveolar nerve.
- Dental anaesthesia:
  - Lower teeth are anaesthetized by a mandibular block—injection of local anaesthetic into the infratemporal fossa lateral to the pterygomandibular ligament anaesthetizes the inferior alveolar and lingual nerves. This anaesthetizes the lower teeth, dorsum of anterior two-thirds of tongue, mucosa of the floor of the mouth, gingiva of the mandibular arch and incisors, and the mucosa of the lower lip. This is augmented by infiltration of local anaesthetic behind the lower 3rd molar, which in addition blocks the long buccal nerve.
  - Upper teeth—require infiltration of anaesthetic on both the inside and outside of the maxillary process, just distal to the tooth to be anaesthetized. This local infiltration provides adequate anaesthesia as the maxilla has a thin layer of cortical bone, and the spongy bone within allows rapid diffusion of the anaesthetic.

5.12.3 Structure of the tooth

See Figure A.5.8.

5.12.4 Hard palate

- Thin, horizontal plate made from:
  - Palatine processes of the maxilla
  - Horizontal plates of palatine bones
- It is continuous with the soft palate behind and forms the floor of the nasal cavities.
- Its blood supply is from the greater palatine artery.
- It is innervated by the greater palatine nerve and nasopalatine nerve.

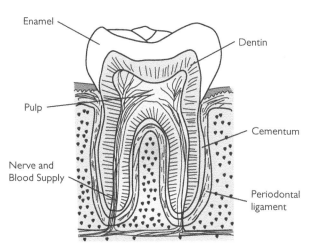

Figure A.5.8 Structure of a tooth

5.12.5 The tongue

- The tongue is divided into 2 parts by the sulcus terminalis (see Figure A.5.9):
  - Anterior two-thirds or oral part
  - Posterior third or pharyngeal part
- Blood supply of the tongue is mainly from the lingual artery. Secondary blood supply is from tonsillar branch of facial artery and ascending pharyngeal artery.
- Nerve supply of tongue:
  - Posterior third:
    - Taste: glossopharyngeal nerve
    - Sensation: glossopharyngeal nerve
  - Anterior two-thirds:
    - Taste: chorda tympani
    - Sensation: lingual nerve (from mandibular nerve)
  - Motor innervation to the whole tongue is from hypoglossal nerve (except palatoglossus, supplied by CN X)
- Lymphatic drainage:
  - Posterior third: drains to deep cervical lymph nodes
  - Anterior two-thirds: drains via submandibular nodes to the deep cervical nodes (tip drains via submental nodes)
- Because the tongue is a midline structure the lymph frequently drains to both sides of the neck (eventually to the jugular lymphatics), meaning it is imperative to detect cancer early. Resection of the tongue is a radical and complicated procedure, and chemo and radiotherapy are frequently used in place of surgery.

5.12.6 Floor of the mouth

- Formed by the anterior two-thirds of the tongue and the mucous membrane from the sides of the tongue to the gum on the mandible.
- In the midline the frenulum connects the under-surface of the tongue to the floor of the mouth.

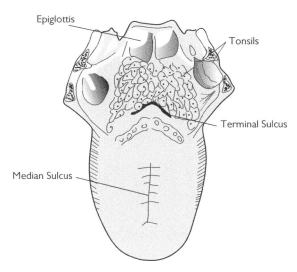

Epiglottis

Tonsils

Terminal Sulcus

Median Sulcus

Figure A.5.9 The structure of the tongue

- The floor contains:
  - Sublingual gland
  - Lingual nerve
  - Submandibular gland
  - Submandibular duct
  - Hypoglossal nerve

5.12.7 The pharynx

- The pharynx is situated posterior to the nasal cavities, mouth, and larynx.
- It is funnel shaped, with the wider end under the skull and the narrow end becoming continuous with the oesophagus at the level of C6.
- Divided into 3 layers—from outside in:
  - Mucous
  - Fibrous
  - Muscular
- Muscular layer arranged as 3 sheets of constrictor muscles, superior, middle, and inferior, whose fibres run in a circular direction.
- Lymph drainage of the pharynx:
  - Direct drainage into deep cervical nodes
  - Indirect drainage into deep cervical nodes via retropharyngeal or paratracheal nodes
- Innervation of pharynx:
  - Main nerve supply is from the pharyngeal plexus formed from branches of:
    - Glossopharyngeal nerve
    - Vagus nerve
    - Sympathetic nerves
  - Motor nerve supply from pharyngeal plexus
  - Sensory nerve supply:
    - Nasopharynx—maxillary nerve
    - Oropharynx—glossopharyngeal nerve
    - Entrance to larynx—internal laryngeal branch of vagus nerve

5.12.8 Interior of pharynx

- The pharynx is arranged into 3 continuous sections (see Figure A.5.10):
  - Nasal part
  - Oral part
  - Laryngeal part

- Nasal part of the pharynx:
  - The adenoids or pharyngeal tonsils are located in the nasal part of the pharynx, high in the submucosa of the posterior wall
  - The opening of the auditory tube is on the lateral wall of the pharynx, at the level of the floor of the nose. This tube equalizes pressure between the pharynx and the middle ear
- Oral part of the pharynx:
  - Contains the palatine tonsils:
    - Lie in the tonsillar fossa on each side of the pharynx
    - Blood supply is via tonsillar branch of facial artery
    - Tonsillar bed is very vascular and there is a risk of postoperative haemorrhage following tonsillectomy
  - Veins drain to the pharyngeal venous plexus and into the facial, external palatine, or pharyngeal vein
  - Lymph drainage is to nodes that drain into the deep cervical nodes

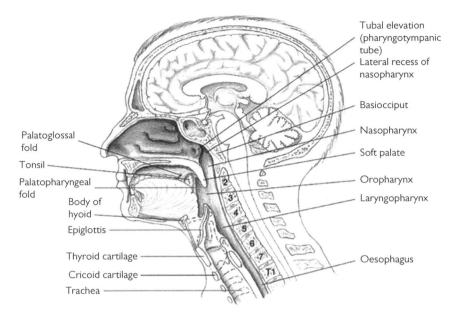

Figure A.5.10 Sagittal section of head and neck to show pharynx

Reproduced with permission from MacKinnon P, Morris J. (2005). *Oxford Textbook of Functional Anatomy*, Vol. 3.
Oxford: Oxford University Press, © 2005.

- ■ The jugulodigastric lymph node, below and behind the angle of the mandible, can become
  particularly swollen and tender in tonsillitis
- ■ The valleculae are situated in the oropharynx, just behind the root of the tongue, on each
  side of the median epiglottic fold, and are an important landmark in intubation
- Laryngeal part of the pharynx:
  - ■ The laryngopharynx lies behind the larynx and the opening into the larynx
  - ■ Its anterior wall comprises the inlet of the larynx, with the piriform fossa on either side.
  - ■ This fossa is a common site for foreign bodies to become lodged and can be viewed with a
    laryngoscope as seen in Figure A.5.11

5.12.9 Soft palate

- The soft palate is a fold of tissue attached to the posterior aspect of the hard palate.
- It is comprised of a mucous membrane and a series of paired muscles, which are able to
  tighten and move the soft palate to aid with speech and closure of the nasopharynx.
- The muscles of the soft palate are innervated by the pharyngeal plexus.
- Sensation of the soft palate is innervated via the maxillary division of the trigeminal nerve
  (via the palatine branches).
- Secretomotor fibres to the soft palate are from the pterygopalatine ganglion.
- The uvula is a small flap of tissue that hangs from the posterior edge of the soft palate.
- The uvula contains fibrous tissue and muscle and is involved in closing off the nasopharynx
  from the mouth during speech and swallowing, and in the gag reflex.

5.12.10 The gag reflex

- This is a reflex contraction of the back of the throat, elicited by touching the soft palate
  or uvula.

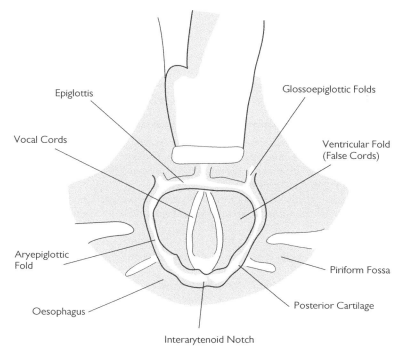

Figure A.5.11 View of the larynx via a laryngoscope

- It plays an important role in preventing material from entering the throat and thus prevents choking.
- The afferent pathway controlling this reflex is from the glossopharyngeal nerve (CN IX).
- The efferent pathway is via the vagus nerve (CN X).
- The gag reflex is absent if there is damage to CNs IX and X and in brainstem death.
- The reflex may also be triggered deliberately to induce vomiting.

5.13 The larynx

- The larynx can be thought of as a valve that protects the entrance to the tracheobronchial tree and allows breath-holding whilst straining.
- It is also important in speech, phonation, and coughing.
- It is situated between the laryngeal part of the pharynx above and the trachea below, with which it is continuous. The larynx lies between the level of C4 and C6.
- The larynx has a cartilaginous framework, connected by a series of ligaments and membranes, and moved by muscles.
- There are 9 cartilages making up the larynx:
  - Cricoid (a complete ring)
  - Thyroid
  - Epiglottis
  - 2 arytenoid (paired)
  - 2 corniculate (paired)
  - 2 cuneiform (paired)

- The articulation of the cartilages is shown in Figures A.5.12 and A.5.13.
- The cuneiform cartilages are very small and rod shaped, and each is situated within one of the aryepiglottic folds.
- The cricoid cartilage is attached to the 1st ring of the trachea by the cricotracheal ligament.
- The cricoid cartilage is attached to the thyroid cartilage by the cricothyroid ligament.
- Movement of the cricothyroid joint changes the tension of the vocal cords.
- Movement of the cricoarytenoid joints abduct and adduct the vocal cords.

5.13.1 Cricothyroid membrane (conus elasticus)

- This structure stretches between the cricoid and thyroid cartilages.
- It is this membrane that is divided during surgical cricothyroidotomy.
- The anterior portion of the superior border of the cricothyroid membrane is thickened at its free edge to form the vocal ligament (vocal cord).
- The vocal cords stretch from the vocal process of the arytenoid cartilages to the thyroid laminae, and movement of these cords together and apart allows phonation.

5.13.2 Laryngeal muscles

- The muscles of the larynx are divided into intrinsic and extrinsic groups.
- Intrinsic muscles:
  - These muscles are responsible for movement of the vocal ligaments
  - They can produce abduction, adduction, tightening, and relaxation of the vocal ligaments
  - They also play a role in controlling the laryngeal inlet
- Extrinsic muscles:
  - Responsible for elevation and depression of the larynx during swallowing
- The motor nerve supply to the muscles of the larynx is via the recurrent laryngeal nerve (except the muscle cricothyroid, which is supplied by the external laryngeal nerve).
- Injury to the recurrent laryngeal nerves (by thyroid surgery, trauma, or tumour) has a profound effect on speech:
  - External laryngeal nerve injury: leads to paralysis of cricothyroid muscle and weakness of the voice
  - Complete recurrent laryngeal paralysis:
    - Unilateral: vocal cord in neutral position (between abducted and adducted position) on affected side. Other vocal cord compensates and voice not greatly affected
    - Bilateral: both vocal cords assume the neutral position, breathing is impaired, and speech is lost

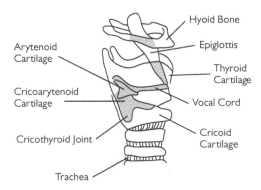

Figure A.5.12 Lateral view of the larynx

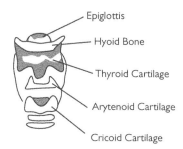

Figure A.5.13 Anterior view of the larynx

- Partial recurrent laryngeal paralysis:
  - Unilateral: vocal cord assumes adducted position, other side can compensate
  - Bilateral: both vocal cords assume the adducted position. Dyspnoea and stridor result and an emergency airway is required

5.14 The orbit and eye

5.14.1 The orbital margin
- Formed from:
  - Superior: frontal bone
  - Lateral: processes of frontal and zygomatic bones
  - Inferior: zygomatic bone and maxilla
  - Medial: process of maxilla and frontal bone

5.14.2 Eyelids
- Situated in front of the eye to protect it.
- Upper lid is larger and more mobile than lower lid.
- The orbital septum forms the framework of the eyelid and attaches to the orbital margin, where it becomes continuous with the periosteum.
- At the lid margins the orbital septum is thickened to form the tarsal plates, and these plates attach medially and laterally to a tubercle just inside the orbital margin.
- The meibomian glands (tarsal glands) are situated along the edges of the eyelids and secrete an oily substance that prevents tear film evaporation, prevents leakage of tears, and helps form an airtight seal when the eye is closed.
- Sensory innervation of the eyelids is via the ophthalmic division of the trigeminal nerve:
  - Upper lid:
    - Infratrochlear
    - Supratrochlear
    - Lacrimal
    - Supraorbital
  - Lower lid:
    - Infratrochlear
    - Infraorbital

5.14.3 Lacrimal apparatus
- Lacrimal gland:
  - Situated above the eyeball in the anterior and upper section of the lateral orbit, surrounding the lateral margin of levator palpebrae superioris

- Serous gland, producing tears
- Ducts open from the gland into the lateral part of the superior fornix of the conjunctiva and tears spread across the eye
● Lacus lacrimalis: tears spread across the eye and accumulate here.
● Canaliculi: tears enter the canaliculi and are transmitted medially to open into the lacrimal sac.
● Lacrimal sac:
  - Lies in the lacrimal groove, behind the medial palpebral ligament
  - Tears collect here before passing into the nasolacrimal duct
● Nasolacrimal duct: travels through a bony canal from the lacrimal sac, downwards, backwards, and laterally, to open into the inferior meatus in the nose.

5.14.4 Orbital muscles

Figure A.5.14 shows the extrinsic muscles of the eyeball and Figure A.5.15 shows the extraocular muscles.

● Levator palpebrae superioris:
  - Origin: lesser wing of sphenoid
  - Insertion: anterior surface and upper border of superior tarsal plate
  - Innervation:
    ● Oculomotor nerve (voluntary)
    ● Sympathetic nerves (involuntary)
  - Action: raises upper eyelid
● Superior rectus:
  - Origin: common tendinous ring
  - Insertion: sclera (6mm behind corneal margin)
  - Innervation: oculomotor nerve

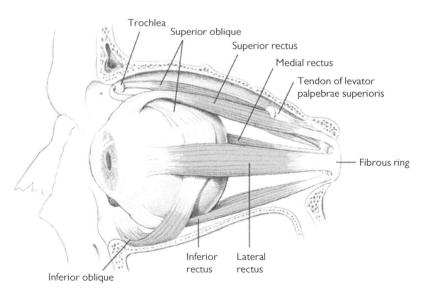

Figure A.5.14 Extrinsic muscles of eyeball
Reproduced with permission from MacKinnon P, Morris J. (2005). *Oxford Textbook of Functional Anatomy*, Vol. 3. Oxford: Oxford University Press, © 2005.

- ■ Action: raises and medially rotates cornea
- ● Inferior rectus:
  - ■ Origin: common tendinous ring
  - ■ Insertion: sclera (6mm behind corneal margin)
  - ■ Innervation: oculomotor nerve
  - ■ Action: depresses and medially rotates cornea
- ● Lateral rectus:
  - ■ Origin: common tendinous ring
  - ■ Insertion: sclera (6mm behind corneal margin)
  - ■ Innervation: abducent nerve
  - ■ Action: moves cornea laterally
- ● Medial rectus:
  - ■ Origin: common tendinous ring
  - ■ Insertion: sclera (6mm behind corneal margin)
  - ■ Innervation: oculomotor nerve
  - ■ Action: moves cornea medially
- ● Superior oblique:
  - ■ Origin: body of sphenoid
  - ■ Insertion: pulley and attached to sclera
  - ■ Innervation: trochlear nerve
  - ■ Action: moves cornea down and laterally
- ● Inferior oblique:
  - ■ Origin: anterior orbital floor
  - ■ Insertion: attached to sclera
  - ■ Innervation: oculomotor nerve
  - ■ Action: moves cornea up and laterally

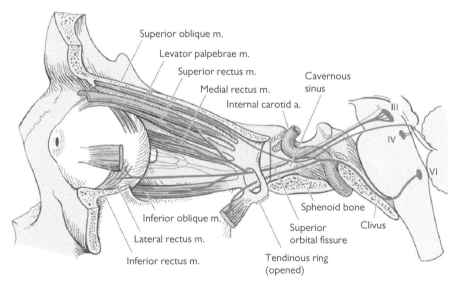

Figure A.5.15 The extraocular muscles

Reproduced with permission from Frotscher, M. and Bahr, M. (2005), *Duus' Topical Diagnosis in Neurology* (4 ed.). Georg Thieme Verlag KG, © 2005.

5.14.5 Orbital stability

- The medial and lateral recti attach the eyeball to the medial and lateral orbital walls (by the medial and lateral check ligaments), providing stability and suspending the eyeball from the orbit, like a hammock.

5.14.6 Optic nerve

- CN II
- Enters the orbit through the optic canal, accompanied by the ophthalmic artery.
- Ensheathed in all 3 dural layers (pia, arachnoid, and dura mater).
- Meninges fuse with sclera, so the subarachnoid space extends into the orbit. When CSF pressure rises, this space fills, and results in papilloedema.
- The optic nerve receives its blood supply from the central artery of the retina, arising from the ophthalmic artery.

5.14.7 Orbital vessels

- The ophthalmic artery and its branches supply the eye, its muscles, and the lacrimal gland.
- Venous drainage of the orbit is via the superior ophthalmic vein (which communicates with the facial vein) and the inferior ophthalmic vein. Both of these veins pass through the superior orbital fissure and drain into the cavernous sinus.
- There are no lymph nodes in the orbit, but drainage of the region occurs via preauricular and parotid groups to the deep cervical nodes.

5.14.8 Structural anatomy of the eye

- The eyeball is coated in 3 layers:
  - Fibrous coat:
    - Sclera: dense fibrous tissue
    - Cornea: transparent area responsible for allowing light to enter
  - Pigmented coat:
    - Choroid: highly vascular
    - Ciliary body: attached to iris and lens and contains ciliary muscle, which alters refractive power of lens
    - Iris: pigmented section of eye; surrounds the pupil. Involuntary muscle fibres control pupillary size
  - Nervous coat: retina
- It has an anterior chamber, filled with aqueous humour, and a posterior chamber, filled with vitreous humour. The lens lies between the humours. See Figure A.5.16.

5.14.9 Corneal reflex

- Consensual reflex in which blinking is stimulated by touching the cornea.
- The sensory innervation of the cornea is:
  - Long ciliary nerves: from the ophthalmic branch of trigeminal nerve
  - Short ciliary nerves: from the oculomotor nerve
- The reflex pathway is:
  - Cornea is touched with cotton wool
  - Afferent limb via long and short nasociliary nerves (trigeminal)
  - Impulse travels through trigeminal ganglion (does not synapse)
  - Impulse reaches trigeminal nucleus in pons
  - Impulse transmitted to facial nerve nucleus in pons
  - Efferent limb via facial nerve
  - Obicularis oculi stimulated—eyes closed

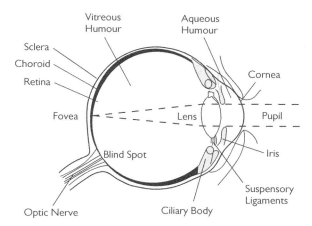

Figure A.5.16 The eye

5.14.10 Control of pupillary size

- The muscle fibres of the iris are involuntary and have circulating and radiating fibres.
- The circular fibres form sphincter pupillae:
  - Supplied by parasympathetic fibres from oculomotor nerve
  - Constricts pupil
- The radiating fibres form dilator pupillae:
  - Supplied by sympathetic fibres that travel with long ciliary nerves
  - Dilates pupil
- The size of the pupil is therefore controlled by the balance of sympathetic and parasympathetic impulses, and this balance may be upset, resulting in pathology:
  - Argyll-Robertson pupil: bilateral small pupils that don't react to light but react to accommodation. Seen in neurosyphillis. Light reactive fibres are damaged but fibres reacting to near vision remain intact.
  - Horner's syndrome: results in unilateral small pupil, due to damage to the sympathetic nervous system fibres that would normally be responsible for pupillary dilation.

5.14.11 Retina

- The retina is the light-sensitive portion of the eye, containing the photosensitive rods and cones.
- The optic nerve enters the retina via the optic disc.
- The optic disc is pierced by the central artery of the retina and also forms the 'blind spot' of the eye as it is devoid of photosensitive cells. See Figure A.5.17.
- The macula lies temporal to the optic disc and has a depressed area within it, called the fovea, which has the most distinct area for vision and the highest density of photosensitive cells.

5.14.12 Oculomotor disorders

- Oculomotor innervation can be remembered using the mnemonic *LR6(SO4)3*:
  - *Lateral Rectus* is supplied by CN *VI*
  - *Superior Oblique* is supplied by CN *IV*
  - The other muscles are supplied by CN *III*

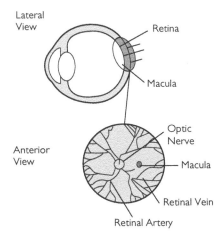

Figure A.5.17 Retina as seen on normal fundoscopy

- Complete IIIrd nerve palsy:
  - Ptosis
  - Inability to move eye superiorly, inferiorly, or medially
  - Eye deviated down and outwards (lateral rectus and superior oblique are spared)
  - Pupil fixed and dilated
- Complete IVth nerve palsy:
  - Paralysis of superior oblique
  - Diplopia, especially on looking down or reading
- Complete VIth nerve palsy:
  - Paralysis of lateral rectus
  - Convergence of the eyes
  - Diplopia maximal on lateral gaze towards the side of the lesion
- Paralysis of individual muscles is summarized in Table A.5.2.

5.15 The ear

- The ear is divided into 3 sections (see Figure A.5.18):
  - External ear
  - Middle ear
  - Inner ear

5.15.1 External ear

- Pinna: folded elastic cartilage, covered with skin
- External auditory meatus: tube leading from the pinna to the tympanic membrane, approximately 3cm long
- Innervation:
  - Auriculotemporal branch of the mandibular division of trigeminal
  - Auricular branch of the vagus nerve

Table A.5.2 Orbital muscle paralysis

Paralysed muscle	Upper eyelid	Eye position at rest	Movements	Images seen
Superior rectus	Ptosis	Normal	Limited elevation, especially on abduction	Diplopia increases on attempted elevation and abduction
Inferior oblique	Normal	Normal	Limited elevation when eye adducted	Diplopia increases on attempted elevation and adduction
Medial rectus	Normal	Abducted	Limited adduction	Diplopia increases on attempted adduction
Inferior rectus	Normal	Normal	Limited depression, especially on abduction	Diplopia increases on attempted depression and abduction
Superior oblique	Normal	Normal	Limited depression when eye adducted	Diplopia increases on attempted depression and adduction (patient may tilt head to 'good' side)
Lateral rectus	Normal	Adducted	Limited abduction	Diplopia increases on attempted abduction (head may be turned to affected side)

- The external auditory meatus ends at the tympanic membrane.
- The long handle of the malleus is attached to the inner surface of the tympanic membrane and can be seen on auriscope examination of the ear as the umbo, a small depression in the membrane. When illuminated this concavity produces a cone of light that radiates anteriorly and inferiorly.

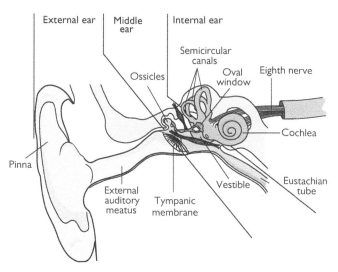

Figure A.5.18 Diagram to illustrate the anatomy of the peripheral auditory system

- The tympanic membrane partitions the external and middle ear and transmits sound from the air to the ossicles.

5.15.2 Middle ear

- The middle ear, or tympanic cavity, is an air-containing cavity in the petrous part of the temporal bone.
- It contains the auditory ossicles, which transmit the vibrations of the tympanic membrane to liquid-borne pulses in the perilymph.
- The malleus transmits vibrations to the incus, the incus to the stapes, and the stapes on to the oval window.
- As well as transmitting the impulses, the ossicles also amplify the vibrations by multiplying the effective pressure on the perilymph by 22 to 1.

5.15.3 Auditory tube (Eustachian tube)

- Extends from the anterior wall of the middle ear downwards, forwards, and medially to the nasopharynx.
- Function is to equalize air pressures in the middle ear and nasopharynx.
- The auditory tube provides a route for pathogenic organisms to gain entry to the middle ear from the pharynx.

5.15.4 Mastoid air cells

- The middle ear also connects with the mastoid air cells via the mastoid antrum.
- These are a series of communicating cavities within the mastoid process of the skull and are clinically significant, as middle ear infections can pass through the mastoid antrum and into the air cells, resulting in mastoiditis.
- From the mastoid air cells infections can spread to the meninges, leading to meningitis and temporal lobe cerebral abscess, or to the inner ear or facial nerve, causing facial nerve palsy, labyrinthitis, and vertigo.

5.15.5 Inner ear

- The inner ear is concerned with 3 functions:
  - Hearing: via the cochlear
  - Static balance: via the utricle and saccule
  - Kinetic balance: via the semi-circular canals

5.16 The temporomandibular joint (TMJ)

- Articulation between:
  - Articular tubercle and anterior portion of mandibular fossa of the temporal bone
  - Condyloid process of the mandible
- Synovial joint: articular disc between the articular surfaces.
- Fibrous capsule surrounds the joint.
- Joint stabilized by:
  - Sphenomandibular ligament: limits posterior movement
  - Temporomandibular ligament: limits inferior movement
  - Stylomandibular ligament: limits excessive opening of the jaw
- Mobile joint—possible movements:
  - Depression: digastrics, geniohyoids, myohyoids
  - Elevation: temporalis, masseter, medial pterygoids
  - Protrusion: lateral and medial pterygoids

- Retraction: posterior fibres of temporalis
- Rotation: alternate protrusion and retraction of mandible using muscles as previously mentioned (e.g. chewing)
- Stability of the joint:
  - The TMJ is much less stable when the mandible is depressed than in the elevated position
  - The condyle of the mandible and the articular disc both move forwards on the articular tubercle
  - A sudden contraction of the pterygoids (yawning) or direct blow can lead to dislocation

5.17 Vertebral column

- A typical vertebra can be seen in Figure A.5.19.
- Vertebral column:
  - 7 cervical vertebrae (C1–C7)
  - 12 thoracic vertebrae (T1–T12)
  - 5 lumbar vertebrae (L1–L5)
  - 5 sacral vertebrae (S1–S5)
  - 4 coccygeal vertebrae

5.17.1 Joints of the vertebrae

- The vertebrae (with the exception of C1 and C2) articulate with each other in a similar way:
  - Secondary cartilaginous joints
  - Each body covered with a thin layer of hyaline cartilage
  - Thick disc of fibrocartilage between them
  - Each disc has an outer fibrous ring—the annulus fibrosus
  - Inside this is a soft nucleus pulposus, with high water content and packed with glycosaminoglycans (see Figure A.5.20)
- Whilst upright, the weight of the body compresses the discs and the central nucleus pulposus is under great pressure.
- With age the water content of the discs diminishes and 'wear and tear' can lead to herniation of the nucleus pulposus through a defect in the annulus fibrosus.
- This herniation usually occurs posteriorly, as the annulus is thinner, and can impinge on a spinal nerve or on the spinal cord.

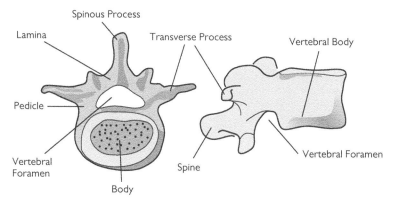

Figure A.5.19 Superior and lateral views of a typical vertebra

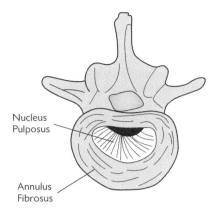

Nucleus
Pulposus

Annulus
Fibrosus

Figure A.5.20 An intervertebral disc

- Because of the way in which the nerve roots emerge, a herniated disc usually presses on the root proximal to its point of exit from the intervertebral foramen, and so a herniation usually causes symptoms at the level 'one below' the lesion (e.g. an L4/5 disc herniation will compress the L5 root and an L5/S1 herniation will compress the S1 root).

5.17.2 Ligaments of the vertebral column

- Anterior and posterior longitudinal ligaments run as continuous bands down the anterior and posterior vertebral surfaces, from skull to sacrum.
- Hold vertebrae firmly together, but allow some movement.
- Anterior ligament:
  - Wide
  - Strongly attached to front and sides of vertebral bodies
  - Also attached to intervertebral discs
- Posterior ligament:
  - Narrow
  - Weak
  - Attached to posterior borders of discs
- Supraspinous ligament:
  - Connects tips of adjacent vertebral spines
- Interspinous ligament:
  - Connects adjacent spines
- In cervical region the supraspinous and interspinous ligaments are joined to form a very strong ligamentum nuchae, from the external occipital protuberance to C7.
- Intertransverse ligament:
  - Connects adjacent transverse processes
- Ligamentum flavum:
  - Connects laminae of adjacent vertebrae

5.17.3 Atlas and axis

- Atlas:
  - The 1st cervical vertebra is called the atlas
  - It is an atypical vertebra:
    - Does not have a body
    - Does not have a spinous process

- Has both anterior and posterior arches
- Has 2 lateral masses to articulate with the occipital condyles
- Has articular surfaces on its inferior surface to articulate with the axis
- Axis:
  - The 2nd cervical vertebra is called the axis
  - It is an atypical vertebra:
    - It has an odontoid peg (process) that projects superiorly
    - This anatomically replaces the absent body of atlas

5.17.4 Atlanto-occipital joints

- Synovial joints formed between occipital condyles (either side of foramen magnum on skull) and the facets on the superior surface of the atlas.
- It is reinforced by ligaments:
  - Anterior atlanto-occipital membrane:
    - Continuation of anterior longitudinal ligament
    - Joins anterior arch of atlas to anterior margin of foramen magnum
  - Posterior atlanto-occipital membrane:
    - Connects posterior arch of atlas to posterior margin of foramen magnum

5.17.5 Atlanto-axial joints

- 3 synovial joints, between odontoid peg and anterior arch of atlas, and between the lateral masses.
- Reinforced by ligaments:
  - Apical ligament: connects apex of peg to anterior margin of foramen magnum
  - Alar ligaments (2): connect peg to occipital condyles
  - Cruciate ligament: connects peg to anterior arch of atlas
  - Membrana tectoria:
    - Continuation of posterior longitudinal ligament
    - Covers posterior surface of odontoid peg and the apical, alar, and cruciate ligaments

5.17.6 Movement of the vertebral column

- The column can move in a number of ways:
  - Flexion
  - Extension
  - Lateral flexion
  - Rotation
  - Circumduction
- Flexion is greatest in the cervical and lumbar regions but restricted in the thoracic region. It is produced by the longus cervicis, scalenus anterior, and sternocleidomastoid in the cervical region, and in the lumbar region by rectus abdominis and psoas.
- Extension is greatest in the cervical and lumbar regions and is produced by the longitudinal erector spinae muscle mass (made up of iliocostalis, longissimus, and spinalis muscles).
- Lateral flexion is produced by the scalenes, trapezius, and sternocleidomastoid in the cervical region, and by longitudinal erector spinae muscle mass, obliques, and quadratus lumborum in the lumbar region.
- Rotation is greatest in the thoracic region and is produced by transversospinalis muscle mass.

5.17.7 Vertebral canal

- Anterior wall: posterior surface of the vertebral bodies and discs.
- Posterior wall: laminae of vertebrae and ligamentum flavum.
- Lateral walls: pedicles of the vertebrae.

- Contents:
  - Canal separated from meninges by epidural space
  - Spinal meninges:
    - Dura mater: external membrane, dense and strong
    - Arachnoid mater: intermediate layer. Separated from pia by subarachnoid space containing CSF, which is continuous with the intracranial subarachnoid space
    - Pia mater: vascular membrane, closely covering spinal cord
  - Spinal cord:
    - Cylindrical structure
    - Begins at foramen magnum
    - Terminates at L1, at the conus medullaris
    - Below this level are the cauda equina and filum terminale (strand of pia mater connecting to coccyx)
  - Nerve roots:
    - 31 pairs of spinal nerve roots along the length of the cord

5.17.8 Lumbar puncture

- This can be performed to access the subarachnoid space and obtain a sample of CSF.
- The patient is placed in the left lateral position, in full flexion (to open the spaces between the lumbar vertebrae).
- The landmarks are the midline and an imaginary line joining the highest points of the iliac crests.
- This identifies the spine of L4 and by passing the spinal needle into the space directly below this, into the L4/5 disc space, it will be well below the termination of the spinal cord.
- The needle is directed towards the umbilicus.
- Aseptic technique is used, and as the needle is inserted a characteristic resistance is felt as the needle passes through the supraspinous ligament (if the needle is inserted just lateral to the midline it will avoid the supraspinous ligament) and fibrous dura, and then a 'give' as it passes into the subarachnoid space.

CHAPTER A6

Central nervous system

CONTENTS

6.1 Overview

- The cerebral hemispheres essentially constitute the developed forebrain.
- The midbrain contains an aqueduct and acts as a connection to the hindbrain (pons, medulla oblongata, and cerebellum).
- The cavity of the hindbrain is the 4th ventricle.
- The brainstem comprises the midbrain, pons, and medulla.
- The medulla passes via the skull's foramen magnum to form the spinal cord, from which cervical nerve roots emerge.
- CSF forms within ventricular choroid plexuses and exits via the foramina in the roof of the 4th ventricle.

6.2 Cerebral hemispheres

- The cerebral hemispheres are covered by a thin outer layer of grey matter—the cerebral cortex. Deeper within the brain are masses of grey matter such as basal nuclei and thalamus.
- The brain surface is comprised of folds (gyri) separated by grooves (sulci). The larger sulci (fissures) divide the brain into lobes (see Figure A.6.1):
  - Frontal lobe—anterior to central sulcus and above lateral sulcus
  - Parietal lobe—behind central sulcus and above lateral sulcus
  - Temporal lobe—below lateral sulcus
  - Occipital lobe—below parieto-occipital sulcus

6.2.1 Structural aspects of the cerebral hemispheres

- The basal nuclei (also called basal ganglia) are situated at the base of the forebrain lying on both sides of the thalamus. The basal nuclei function as a supraspinal control centre over voluntary movement and movement coordination.

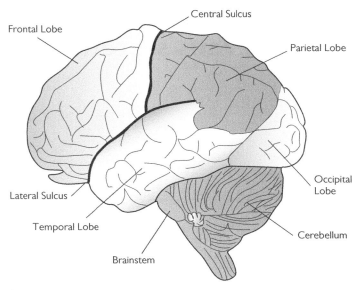

Figure A.6.1 Lobes of the brain

- The white matter can be divided into 3 major groups:
  - Association (arcuate) fibres (forming cortical connections within the same hemisphere)
  - Commissural fibres (interconnect the 2 hemispheres)
  - Projection fibres (from the cerebral cortex to other parts of the CNS, e.g. thalamus)—these projection fibres located between the basal ganglia and the thalamus are termed the *internal capsule*
- A thrombosis or haemorrhage occurring in the internal capsule results in a contralateral hemiparesis or hemiplegia. This is the most common site of intracerebral haemorrhage.
- The corpus callosum is a structure composed of commissural fibres, in the longitudinal fissure that connects the left and right cerebral hemispheres, and facilitates communication between the two.

6.2.2 Cortical areas

- Appreciation of the key areas within which bodily function is determined is a fundamental part of the rationale for knowledge of CNS anatomy.
- The effects of traumatic and atraumatic brain lesions can be predicted based upon a working knowledge of the likely clinical signs, and this works in reverse such that typical neurological presentations infer typical areas of central damage.
- Broca's area lies in the inferior frontal gyrus in the left frontal lobe. It is important for speech production, language processing, and language comprehension. See Figure A.6.2.
- Wernicke's area is located at the posterior section of the superior temporal gyrus in the left hemisphere. It is important for language comprehension, recognition, and interpretation.
- The auditory area (or cortex) is located in the floor of the lateral sulcus and on the dorsal surface of the superior temporal gyrus in the temporal lobe. It is responsible for the processing of auditory information.
- The visual area (or cortex) occupies the entire surface of the occipital lobe. It is responsible for processing visual information (see Chapter A6, Section 6.2.3).

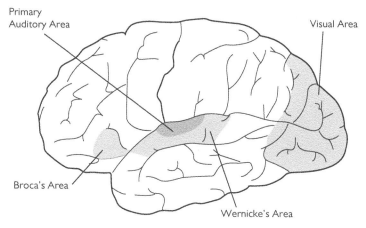

Primary
Auditory Area

Visual Area

Broca's Area

Wernicke's Area

Figure A.6.2 Areas of the brain

6.2.3 Visual fields and pathways

- As a part of the retina, the *bipolar cells* exist between photoreceptors (rod and cone cells) and *ganglion cells*. They act, directly or indirectly, to transmit signals from the photoreceptors to the ganglion cells.
- Retinal ganglion cells collectively transmit visual information from the retina to several regions in the brain. They do this by the defining property of a long axon extending into the brain—the *optic nerve*.
- The optic nerve (CN II) transmits visual information from the retina to the brain. It leaves the orbit via the optic canal and runs posteromedially toward the *optic chiasm* where the nasal visual field crosses over. This allows for parts of both eyes that attend to the right visual field to be processed in the left visual system in the brain, and vice versa.
- The optic chiasm is located in the bottom of the brain, immediately below the hypothalamus. The optic nerve then continues as the *optic tract* to the *lateral geniculate nucleus*.
- Most of the axons of the optic nerve terminate in the lateral geniculate nucleus, from where information is relayed to the visual cortex. This is the primary processing centre for visual information and is found in the thalamus.
- From the lateral geniculate body, fibres of the *optic radiation* (forming part of the internal capsule) pass to the *visual cortex* in the occipital lobe of the brain. See Figure A.6.3.
- The *internal carotid artery* supplies the optic chiasm and optic nerve. The *posterior communicating artery* supplies optic chiasm and optic tract. The *anterior cerebral artery* supplies the optic chiasm.

6.2.4 Olfactory pathways

Knowledge *not* required.

6.2.5 Limbic system

Knowledge *not* required.

6.2.6 Ventricles

- The ventricular system is composed of 2 lateral ventricles and 2 midline ventricles, referred to as the 3rd and 4th ventricles.

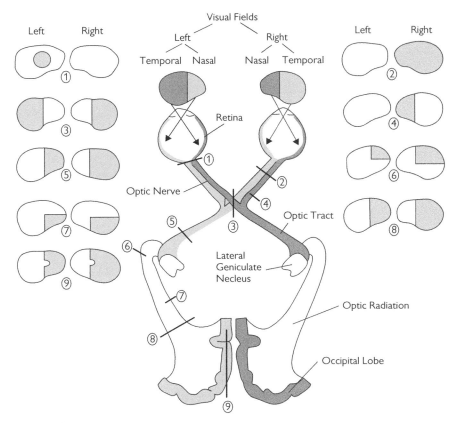

Figure A.6.3 The optic pathway

- The chambers are connected to allow the flow of CSF via 2 interventricular foramen (referred to as the foramen of Monro) between the lateral and 3rd ventricles; and the cerebral aqueduct (referred to as the aqueduct of Sylvius) between the 3rd and 4th ventricles. See Figure A.6.4.
- The ventricles are the source of CSF. CSF is secreted by the choroid plexuses, which are vascular conglomerates of capillaries, pia, and ependyma cells. The bulk of CSF arises from the plexuses of the lateral ventricles.
- In cross-sectional radiology, the midline cavities (3rd and 4th ventricles and the aqueduct) are symmetrical, but the lateral ventricles (the cavities of the hemispheres) are not.
- The 2 lateral ventricles, located within the cerebrum, are relatively large and C-shaped, roughly wrapping around the dorsal aspects of the basal ganglia. Each lateral ventricle has 3 horns:
  - The *anterior* horn extends into the frontal lobe
  - The *posterior* horn extends into the occipital lobe
  - The *inferior* horn extends into the temporal lobe
- The body of the lateral ventricle is the central portion, just posterior to the frontal horn.
- The 3rd ventricle is a slit-like space in the sagittal plane. It is bordered on each side by thalami, and lies directly above the hypothalamus. The 3rd ventricle contains the choroid plexus, which is responsible for CSF production; this in turn helps protect the brain from trauma.
- The 4th ventricle has a characteristic diamond shape in cross-sections of the human brain. It is located within the pons or in the upper part of the medulla.

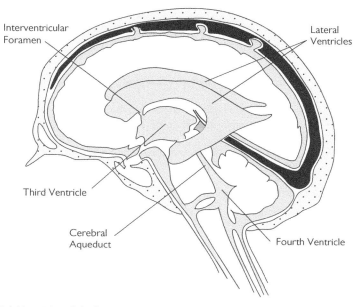

Figure A.6.4 Ventricles of the brain

6.2.7 Thalamus

- The thalamus lies between the cerebral cortex and the midbrain and is a wedge-shaped structure that surrounds the 3rd ventricle. It consists of clusters of cell groups (nuclei).
- The thalamus is known to have multiple functions:
  - The thalamus is believed to both process and relay sensory information selectively to various parts of the cerebral cortex
  - It also plays an important role in regulating states of sleep and wakefulness by strong reciprocal connections with the cerebral cortex that are believed to be involved with consciousness
  - The thalamus plays a major role in regulating arousal, the level of awareness, and activity
  - Damage to the thalamus can lead to permanent coma

6.3 Cerebral blood supply

- The blood supply to the brain is from branches of the internal carotid and vertebral arteries.
- The internal carotid arteries branch into the *anterior* and *middle cerebral arteries*.
- The vertebral arteries originate from the subclavian arteries and unite to form the *basilar artery*. This then ends by dividing into the 2 *posterior cerebral arteries*.
- These arteries are end-arteries, therefore if one of these branches becomes blocked, the brain tissue served by that artery becomes infarcted and dies:
  - Anterior cerebral artery:
    - Medial surface
    - Superior surface
    - Frontal pole
  - Middle cerebral artery:
    - Lateral surface
    - Temporal pole

- Posterior cerebral artery:
  - Inferior surface
  - Occipital pole
- However, anastomoses do occur between the branches of the 3 cerebral arteries across the pia.
- The *cerebral arterial circle (of Willis)* is located at the base of the brain around the optic chiasm.
- It is an important anastamosis between the 4 arteries supplying the brain (vertebrals and internal carotids). It is an important means of collateral circulation in the event of one of the arteries becoming obstructed.
- This is a common location for aneurysms (particularly berry aneurysms). If this aneurysm ruptures it will allow blood to enter the subarachnoid space.

6.3.1 Internal carotid artery

- Originates from the common carotid artery and has no branches in the neck before entering the cranial cavity via the carotid canal in the petrous temporal bone.
- It has 3 terminal branches:
  - Ophthalmic artery
  - Anterior cerebral artery
  - Middle cerebral artery

6.3.2 Middle cerebral artery

- The middle cerebral artery is the artery most often occluded in stroke.
- Occlusion yields:
  - Contralateral hemiplegia or hemiparesis
  - Eye deviation toward the side of the infarct
  - Contralateral hemianopia
  - Contralateral hemianaesthesia
  - Occlusion involving the dominant hemisphere causes global aphasia
  - Occlusion of the nondominant hemisphere causes impaired perception of deficits (anosognosia) resulting from the stroke and more qualitative deficits of speech such as Wernicke's aphasia

6.3.3 Anterior cerebral artery

- The left and right anterior cerebral arteries are connected by the anterior communicating artery.
- Occlusion of the anterior cerebral artery may result in:
  - Paralysis of the contralateral foot and leg
  - Sensory loss in the contralateral foot and leg
  - Left-sided strokes may develop aphasia
  - Gait apraxia
  - Urinary incontinence usually occurs with bilateral damage
  - Confused language may also occur

6.3.4 Posterior cerebral artery

- The posterior cerebral artery supplies the occipital lobe, thus has a key role in the supply of the visual areas.
- Occlusion may result in:
  - Contralateral loss of pain and temperature sensations
  - Visual field defects (contralateral hemianopia with macular sparing)

- Macular sparing can occur if the occipital pole remains intact through collateral blood supply from a branch of the middle cerebral artery and preservation of the optic radiations.

6.4 Cerebral venous drainage

- Veins that drain the brain ultimately empty into the internal jugular vein. The veins can be categorized into superficial and deep.
- Some of the superficial veins have to bridge the subarachnoid space before emptying. This is a site of weakness and blows to the head can tear these and causing bleeding into the subdural space.

6.5 Brainstem

- This area comprises the midbrain, pons, and medulla.
- It extends from the tentorial aperture to the level of C1. The medulla passes out via the foramen magnum and becomes the spinal cord as C1 roots emerge.

6.5.1 Anatomy I: nuclei

- The brainstem has a number of neural centres where cells are clumped together, called nuclei, which manage many automatic aspects of physiology and behaviour.
- Nerves with mixed sensory and motor fibres must have more than one nucleus of origin—at least one sensory (afferent) and one motor (efferent). Sometimes more than one nerve will originate from a single nucleus: for example, the sense of taste is spread across at least 2 nerves but merges into a single nucleus.
  - Oculomotor:
    - Motor: most eye movements
  - Trochlear:
    - Motor: superior oblique only
  - Trigeminal:
    - Motor: muscles of mastication
    - Motor: tensor tympani
    - Sensory: ipsilateral face crude touch, pain, temperature
    - Sensory: proprioception of the jaw
  - Abducens:
    - Motor: lateral rectus only
  - Facial:
    - Motor: muscles of facial expression
    - Sensory: taste (anterior two-thirds of tongue)
  - Vestibulocochlear:
    - Sensory: auditory information
  - Glossopharyngeal:
    - Sensory: taste (posterior third of tongue)
    - Sensory: touch from back of throat (gag reflex)
  - Vagus:
    - Motor: muscles of palate, pharynx, and larynx
    - Somatic: parasympathetic to heart, GI tract, and lungs
  - Accessory:
    - Motor: trapezius and sternocleidomastoid
  - Hypoglossal:
    - Motor: muscles of the tongue

6.5.2 Anatomy II: midbrain

- The midbrain lies predominantly within the posterior cranial fossa. The cerebellum is separated from the occipital lobes by the tentorium cerebelli (an extension of dura mater). The aperture in this lies on the dorsal surface of the midbrain.
- The blood supply to the midbrain is via the posterior cerebral and superior cerebellar arteries (a branch of the basilar artery).
- A part of the midbrain called the *substantia nigra* is responsible for the production of dopamine. This is critical for normal movement. Loss of these dopaminergic neurons is the basis of Parkinson's disease.

6.5.3 Anatomy III: pons

- The pons houses the following cranial nerve nuclei:
  - Trigeminal (sensory and motor)
  - Abducens
  - Facial
  - Vestibulocochlear
- Pontine haemorrhage therefore leads to a classical picture. The patient complains of a severe headache and rapidly becomes unconscious, and then develops periodic respiration, pinpoint pupils, loss of 'doll's head' horizontal ocular movements, hyperthermia, and bilateral bulbar muscle weakness. There is no flaccidity and the patient may rapidly go into decerebrate posturing. This presentation is seen most often in patients with uncontrolled hypertension.
- The blood supply to the pons is via multiple pontine branches of the basilar artery.

6.5.4 Anatomy IV: medulla oblongata

- The medulla oblongata is the lowest part of the brainstem and can be seen as an upward continuation of the spinal cord past the foramen magnum.
- The blood supply is via:
  - Anterior spinal artery
  - Posterior inferior cerebellar artery (PICA)
  - Direct branches of the vertebral artery
  - Direct branches of the basilar artery
- An infarct in the anterior spinal artery will result in '*medial medullary syndrome*':
  - A deviation of the tongue to the ipsilateral side of the infarct on attempted protrusion (caused by muscle weakness due to the death of hypoglossal nerve fibres)
  - Limb weakness (or hemiplegia, depending on severity) on the contralateral side of the infarct
  - A loss of discriminative touch, conscious proprioception, and vibration sense on the contralateral side of the infarct
  - Sensation to the face is preserved due to the sparing of the trigeminal nucleus
- An infarct in the PICA will result in '*lateral medullary syndrome*'. This syndrome is characterized by sensory deficits affecting the trunk and extremities on the opposite side of the infarct and sensory and motor deficits affecting the face and cranial nerves on the same side as the infarct. Other clinical symptoms and findings are:
  - Ataxia
  - Absence of facial touch, pain, and temperature on ipsilateral side of face
  - Absent corneal reflex
  - Loss of contralateral pain and temperature sensation
  - Vertigo
  - Nystagmus
  - Ipsilateral Horner's syndrome
  - Diplopia

- Dysphagia
- Dysarthria and hoarseness

6.6 Cerebrospinal fluid

- CSF is produced in the brain by modified cells in the choroid. Total CSF volume is about 130–150mL, of which the majority is in the subarachnoid space. CSF then returns to the vascular system via the arachnoid granulations.
- There is small but significant CSF drainage via the cribriform plate of the ethmoid into the nasal lymphatics. Thus with head trauma and fracture to this area (base of skull) there can be CSF leakage into the nose (rhinorrhoea).
- Because the brain and spinal cord are suspended in the CSF, it cushions the CNS and protects it from traumatic injury. It is also involved in distribution of neuroendocrine factors, and in the prevention of brain ischaemia (by dropping the volume of CSF and so decreasing intracranial pressure).

6.7 Cerebellum

- The cerebellum is located in the hindbrain, in the posterior cranial fossa.
- The cerebellum is involved in the coordination of voluntary motor movement, balance and equilibrium, and muscle tone. Postural reflexes, truncal stability, and synergistic muscular movements all depend upon an intact cerebellum.
- Cerebellar injury does not cause paralysis, but results in movements that are slow and uncoordinated. Individuals with cerebellar lesions tend to sway and stagger when walking.
- Damage to the cerebellum can lead to:
  - Loss of coordination of motor movement (asynergia)
  - The inability to judge distance and when to stop (dysmetria)
  - The inability to perform rapid alternating movements (dysdiadochokinesia)
  - Movement tremors (intention tremor)
  - Staggering, wide-based walking (ataxic gait)
  - Tendency toward falling
  - Weak muscles (hypotonia)
  - Slurred speech (ataxic dysarthria)
  - Abnormal eye movements (nystagmus)
- Knowledge of the blood supply of the cerebellum facilitates understanding of the clinical effects of occlusion. Interruption of flow through any of the following will lead to 'cerebellar signs' (HANDS Tremors):
  - *H*ypotonia and truncal ataxia
  - *A*synergy (lack of coordination with dysdiadochokinesia)
  - *N*ystagmus
  - *D*ysarthria (both scanning and explosive speech)
  - *S*tance and gait (postural instability and broad-based gait)
  - *T*remor (intentional tremor)
- 3 arteries supply blood to the cerebellum:
  - Posterior inferior cerebellar artery (see Chapter A6, Section 6.5.4 for effects of occlusion)
  - Anterior inferior cerebellar artery:
    - Ipsilateral ataxia
    - Contralateral weakness
    - Contralateral loss of pain and temperature

- Superior cerebellar artery:
  - Ipsilateral ataxia
  - Nausea and vomiting
  - Slurred speech (pseudobulbar)
  - Contralateral loss of pain and temperature

6.8 Spinal cord anatomy

6.8.1 Extent

- At birth, the terminal end of the spinal cord (the conus medullaris) lies around the level of L3. By the age of 21 it sits at L1 or 2.

6.8.2 Enlargements

- There are 2 regions where the spinal cord enlarges:
  - Cervical—corresponds roughly to the brachial plexus nerves:
    - Spinal cords = C4–T1
    - Vertebral level = C3–T1
  - Lumbosacral—corresponds to the lumbosacral plexus nerves:
    - Spinal cords = L2–S3
    - Vertebral level = T9–L1

6.8.3 Spinal nerve roots

- Rootlets emerge from the cord in the subarachnoid space and amalgamate shortly afterwards into roots.
- Anterior and posterior roots then emerge from their individual intervertebral foramina. After invaginating the dura they combine into mixed spinal nerves, which then go off to their respective destinations.
- The cord is shorter than the space available to it: below L1 level, the roots from the lumbar and sacral levels pass down near-vertically to form the *cauda equina*.
- The lower a nerve root, therefore, the more steeply it slopes down before gaining its intervertebral foramen: this is an important anatomical fact when interpreting potential clinical signs in spinal trauma with differing heights of injury.

6.8.4 Internal anatomy

- The interior of the cord is formed by grey matter, which is surrounded by white matter. In transverse sections, the gray matter is conventionally divided into dorsal (posterior) lateral and ventral (anterior) 'horns'. The grey matter is composed of various afferent and efferent cell bodies, whilst the white matter comprises various nerve fibres.
- Figure A.6.5 illustrates the locations of the important white matter tracts:
  - Gracile/cuneate (dorsal columns)
  - Lateral corticospinal (LCST)
  - Anterolateral (spinothalamic) (STT)
  - Spinocerebellar (DSCT + VSCT)

6.8.5 Projectional tracts: impulse transmission

- Like most brain functions, motor controls are crossed. The axons of the neurons must therefore bifurcate and cross over.

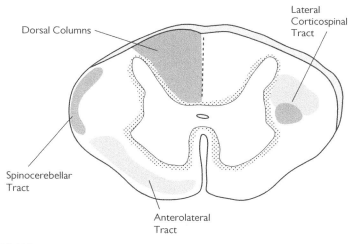

Figure A.6.5 White matter tracts

- This decussation occurs just before the junction between the medulla oblongata and the spinal cord. This decussation of the pyramidal tract is the reason that brain injuries and strokes on one side of the head typically cause paralysis on the contralateral side of the body.
- The dorsal roots contain *afferent sensory* axons to the dorsal root ganglion, which contains the cell bodies of the nerve fibres. These roots transmit information from receptors to the CNS.
- The ventral roots contain *efferent motor* axons. These roots transmit impulses away from the CNS to effectors.
- Distally these 2 roots join to form a mixed spinal nerve.

6.9 Division of the cord

6.9.1 Complete transection

- This is damage to the cord that leads to paraplegia or quadriplegia depending on the height of the lesion.
- Transection most frequently results from trauma but it can be associated with vascular infarction or haemorrhage, compression, demyelinating, or inflammatory lesions. Shearing or compressing the cord produces destruction of the grey and white matter.
- Pathological changes are maximal at the level of the lesion but injury extends above and below the lesion for a segment or two. The final clinical outcome is a result of the irreversible structural damage.
- The classic syndrome of complete spinal cord transection at the high cervical level consists of:
  - Respiratory insufficiency
  - Quadriplegia
  - Upper and lower extremity areflexia
  - Bilateral loss of all sensation below the affected level
  - Neurogenic shock (hypotension without compensatory tachycardia)
  - Loss of rectal and bladder sphincter tone

■ Urinary and bowel retention leading to abdominal distension, ileus, and delayed gastric emptying
- This constellation of symptoms is called spinal shock.
- Horner's syndrome (i.e. ipsilateral ptosis, miosis, and anhydrosis) is also present with higher lesions because of interruption of the descending sympathetic pathways originating from the hypothalamus. Patients experience problems with temperature regulation because of the sympathetic impairment, which leads to hypothermia.
- Lower cervical level injury spares the respiratory muscles. High thoracic lesions lead to paraparesis instead of quadriparesis, but autonomic symptoms are still marked. In lower thoracic and lumbar lesions, hypotension is not present but urinary and bowel retention are.

6.9.2 Hemisection

- This incomplete cord lesion is also known as Brown-Séquard syndrome and results from injury to one side of the spinal cord.
- It causes ipsilateral weakness, loss of proprioception, vibration, and light touch, spacticity and hyperreflexia (lateral corticospinal tract), and contralateral loss of pain and temperature sensation (lateral spinothalamic tract fibres cross from opposite side) about 1 dermatomal segment below the level of the lesion.
- Bladder function may be spared since bilateral lesions are required to interfere with bladder function.
- Common injury mechanisms include penetrating trauma or unilateral facet fracture or dislocation. This has a good prognosis for recovery—more than 90% of patients regain bladder and bowel control and ability to walk.

6.9.3 Central cord syndrome

- This is the most common form of incomplete spinal cord injury characterized by greater impairment in upper limb function compared to lower limbs as well as bladder dysfunction, and with variable sensory loss.
- This syndrome is associated with variable sensory and reflex deficits; often the most affected sensory modalities are pain and temperature because the lateral spinothalamic tract fibres cross just ventral to the central canal.
- Most often the damage is to the cervical or upper thoracic regions of the spinal cord—indeed, central cord syndrome most often occurs after a hyperextension injury in an individual with longstanding cervical spondylosis.
- This condition is associated with ischemia, haemorrhage, or necrosis involving the central grey matter of the spinal cord where fibres controlling the upper extremity and voluntary bowel and bladder function are more centrally located. Corticospinal fibres responsible for lower extremity motor and sensory functions and sacral tracts are spared due to their more peripheral location in the spinal cord.
- This clinical pattern may emerge during recovery from spinal shock due to prolonged swelling around or near the vertebrae, causing pressures on the cord. Central cord syndrome is observed most often in syringomyelia, hydromyelia, and trauma. The symptoms may be transient or permanent. Considerable recovery is common.
- Lateral extension can result in ipsilateral Horner syndrome (because of involvement of the ciliospinal centre), kyphoscoliosis (because of involvement of dorsomedian and ventromedian motor nuclei supplying the paraspinal muscles), and spastic paralysis (because of corticospinal tract involvement). Dorsal extension can result in ipsilateral position sense and vibratory loss due to involvement of dorsal column.

6.9.4 Anterior spinal artery syndrome

- Symptoms are caused by the blockage of the anterior spinal artery. The blockage may be caused by such things as trauma, cancer, thrombosis, and arterial disease. Ischemia or infarction of the spinal cord is in the distribution of the anterior spinal artery, which supplies the ventral two-thirds of the spinal cord and medulla.
- The sensory signs (i.e. bilateral loss of pain and temperature sense) are indicative of injury to the spinothalamic tracts in the lateral white funiculi with sparing of the posterior white columns (relative sparing of position and vibratory sensation), which are supplied by the posterior spinal arteries.

6.10 Cord blood supply

- The arterial supply of the spinal cord is by 3 arteries that are branches of the 2 vertebral arteries (left and right). Each vertebral artery gives rise to a posterior spinal artery, which proceeds along the line of attachment of the dorsal roots. Each vertebral artery also gives rise to an anterior spinal artery. These 2 anterior spinal arteries (left and right) fuse to form a single midline vessel. This leaves a single anterior artery and 2 posterior arteries.
- The very long anterior spinal artery is usually a continuous vessel for the length of the spinal cord. It supplies 75% of the blood to the spinal cord—the anterior two-thirds of the spinal cord, the base of the posterior horn, and a variable portion of the lateral corticospinal tract.
- The posterior spinal arteries supply 25% of the blood to the spinal cord—the posterior columns, dorsal root, and a variable portion of the lateral corticospinal tract.

Cranial nerve lesions

CONTENTS

7.1 Olfactory (I) nerve

- Anatomy: olfactory cells are a series of bipolar neurons that pass through the cribriform plate to the olfactory bulb.
- Signs: reduced taste and smell (but not to ammonia, which stimulates the pain fibres carried in the trigeminal nerve).
- Causes:
  - Blunt trauma (e.g. coup–contrecoup)
  - Frontal lobe tumour
  - Meningitis

7.2 Optic (II) nerve

- Anatomy:
  - The optic nerve fibres are the axons of the retinal ganglion cells
  - At the optic chiasm, only the fibres derived from the nasal parts of the retina decussate, join with the non-decussating fibres and pass backwards in their respective optic tracts to the lateral geniculate bodies, where fibres of the optic radiation pass to the visual cortex
- Visual field defects: field defects start as small areas of visual loss (scotomas) (see Figure A.7.1).
  - Monocular blindness:
    - Lesions of one eye or optic nerve
    - For example, MS, giant cell arteritis
  - Bilateral blindness:
    - Methyl alcohol, tobacco amblyopia, neurosyphilis
  - Bitemporal hemianopia:
    - Optic chiasm compression
    - For example, internal carotid artery aneurysm, pituitary adenoma, or craniopharyngioma

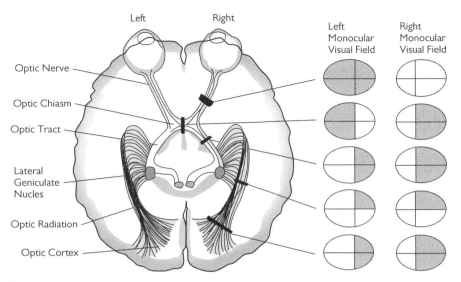

Figure A.7.1 Visual field defects

- Homonymous hemianopia:
  - Affects half the visual field contralateral to the lesion in each eye
  - Lesions lie beyond the optic chiasm in the tract, radiation, or occipital cortex (macular sparing if cortex)
  - For example, stroke, abscess, tumour
- Optic neuritis:
  - Pain on moving eye
  - Loss of central vision
  - Afferent pupillary defect
  - Papilloedema
  - For example, demyelination; rarely sinusitis, syphilis, collagen vascular disorders
- Optic atrophy:
  - Pale optic discs
  - Reduced acuity
  - For example, MS, frontal tumours, Friedreich's ataxia, retinitis pigmentosa, syphilis, glaucoma, Leber's optic atrophy, optic nerve compression
- Papilloedema:
  - Swollen discs
  - For example, raised ICP (tumour, abscess, encephalitis, hydrocephalus, benign intracranial hypertension), retro-orbital lesion (e.g. cavernous sinus thrombosis), inflammation (e.g. optic neuritis), ischaemia (e.g. accelerated hypertension)

7.3 Oculomotor (III) nerve

- Anatomy:
  - This nerve emerges from the brainstem on the medial aspect of the crus cerebri and then passes forwards between the posterior cerebral and superior cerebellar arteries, very close to the posterior communicating artery

- It pierces the dura near the edge of the tentorium cerebelli and passes through the lateral part of the cavernous sinus with the IV and VI nerves to enter the orbit
- Signs:
  - The initial sign is often a fixed, dilated pupil that doesn't accommodate
  - Then ptosis develops before a complete internal ophthalmoplegia (masked by ptosis)
  - Unopposed lateral rectus causes outward deviation of the eye
  - If the ocular sympathetic fibres are also affected behind the orbit, the pupil will be fixed but not dilated
- Causes:
  - Diabetes mellitus
  - Direct trauma
  - MS
  - Giant cell arteritis
  - Syphilis
  - Posterior communicating artery aneurysm
  - Idiopathic
  - Raised ICP (if causes uncal herniation through the tentorium—this compresses the nerve)
- IIIrd nerve palsies without a dilated pupil are due to diabetes mellitus or another vascular cause.
- Early dilatation of a pupil implies a compressive lesion.
- Diplopia from a IIIrd nerve lesion may cause nystagmus.

7.4 Trochlear (IV) nerve

- Anatomy:
  - Passes backwards in the brainstem, decussates in the anterior medulla, and emerges to pass round the cerebral peduncle between it and the temporal lobe, passing over the tentorium to enter the cavernous sinus with II and VI, and enters the orbit to supply the superior oblique
- Signs:
  - Diplopia due to weakness of downward and inward eye movement
  - Commonest cause of a pure vertical diplopia
  - Patient tends to compensate by tilting head downwards (tuck chin in) and towards the opposite side
- Causes:
  - Rare and most commonly due to trauma to the orbit
  - Infarction secondary to hypertension
  - A generalized increase in intracranial pressure—hydrocephalus, pseudotumor cerebri, haemorrhage, oedema
  - Infections (meningitis, herpes zoster)
  - Demyelination (MS)
  - Diabetic neuropathy
  - Cavernous sinus disease
  - Orbital tumours
  - The most common cause of *chronic* IVth nerve palsy is a congenital defect

7.5 Trigeminal (V) nerve

- Anatomy:
  - Forms 3 trunks: ophthalmic, maxillary, and mandibular divisions
  - The latter contains both sensory and motor fibres
  - There may be considerable individual variation in the exact areas of skin supplied

- Ophthalmic division lies with III, IV, and VI in the cavernous sinus and supplies the skin over the medial nose, forehead, eye (including corneal reflex)
- Maxillary division passes through the inferior part of the cavernous sinus and the foramen rotundum and joins with parasympathetic fibres to form the sphenopalatine ganglion (lacrimation)
- It then enters the orbit as the infraorbital nerve, eventually supplying the skin of the upper lip, cheek, and triangle of skin extending from the angle of eye and mouth to an apex in the midtemporal region
- Mandibular division leaves the skull through the foramen ovale carrying sensory fibres from the skin of the lower lip and chin up to and including the tragus and upper part of the pinna, and mucus membranes of floor of the mouth, cheek, and anterior two-thirds of the tongue (taste fibres joining it from the chorda tympani branch of the facial nerve)
- Motor fibres supply the masseter, temporalis, and pterigoids
- Signs:
  - Reduced sensation or dysasthesia over affected area
  - Weakness of jaw clenching and side-to-side movement
  - If there is a LMN lesion, the jaw deviates to the weak side when the mouth is opened
  - There may be fasiculation of temporalis and masseter
- Causes:
  - Sensory:
    - Trigeminal neuralgia
    - Herpes zoster
    - Nasopharyngeal carcinoma
  - Motor:
    - Bulbar palsy
    - Acoustic neuroma

7.6 Abducens (VI) nerve

- Anatomy:
  - From the nucleus in the floor of the 4th ventricle fibres pass forward in the pons and emerge to follow a long extracerebral course on the base of the brain, across the apex of the petrous temporal, through the cavernous sinus, and thence to the orbit and lateral rectus
- Signs:
  - Inability to look laterally
  - Eye is deviated medially because of unopposed action of medial rectus
- Causes:
  - Perhaps the most common overall cause is diabetic neuropathy
  - Demyelination (MS)
  - TB
  - Pontine CVA
  - Cavernous sinus disease
  - Infections (meningitis)
  - Wernicke–Korsakoff syndrome
- Indirect damage to the VIth nerve can be caused by any process (brain tumour, hydrocephalus, haemorrhage, oedema) that exerts downward pressure on the brainstem, causing the nerve to stretch. This type of traction injury can affect either side first.
- A right-sided brain tumour can produce either a right-sided or a left-sided VIth nerve palsy as an initial sign. Thus a right-sided VIth nerve palsy does not necessarily imply a right-sided cause. VIth nerve palsies are infamous as 'false localizing signs'.

7.7 Facial (VII) nerve

- Commonest of all cranial nerve lesions.
- Anatomy:
  - Mainly motor (some sensory fibres from external acoustic meatus, fibres controlling salivation, and taste fibres from the anterior tongue)
  - Fibres loop around the VI nucleus before leaving the pons medial to VIII and passing through the internal acoustic meatus
  - It passes through the petrous temporal in the facial canal, widens to form the geniculate ganglion (taste and salivation) on the medial side of the middle ear, whence it turns sharply (and the chorda tympani leaves) to emerge through the stylomastoid foramen, and passes through the parotid gland to supply the muscles of facial expression
- Signs:
  - Facial weakness
  - In a LMN lesion the forehead is paralysed—the final common pathway to the muscles is destroyed; whereas the upper facial muscles are partially spared in an UMN lesion because of bilateral innervation in the brainstem
- Causes:
  - LMN:
    - Bell's palsy
    - Polio
    - Otitis media
    - Skull fracture
    - Cerebello-pontine angle tumours
    - Parotid tumours
    - Herpes zoster (Ramsay Hunt syndrome)
    - Lyme disease
  - UMN:
    - Stroke
    - Tumour

7.8 Vestibulocochlear (VIII) nerve

- Anatomy:
  - Carries 2 groups of fibres: those to the cochlea (hearing) and to the semi-circular canals, utricle, and saccule (balance and posture)
  - They pass, together with the facial nerve, from the brainstem across the posterior fossa to the internal acoustic meatus
- Signs:
  - Unilateral sensorineural deafness
  - Tinnitus
  - Nystagmus
  - Vertigo
- Causes:
  - Loud noise
  - Paget's disease
  - Ménière's disease
  - Herpes zoster
  - Neurofibroma
  - Acoustic neuroma

- Brainstem CVA
- Lead
- Aminoglycosides
- Furosemide (frusemide)
- Aspirin

7.9 Glossopharyngeal (IX) nerve

- Anatomy:
  - Contains sensory, motor (stylopharyngeus only), and parasympathetic fibres (salivary glands)
  - Passes across the posterior fossa, through the jugular foramen, and into the neck supplying tonsil, palate, and posterior third of tongue
- Signs:
  - The gag reflex, as it is responsible for the afferent limb of the reflex
- Causes:
  - Single nerve lesions exceedingly rare
  - Trauma
  - Brainstem lesions
  - Cerebello-pontine angle and neck tumours
  - Polio
  - GBS

7.10 Vagus (X) nerve

- Anatomy:
  - Contains motor fibres (to the palate and vocal cords), sensory components (posterior and floor of external acoustic meatus), and visceral afferent and efferent fibres
  - It leaves the skull through the jugular foramen, passes within the carotid sheath in the neck (giving off cardiac branches and the recurrent laryngeal nerves supplying the vocal cords), through the thorax supplying lungs, and continues on via the oesophageal opening to supply the abdominal organs
- Signs:
  - Palatal weakness can cause 'nasal speech' and nasal regurgitation of food
  - The palate moves asymmetrically when the patient says 'ah'—uvula deviates away from the side of lesion
  - Recurrent nerve palsy results in hoarseness, loss of volume, and 'bovine cough'
  - There is also dysphagia and loss of gag reflex
- Causes:
  - Single nerve lesions exceedingly rare
  - Trauma
  - Brainstem lesions
  - Tumours in cerebello-pontine angle, jugular foramen, and neck
  - Polio
  - GBS

7.11 Accessory (XI) nerve

- Anatomy:
  - Unique in that it originates outside the skull, enters via foramen magnum, and leaves via jugular foramen to supply motor to sternocleidomastoid and trapezius

- Signs:
  - Weakness and wasting of these muscles
- Causes:
  - As for vagus nerve (see Chapter A7, Section 7.10)

7.12 Hypoglossal (XII) nerve

- Anatomy:
  - It passes briefly across the posterior fossa, leaves the skull through the hypoglossal canal, and supplies motor fibres to the tongue and most of the infrahyoid muscles
- Signs:
  - Wasting of the ipsilateral side of the tongue
  - Fasiculation
  - On attempted protrusion tongue deviates towards affected side
- Causes:
  - Rare
  - Polio
  - Syringomyelia TB
  - Median branch thrombosis of the vertebral artery

7.13 Combined cranial nerve lesions

- VII, VIII, then V, and sometimes IX: cerebello-pontine angle tumours.
- V, VI (Gradenigo's syndrome): lesions within petrous temporal bone.
- Combined III, IV, VI:
  - Stroke
  - Tumours
  - Wernicke's encephalopathy
  - Aneurysms
  - MS
  - Myasthenia gravis
  - Meningitis
  - Muscular dystrophy
  - Myotonic dystrophy
  - Cavernous sinus thrombosis
  - GBS
  - Cranial arteritis
  - Trauma and orbital pathology

7.14 Conditions that can affect any cranial nerve

- Diabetes mellitus
- MS
- Tumours
- Sarcoid
- Vasculitis (e.g. polyarteritis nodosa)
- Systemic lupus erythematosus
- Syphilis
- Chronic meningitis (malignant, TB, or fungal)

MEDICAL MICROBIOLOGY: PRINCIPLES OF MICROBIOLOGY

Natural and innate immunity

CONTENTS

1.1 Barriers to infection

1.1.1 Skin
- Anatomical barrier physically preventing invasion of microorganisms.
- Chemical barrier providing unfavourable conditions for most organisms to survive due to:
  - Free fatty acids produced by the sebaceous glands and skin flora
  - Lactic acid in the sweat
  - Low pH
  - Relatively dry environment.
- If the skin is damaged it loses its ability to act as an anatomical barrier (e.g. transmission of HIV or hepatitis through a needle-stick injury).
- Psoriasis and eczema reduce the skin's ability to act as a chemical barrier leading to more favourable conditions for bacterial infection.
- Burns reduce the skin's ability to act as an anatomical and chemical barrier.

1.1.2 Mucociliary clearance
- Occurs in the respiratory tract.
- Mucus is produced by goblet cells and submucosal mucus-secreting glands.
- Ciliated columnar epithelial cells are present. Each cell contains approximately 200 cilia beating at 1000 beats per minute.
- There is continual movement of mucus towards the oropharynx where it is swallowed.
- Smaller particles reaching the alveoli are phagocytosed by macrophages and transported out of air spaces to the mucus stream.
- Nasal secretions containing antibodies, lysozyme, and interferon are moved to the oropharynx and swallowed.
- This can be disrupted by pollutants (such as cigarette smoke) and microorganisms (such as rhinovirus), which attach to receptors on epithelial cells, damaging them and disrupting cilia motility.

1.1.3 Secreted antibacterial compounds

- Lysozyme: found in tears, saliva, and mucus. Enzyme that attacks peptidoglycans in bacterial cell walls.
- Lactic acid: found on the skin and vagina leading to an acidic environment.
- Free fatty acids: found on the skin leading to an acidic environment.
- Hydrochloric acid: found in the stomach leading to an acidic environment.
- Lactoperoxidase: found in breast milk and saliva. Inhibitory to many microorganisms.

1.1.4 The urinary tract

- There are 2 main barriers to infection in the urinary tract:
  - Passing of urine acts to flush any microorganisms out of the urinary tract, limiting the establishment of infections.
  - Relatively acidic environment provides unfavourable conditions.

1.2 Normal bacterial flora

- These are microbes that are adapted to life on our skin and mucous membranes and consistently inhabit the human body.
- The presence of normal flora uses up a niche in which they are well established that cannot subsequently be used by a pathogen, for example, in the gut.
- Some microorganisms in the normal flora naturally produce antibiotics and bacteriocins, inhibiting the proliferation of pathogens.
- Normal bacterial flora also stimulates the production of IgA (an important surface antibody), protecting us from invasion of deeper tissues by the flora and pathogenic microorganisms.
- When systemic antibiotic therapy removes normal flora, resistant organisms are able to occupy that niche and can lead to pathological conditions. For example, *Clostridium difficile* leading to enterocolitis and *Candida albicans* leading to oral thrush.

1.3 Phagocytes and complement

- Phagocytosis describes the process by which neutrophils and tissue macrophages find, engulf, and destroy microbes.

1.3.1 Neutrophils

- The most abundant granulocyte.
- Attracted to the site of infection where microbes are adhesed and ingested, forming phagosomes.
- Granules contain numerous microbicidal molecules, which kill then break down microbes.
- An increase of neutrophils in the blood indicates likely bacterial infection.
- They enter the tissues when a chemotactic factor is produced as a result of injury or infection.

1.3.2 Macrophages

- As well as being involved with phagocytosis, macrophages trigger the acute-phase response by releasing interleukins, tumour necrosis factor, and chemokines in response to bacterial cell wall components.

1.3.3 Opsonins

- Co-factors that coat microbes, enhancing the ability of phagocytes to bind to them.
- Examples include complement C3b and C-reactive protein.

- As well as having a role in removing old blood cells and antigen recognition, the spleen is also an important store of monocytes and macrophages.
- Splenectomized patients lose this reserve, and should be immunized against encapsulated organisms such as *Haemophilus influenzae* and *Streptococcus pneumoniae* and receive prophylactic antibiotics.

1.3.4 Complement

- The complement system is a group of about 20 serum proteins involved in a cascade where the product of one reaction is an enzyme catalysing the next.
- It is activated in response to a stimulus such as invading microorganisms (infection).
- The cascade contains an amplification loop, which increases the overall quantity of proteins within the cascade, enhancing its effectiveness.
- It has 3 pathways: the alternative, the classical, and the lectin.
- It leads to the formation of the membrane attack complex, which lyses bacteria by forming water-permeable channels within their cell membranes.
- It also plays a role in enhancing phagocytosis, migration of phagocytes to the site of infection, and increasing vascular permeability.
- Congenital complement deficiencies can affect any of the components:
  - Because of the alternative pathways, deficiencies of C1, C2, and C4 have little clinical relevance.
  - Defects in C3 and C5–8 affect both opsonization and the membrane attack complex, making patients susceptible to infections with encapsulated organisms such as *Streptococcus pneumoniae, Neisseria meningitidis, N. gonorrhoeae* (gonococci), and *Haemophilus influenza*.

Mechanisms of disease

CONTENTS

2.1 Basic terminology

- Colonization: the continuing presence of microorganisms without injury or invasion of our tissues (e.g. MRSA in the nostrils, normal gut flora).
- Pathogen: a microorganism that parasitizes a human and causes disease.
- Infection: injury to or invasion of tissue by microorganisms (pathogens) resulting in a state of disease.
- Obligate pathogen: microorganisms that must cause disease in order to spread (e.g. HIV, hepatitis B).
- Conditional pathogen: microorganisms that can invade tissues and cause disease when ideal conditions are met; commonly the normal flora (e.g. *Staphylococcus aureus* infecting a surgical wound).
- Opportunistic pathogen: microorganisms that would not normally cause disease but become pathogenic when the host defences are impaired (e.g. *Pneumocystis jirovecii* in AIDS).

2.2 Mechanisms of attachment, invasion, and persistence

2.2.1 Invasion

- Microorganisms invade the body by 4 main routes:
  - Mouth and GI tract
  - Respiratory tract
  - Skin (insect bite; incision and implantation; injection and inoculation)
  - Genital tract.

2.2.2 Attachment in viruses

- A virus's initial interaction with a host cell is by random collision.
- Viruses are adsorbed through specific binding sites on the virus (antigen) and receptors on the plasma membrane of the host cell.
- This is a temperature- and energy-dependent process.
- Presence of the receptor determines susceptibility.

2.2.3 Adhesion in bacteria

- Interactions between specific receptors on the plasma membrane of the host cell and ligands on the bacterial cell.
- Involves bacterial use of adhesins, which may be fimbrial or non-fimbrial.
- Adhesion not only prevents loss of the pathogen from the host, it can also induce functional and structural change within the mucosa that may contribute to pathology.

2.2.4 Clinically relevant type examples

- Influenza virus: attaches via the haemagglutinin antigen interacting with cell membrane receptors containing sialic acid (N-acetylneuraminic acid).
- *Giardia lamblia*: attaches to gut mucosa using ventral sucking discs causing local damage.
- *Plasmodium falciparum*: causes red cell protein expression enhancing adhesion of parasitized red cells to the epithelium of brain capillaries. Facilitates cerebral malaria.
- HIV: binds strongly to the CD4 antigen, infecting T lymphocytes that express it.

2.2.5 Ability of microbes to survive and flourish once beyond natural barriers

- *N. meningitidis*: produces IgA protease leading to barrier breakdown.
- *S. aureus*: expresser of protein A, which inhibits complement activation.
- *S. pneumoniae*: has a specialized capsule that inhibits phagocytosis by neutrophils.
- *Vibrio cholerae*: a flagellated motile microbe, enhancing its virulence.

2.2.6 Toxins

- Some microbes have the ability to produce toxins. These are most commonly protein exotoxins but many Gram-negative organisms contain important lipopolysaccharide endotoxins:
  - Cholera toxin: stimulates diarrhoea via epithelial irritation of the gut.
  - Tetanus toxin: disrupts neurological signalling and integrity.

Controlling infection

CONTENTS

3.1 Endogenous and exogenous infection sources

3.1.1 Endogenous infection

- Invasion under specific conditions by the normal flora (making them opportunistic pathogens).
- For example: aspiration pneumonia, neutropenic sepsis, and cannulation.

3.1.2 Exogenous infection

- Organisms acquired from a non-host origin.
- For example: *Legionella* with infected water supply and aerosol transmission; *Clostridium*, which can proliferate in the gut during antibiotic therapy; and *Salmonella* from unclean food and polluted water.

3.2 How infection spreads

- Droplet spread: organisms are acquired via inhalation (e.g. influenza, *N. meningitides*).
- Faecal–oral route: organisms are acquired via ingestion (e.g. *Salmonella*).
- Invasion of intact skin: some organisms can penetrate intact skin (e.g. *Leptospira*).
- Invasion of breached skin: organisms can be acquired by incision and implantation (e.g. *Staphylococcus epidermidis* wound infection) or by injection by needle (e.g. transmission of hepatitis B in a needle-stick injury).
- Sexual intercourse: organisms acquired via sexual intercourse (e.g. HIV, *N. gonorrhoeae*).

3.3 Hospital-acquired infection

- Defined as an infection that was not present or incubating at the time of hospital admission.

3.3.1 Predispositions

- Air conditioning and piped air supplies (e.g. contamination by *Legionella*).

- Fomites are objects that have been used or handled by someone with a communicable disease, thereby contaminating them (e.g. contaminated light boxes, fans, viewing boxes, door handles, and bed sheets).
- Hospital food can transmit infection through inadequate temperature and issues with transporting it to the ward.
- Water supplies can be a source of *Legionella*, especially if pipework is lukewarm.

3.3.2 Patient-centred factors

- Restricted ability to access washing facilities.
- Effects of disease or treatment lowering resistances (e.g. antibiotics and *C. difficile*).
- Effects of close patient contact in a busy ED (e.g. allowing easier spread of airborne pathogens such as influenza A (H1N1) virus).

3.3.3 Cannulation

- Commonest cause of hospital bacteraemia.
- Infection risk is a direct effect of length of time *in situ* (current guidance states cannulae should not remain *in situ* for longer than 48 hours).
- Typical organisms are skin commensals such as *S. aureus* and *S. epidermidis*.

3.3.4 Urinary catheters

- Can act as a source of ascending infection.
- Urinary stasis relating to a blocked catheter is a risk factor for colonization and subsequent infection.

3.3.5 Staff clothing

- The 'bare below the elbow' approach is important as otherwise staff clothing can act as a fomite.

3.4 Control of hospital-acquired infection

- Good clinical practice: the correct method of handwashing should be known, ensuring no areas are missed.
- Isolation of patients: patients with communicable disease (e.g. *C. difficile*, MRSA) should be nursed in a cubicle with aprons, gloves, sink, and alcohol gel available (barrier nursing).
- Disinfection: this results in a reduction in the number of infectious particles.
- Disinfectants: substances that kill or inhibit microbes, for example, iodine acts as a slow-acting antibacterial disinfectant and chlorhexidine as an anti-staphylococcal agent.
- Sterilization: the inactivation of all infectious agents, usually by irradiation or autoclaving.

Principles of investigation

CONTENTS

4.1 Specimen types

- UTI: MSU/CSU
- Skin wounds: wound swab
- Meningitis: CSF and blood
- Non-specific pyrexia: blood and serology
- Pneumonia: blood and sputum
- Severe diarrhoea: stool ± *C. difficile* toxin

4.2 Specimen culture

- Culture of microbes in specimens involves adding that specimen to a culture medium.
- It allows the cultivation of increased numbers of the organism.
- It produces live organisms allowing for full identification and sensitivity testing.
- Media may be:
  - Liquid in order to maximize growth
  - Solid to separate different organisms.

4.3 Specimen examination

4.3.1 Light microscopy

- Direct: wet mount for stool parasites.
- Gram stain: quick and easy stain showing the shape and cell wall type of common bacteria (e.g. CSF).
- Ziehl–Neelsen stain: used for *Mycobacteria*, *Nocardia*, and *Cryptosporidium* spp. (e.g. sputum in TB).
- Giemsa stain: used to detect malaria on blood films.

4.3.2 Fluorescent microscopy

● Used for RSV in sputum samples.

4.4 Serology

● Involves the investigation of blood serum whereby pathogens can be identified by the immune response that they invoke.
● Serological diagnosis rests upon increasing and decreasing concentrations of antibodies in serial specimens. For example, an atypical pneumonia screen should be performed at least 7 days after the onset of illness in order to allow the body to produce antibodies.
● Specific antigen detection is an alternative method looking specifically for pathological antigens. For example, CSF can be examined for bacterial capsular antigens, which would indicate *N. meningitides*.

4.5 Molecular techniques

● These use nucleic acid amplification technology, such as the polymerase chain reaction.
● This exponentially increases the amount of nucleic acid, allowing for identification of organisms that grow slowly.
● This is useful for organisms such as *M. tuberculosis* and *C. trachomatis*.

Principles of immunization

CONTENTS

5.1 Normal childhood immunization schedule

See Table B.5.1.

5.1.1 Varicella

- Only given to immunosuppressed children who have been exposed.
- If they are asymptomatic they are given varicella immunoglobulin.
- If they are symptomatic they receive full vaccination.
- It is currently recommended that non-immune healthcare workers are immunized against varicella.
- If a non-immune pregnant woman comes into contact with varicella she should be given varicella immunoglobulin.
- If a pregnant woman develops chickenpox a week before or after delivery, the baby should be given varicella immunoglobulin.

5.2 Additional immunization schedules

5.2.1 Hepatitis B

- Vaccine is given to all healthcare workers and other professionals considered at high risk (e.g. police officers, prison officers).
- Can be given to anyone who has, or may have, been exposed.
- Can be given to all babies with mothers or close relatives who are infected with hepatitis B.
- Consists of 3 injections given at 1-month intervals followed by a booster at 12 months.
- Further boosters can be given if the patient is subimmune (has not had a satisfactory response to vaccination) or following suspected exposure.

5.2.2 Tetanus

- Tetanus immunization was introduced in the UK in 1961; therefore, most people born after this time are likely to be fully immunized.

Table B.5.1 Childhood immunization schedule

	2 months	3 months	4 months	12–13 months	3 years and 4 months	13–18 years
Diphtheria, tetanus, pertussis	Yes	Yes	Yes		Booster	Booster (not pertussis)
Haemophilus influenzae type b	Yes	Yes	Yes	Yes		
Polio (inactivated)	Yes	Yes	Yes		Booster	Booster
Pneumococcal infection	Yes		Yes	Yes		
MMR				Yes	Booster	
Meningitis C		Yes	Yes	Yes		
HPV (girls)						Yes

- People with tetanus-prone wounds born before this time or who are uncertain of their immunity should have a booster if they have not received one within the last 10 years.
- Tetanus is most common in people aged over 65.

5.2.3 Influenza

- The influenza virus contains 3 types, A, B, and C, of which A and B cause disease in humans.
- The virus continually changes and a new vaccine is released each year.
- It is offered to at-risk groups including those over the age of 65, those with severe cardiac or respiratory disease, and those who are immunosuppressed.
- Healthcare workers are also offered the vaccine in order to protect patients and other healthcare staff.

5.3 Sources of information

Public Health England publishes up-to-date information at the following website: https://www.gov.uk/government/collections/immunisation.

MEDICAL MICROBIOLOGY: SPECIFIC PATHOGEN GROUPS

Streptococci and staphylococci

1.1 Streptococci

- Gram-positive cocci.
- Facultative anaerobes.

1.1.1 *Streptococcus pneumoniae*

- Encapsulated, alpha-haemolytic cocci.
- Methods of spread:
  - *Streptococcus pneumoniae* is a common nasopharyngeal commensal
  - Spread is by droplet
  - Exogenous (respiratory droplet spread from carrier infecting another host) or endogenous (carrier develops impaired resistance to organism) infection may occur
- Clinical features:
  - Most common cause of pneumonia and otitis media
  - An important cause of meningitis, resulting in high mortality
  - Frequent agent in bacteraemia and sepsis in the absence of an obvious focus of infection
  - Also responsible for sinusitis, osteomyelitis, septic arthritis, endocarditis, peritonitis, cellulitis, and brain abscesses

1.1.2 *Streptococcus pyogenes*

- Group A, beta-haemolytic *Streptococcus*l.
- Methods of spread:
  - *S. pyogenes* is one of the most common human bacterial pathogens
  - Invades apparently intact skin and mucous membranes, rapidly and progressively
  - Resides on skin/mucous membranes (especially nasopharynx) of infected patients and healthy carriers
  - Respiratory droplet or skin contact spread
- Clinical features:
  - Acute pharyngitis/tonsillitis:
    - *S. pyogenes* is the most common bacterial cause of sore throats
    - Induces purulent inflammation in the posterior oropharynx and tonsils, and may lead to scarlet fever

- Impetigo:
  - A highly contagious, localized, superficial spreading, crusty skin lesion common in children
- Erysipelas:
  - A superficial skin infection with fiery red advancing erythema on face/lower limbs
- Necrotizing fasciitis:
  - Deep infection involving fascia and subcutaneous tissues, which may progress to pyogenic myositis/myconecrosis
  - Spreads rapidly causing bacteraemia and sepsis
  - Presents with fever and severe pain disproportionate to examination findings
  - Skin signs include slight erythema, tenderness, and swelling
  - In later stages skin becomes discoloured and haemorrhagic blisters and skin necrosis develop
  - Toxic shock may occur and mortality is high
  - Requires rapid surgical debridement
- Puerperal sepsis:
  - Endometrial infection postpartum, presenting with purulent vaginal discharge, high fever, and systemic upset
- Streptococcal toxic shock-like syndrome:
  - Due to streptococcal exotoxins commonly associated with necrotizing fasciitis and packing of cavities (such as tampons, wounds)
  - Can also be caused by staphylococcal species
  - Causes septic shock/multiorgan failure
- Scarlet fever:
  - Also due to streptococcal exotoxins
  - Diffuse erythematous sunburn-like rash
  - Initially white tongue then strawberry red
  - Complete recovery is usual with antibiotics
- Acute rheumatic fever:
  - Autoimmune disease, occurs 2–3 weeks following pharyngitis
  - Presents with fever, rash, carditis, arthritis
- Acute glomerulonephritis:
  - Rare, autoimmune mediated
  - Can follow any streptococcal infection

1.1.3 Alpha-haemolytic streptococci

- 'Viridans streptococci'.
- A nasopharyngeal commensal.
- Most common cause of bacterial endocarditis.
- Risk of introduction to bloodstream during interventional procedures.
- People at risk of infective endocarditis include those with:
  - Valve replacements
  - Valvular heart disease
  - Structural congenital heart disease
  - Hypertrophic cardiomyopathy
  - Previous infectious endocarditis
- In the past, antibiotic prophylaxis was given routinely to those at risk of endocarditis undergoing interventional procedures. This practice has been recently reviewed, and

NICE Guidelines (CG64) currently recommend antibiotic prophylaxis is *not* routinely given in dental procedures, GI, genitourinary, gynaecological, or respiratory tract intervention.

1.2 Staphylococci

- Gram-positive cocci.
- One of the most common causes of bacterial infections.

1.2.1 *Staphylococcus aureus*

- Methods of spread:
  - Part of normal skin/mucous membrane flora
  - Survives for long periods on inanimate objects
  - Transmission via direct contact, contaminated objects/food
  - Infects via both exogenous and endogenous route
  - *S. aureus* produces toxins that can cause disease in the absence of invasive infection
- Clinical features:
  - Common cause of nosocomial infections
  - In immunocompetent patients, usually remains localized at portal of entry by host defences
  - Skin infections include folliculitis, abscess, wound infection, cellulitis, and impetigo (although impetigo is more commonly caused by *Streptococcus pyogenes*)
  - Osteomyelitis and septic arthritis
  - Endocarditis occurs in IVDUs due to contaminated needles
  - Necrotizing pneumonia
- Toxinoses:
  - Scalded skin syndrome:
    - Epithelial desquamation resulting from exfoliative toxin production
  - Toxic shock syndrome:
    - Caused by *S. aureus* exotoxins
    - Associated with *Staphylococcus* wound infection, tampon use, cellulitis, osteomyelitis, postpartum
    - Presents as high fever, confusion, vomiting, diarrhoea, skin rash
    - Septic shock and multiorgan failure may develop, resulting in a high mortality
  - Staphylococcal gastroenteritis:
    - Develops following ingestion of food containing enterotoxin-producing *S. aureus*
    - Incubation period less than 6 hours
    - Clinical features are enterotoxin-mediated, rather than invasive infection

1.2.2 MRSA

- Methicillin-resistant *Staphylococcus aureus*.
- A nasopharyngeal/skin commensal.
- Resistant to multiple antibiotics.
- Associated with worse outcomes:
  - Longer hospital stay
  - Longer ITU stay
  - Higher mortality rates

1.2.3 *Staphylococcus epidermidis*

- Coagulase-negative staphylococci.
- Facultative anaerobe.
- Frequently a contaminant of blood cultures.
- Methods of spread:
  - Part of normal skin flora
  - Transmitted via direct contact
  - Opportunistic pathogen, usually hospital acquired
- Clinical features:
  - Prosthetic implant infections—catheters, heart valves
  - Produces an extracellular polysaccharide 'slime' that facilitates adherence to bioprosthetic material

CHAPTER C2

Tuberculosis

CONTENTS

- *Mycoplasma tuberculosis*
- Gram-negative, acid fast bacilli, obligate aerobe
- 95% of all cases of TB worldwide occur in developing countries

2.1 Transmission and establishment in host

- Large numbers of organisms are released by coughing, therefore transmission is primarily via respiratory droplet (aerosol), and frequently the initial site of infection is pulmonary.
- Initial phase:
  - Bacilli inhaled, ingested by macrophages but not killed, and initiate inflammatory reaction
  - Bacilli multiply within macrophages and drain to local lymph nodes, disseminating infection
- Tubercle formation:
  - Additional macrophages migrate to the area and form tubercle
  - Central macrophages die, releasing bacilli into caseous centre
  - At this point the disease may become dormant or spread
- Dormant:
  - Fibrosis and calcification of tubercle
- Spread:
  - Tubercle matures, may invade blood vessels/bronchi enabling spread
  - Enlarging caseous centre liquefies, forming a 'tuberculous cavity' in which the bacilli multiply
  - The tubercle eventually ruptures, allowing bacilli to be disseminated to almost any organ in the body
- Reactivation:
  - *M. tuberculosis* survives in dormant tubercle (most commonly in lung apices where high oxygen tension favours mycobacterial growth)
  - Reactivation is caused by an impairment in immune status (e.g. elderly, malnutrition, alcoholism, stress, immunosuppressive medication, diabetes, AIDS)

- *M. tuberculosis* resistance relies on cell-mediated immune response from CD4 + T cells. Although antibodies may be generated, they do not convey resistance because *M. tuberculosis* is intracellular.

2.1.1 Clinical features

- Active TB has a broad spectrum of clinical presentations.
- Primary TB is usually pulmonary and asymptomatic.
- Post-primary TB may present with fever, sweats, malaise, anorexia, weight loss.
- Pulmonary TB results in cough, sputum, haemoptysis, pneumonia, pleural effusion.
- Miliary TB:
  - Disseminated infection
  - May occur as primary TB or develop after initial infection, and therefore may occur in the absence of active lung infection
  - Presents with fever, weight loss, malaise, breathlessness, and symptoms specific to the organs affected
  - Classic miliary TB shows 'millet-like' seeds of TB on CXR
  - Common in immunocompromised hosts
- Genitourinary tract TB:
  - The most common site after the lungs to be infected
  - Scarring, fibrosis, and tubercles occur resulting in vesicoureteric reflux, hydronephrosis, and secondary infections
  - May be asymptomatic. May present with dysuria, haematuria, and frequency. In men, prostatitis, orchitis, and epididymitis may be present
- Gastrointestinal TB:
  - Results in fibrosis and inflammation of the GI tract, ulcerative lesions, granulomas, strictures, and fistulas
  - Symptoms include weight loss, fevers, abdominal pain, nausea, vomiting, and constipation
  - May lead to obstruction, GI haemorrhage, and perforation
- 'Potts disease'/tuberculous spondylitis:
  - Osteomyelitis/arthritis involves multiple vertebrae, causing progressive bone destruction, vertebral collapse, and kyphosis
  - Rare in developed countries
  - Presents with back pain and constitutional symptoms
  - Neurological defects may develop including spinal cord compression
- CNS TB:
  - Meningitis, tuberculoma, cerebral abscess, and hydrocephalus

2.1.2 Laboratory identification

- Isolation of *Mycobacterium tuberculosis* is essential to confirm species and strain of *Mycobacterium*, and to obtain sensitivities.
- Specimens—blood, sputum, urine, and CSF should be sent for:
  - Microscopy and staining, e.g. Ziehl-Neelsen staining will detect acid fast bacilli—but cannot differentiate between *Mycobacteria*. May be false negative
  - Culture on specialist Lowenstein–Jensen agar (very slow growing, may take 2–8 weeks)
  - Nucleic acid amplification techniques expedite detection—PCR and the Amplified *Mycobacterium tuberculosis* Direct test.

2.1.3 Management

● Combination antibiotics used to delay/prevent emergence of antibiotic-resistant organisms.
● 3–4 drugs are used for the first 2 months then 2 drugs for 4 months.
● Rifampicin, isoniazid, pyrazinamide, ethambutol, and streptomycin are first-line therapy.

2.1.4 Immunosuppression and TB

● TB prophylaxis is recommended for all patients with significant immunosuppression (e.g. HIV infection) and latent TB infection, because of the high risk of developing active TB.

CHAPTER C3

Clostridial infection

CONTENTS

- Clostridial bacteria are Gram-positive, anaerobic, spore-forming rods.
- Commonly found in GI tract, dust, soil, and vegetation.
- Potent exotoxins cause botulism, tetanus, gas gangrene, and pseudomembranous colitis.

3.1 Clostridial colitis

- Pseudomembranous colitis.
- Caused by *Clostridium difficile*.

3.1.1 Source
- Minor component of intestinal flora located in GI tract.
- Antibiotic therapy depletes other bacterial flora leading to overgrowth of *C. difficile*.
- *C. difficile* produces 2 major toxins:
  - Toxin A, an enterotoxin, stimulates excess fluid secretion and inflammatory response
  - Toxin B, a cytotoxin, causes lysis of host cells
  - Binary toxin is produced by a small percentage of *C. difficile* isolates and may be associated with increased disease severity

3.1.2 Clinical features
- Disease spectrum caused by *C. difficile* varies from an asymptomatic carrier state, through mild self-limiting diarrhoea, to pseudomembranous colitis and fulminant colitis.
- Variable disease severity depends partly on strain and partly on patient co-morbidity.
- Pseudomembranous colitis is caused by enterotoxin effects on GI tract.
- Presents with profuse watery diarrhoea, which may be bloody.
- Rare complications include toxic megacolon, colonic perforation, and death.

3.1.3 Principles of isolation and drug therapy
- Discontinue causative drug if possible.
- Supportive therapy—rehydrate, correct electrolyte disturbance.
- Oral metronidazole is the first-line therapy, with vancomycin for resistant strains.

- Relapse following treatment is common, occurring in up to a third of patients.
- Isolate patients to prevent spread and *C. difficile* outbreaks. Spores are very hardy and can survive alcohol-based disinfectants; therefore hypochlorite bleach is required to clean surfaces. Alcohol hand gel is not sufficient for hand decontamination.

3.2 Clostridial gas gangrene

- Causative agent is Clostridium perfringens.

3.2.1 Source

- Part of the normal flora of vagina and GI tract; also found in soil.
- Clostridial spores enter tissue via infected soil or endogenous transfer from the vagina or GI tract.
- Spores germinate in open wounds, particularly those associated with GI tract, or devitalized tissue.
- Exotoxins are produced that kill cells and hydrolytic enzymes facilitate spread of infection.
- Fermentation of tissue carbohydrate creates gas, which accumulates as bubbles in subcutaneous tissue, causing crepitations felt on palpation.
- Exudates are copious and foul smelling.
- Exotoxins spread in the systemic circulation to end organs, causing renal failure, shock, and haemolysis.

3.2.2 Clinical features

- Clostridial myonecrosis (gas gangrene):
  - Untreated causes septicaemia and is fatal within days of initial gangrene
- Enteritis necroticans:
  - Necrotizing bowel disease, rare, high mortality
- Anaerobic cellulitis:
  - Infection of connective tissue
  - Spreads along fascia; may be necrotizing
  - Prompt aggressive surgical intervention essential due to rapid spread
- Clostridial endometritis:
  - Complication of retained products following abortion or inadequately sterilized instruments
  - Gangrenous infection of uterine tissue, causes toxaemia, bacteraemia
- Food poisoning:
  - Due to *C. perfringens* enterotoxin
  - Incubation period 8–18 hours
  - Nausea, abdominal cramps, diarrhoea
  - Self-limiting, lasting 1–2 days rarely may be fatal

3.2.3 Principles of treatment and prevention

- Gas gangrene:
  - Urgent thorough debridement
  - Amputation may be required
  - Expose wound to oxygen—hyperbaric oxygen chambers increase oxygen tension and inhibit the pathological process
  - High-dose broad-spectrum IV antibiotics (metronidazole with penicillins or clindamycin)
- Food poisoning:
  - Self-limiting, only supportive treatment generally required

3.3 Tetanus

- Caused by *Clostridium tetani*.
- Rare in the UK due to vaccination.

3.3.1 Source

- *C. tetani* commonly found in soils.
- Infects contaminated wounds, dirty and devitalized tissues harbour spores.
- Tetanus-prone injuries:
  - Burn/wound sustained 6 hours before treatment
  - Significant amount of dead/devitalized tissue
  - Deep puncture wounds create a small area of devitalized tissue where *C. tetani* germinates
  - Illicit drugs injection sites
  - Wounds heavily contaminated with soil/manure
  - Wounds or burns with clinical evidence of sepsis

3.3.2 Clinical features

- *C. tetani* produces tetanospasmin, a potent neurotoxin:
  - Transported to CNS by retrograde neuronal flow or via bloodstream
  - Blocks the release of inhibitory neurotransmitters
  - Causes prolonged, unrestrained excitation of motor neurons, spasmodic muscle contraction, and spastic paralysis
- Tetanus usually presents as a spastic paralysis:
  - Muscle spasms often first involve the site of infection
  - Early in the disease the jaw muscles are affected causing 'lockjaw'
  - Gradually other muscles become involved
  - Any sudden stimulus can precipitate painful spasms/convulsions
- High mortality (40%), usually a result of paralysis of chest muscles causing respiratory failure.
- Incubation period 2–50 days.

3.3.3 Principles of treatment

- Urgent administration of antitoxin to neutralize any toxins not yet bound to neurons.
- Intravenous penicillin and metronidazole.
- Human tetanus immunoglobulin.
- Debridement of necrotic tissue at entry site.
- Supportive measures:
  - Sedatives
  - Muscle relaxants to minimize spasms
  - Attention to maintaining adequate ventilation

3.3.4 Principles of prevention

- Wound care, i.e. thorough irrigation and debridement of devitalized tissue.
- Active tetanus immunization should be commenced/boosted if appropriate.
- Tetanus immunoglobulin should be given if unimmunized, or to those with tetanus prone wounds, as it provides immediate passive immunity.
- Antibiotic cover may also be required for some wounds.

3.3.5 Vaccination schedule for tetanus toxoid

- Primary vaccination—3 doses of vaccine 1 month apart (in children at 2, 3, and 4 months of age).

- Initial booster required 3 years after primary course for preschool children, or 10 years after primary course if an adult.
- Further booster after 10 years.
- If an adult has already received more than 5 doses in total, further routine boosters are not recommended.

Neisseria

CONTENTS

- Gram-negative aerobic cocci.
- 'Pyogenic cocci'—produce purulent material comprised largely of white blood cells.

4.1 Neisseria meningitidis

4.1.1 Epidemiology

- 'Meningococcus', the most frequent cause of meningitis.
- Affects young, healthy individuals.
- Outbreaks of meningitis in winter/early spring occur particularly in schools, institutions, and amongst the military.
- N. meningitidis colonizes nasopharyngeal mucosa.
- Transmission: inhalation of respiratory droplets from carrier/infected host.

4.1.2 Pathogenesis

- Different serogroups:
  - Serotype A causes epidemics
  - Serotype B causes most morbidity and mortality followed by serotype C
- N. meningitidis is encapsulated with a lipooligosaccharide (LOS) outer core, which mediates immune system evasion. It is antiphagocytic and resists complement-mediated lysis.
- When complement-mediated lysis occurs, LOS is released and functions as an endotoxin, responsible for many of the toxic effects found in disseminated meningococcal infection.
- Pili, hair-like surface appendages, enhance attachment of organism to host cells.
- Attaches to nasopharyngeal mucosa where it colonizes or infects.
- If meningococci penetrate the nasopharynx and enter bloodstream they rapidly multiply, causing septicaemia, and if they penetrate the blood–brain barrier, meningitis develops.

4.1.3 Clinical features

- Meningitis, meningococcaemia with DIC, septic shock without meningitis.
- Symptoms can occur rapidly with great intensity, with death after a matter of hours.

- Incubation period 2–10 days.
- Meningitis features include fever, malaise, severe headache, neck stiffness, vomiting, photophobia, joint symptoms, and a petechial and/or purpuric rash.
- 30% of patients with meningitis develop fulminant septicaemia.
- Meningococcal septicaemia may be fatal in less than 12 hours—bacterial endotoxin largely responsible.
- Waterhouse–Friderichsen syndrome affects very young children and can cause death within 10–12 hours. It is characterized by:
  - Large, blotchy purple skin haemorrhages
  - Vomiting
  - Diarrhoea
  - Circulatory collapse
  - Adrenal necrosis

4.1.4 Basis of diagnosis

- Gold standard for diagnosis is isolation of N. meningitidis from blood/CSF.
- Can also isolate from rash aspirates and nasopharyngeal swabs.
- Microscopy and staining: Gram-negative cocci.
- Culture:
  - Chocolate agar with increased carbon dioxide
  - Plain chocolate agar for CSF or blood as usually sterile
  - Thayer–Martin agar for nasopharyngeal/skin lesions to eliminate contaminants

4.1.5 Medical management

- Medical emergency.
- Antibiotic therapy cannot wait for definitive bacteriologic diagnosis.
- If clinically suspicious, treat immediately.
- Intravenous antibiotics (e.g. cefotaxime 2g) pending culture result.
- Prompt treatment significantly reduces mortality.

4.1.6 Principles of prevention

- Meningococcal vaccine—targets meningococcal serogroups A, C, W-135, and Y, but is not effective against serogroup B.
- Rifampicin prophylaxis is used to treat close contacts and eliminate carrier state.

4.2 Neisseria gonorrhoeae

- 'Gonococcus'.
- Gram-negative diplococci.

4.2.1 Epidemiology

- Transmitted sexually or vertically through infected birth canal.
- Asymptomatic/untreated patients act as reservoir for maintaining and transmitting infection.
- Second most common STI after chlamydia.
- Highest rates of infection amongst the young.

4.2.2 Basis of infection

- Pili enhance attachment of organism to host cells, provoke localized inflammation, and resist phagocytosis.
- Gonococci most often colonize the mucous membranes of genitourinary tract or rectum.

- Cause localized infection with production of pus or lead to tissue invasion, chronic inflammation, and fibrosis.
- Incubation period 1–12 days.

4.2.3 Clinical features

- May be asymptomatic, especially in females.
- Greenish-yellow urethral/cervical discharge, dysuria, intermenstrual bleeding.
- In females, infection occurs in the endocervix, urethra and vagina. If it progresses to the uterus causes salpingitis, PID, and fibrosis.
- Infertility occurs in 20% with gonococcal salpingitis as a result of tubal fibrosis.
- Rectal infections are prevalent in sexually active homosexuals and cause constipation, painful defecation, and purulent discharge.
- Pharyngitis:
  - Caused by oral–genital contact
  - Sore throat, purulent exudates
- Opthalmia neonatorum.
- Disseminated infection:
  - Gonococcal bacteraemia is rare
  - Gonococci have limited ability to replicate in the bloodstream as opposed to meningococci
  - Gonococcal arthritis presents as fever, painful septic joints, and rash (small pustules with erythematous base, which may become necrotic)

4.2.4 Basis of diagnosis

- Swab:
  - Urethra (men)
  - Endocervix (women)
  - Rectum
  - Oropharynx
- If disseminated:
  - Blood
  - Joint aspirate
  - Skin lesions
- Microscopy and Gram stain: Gram-negative cocci.
- Culture on Thayer–Martin agar—allows selective growth of *Neisseria*, otherwise overgrowth of normal flora on non-selective media.

4.2.5 Medical management

- Often antibiotic resistant:
  - Recommend 3rd-generation cephalosporins
- Patients with gonorrhoea are at risk for other STDs:
  - Treat for both gonorrhoea and chlamydia (i.e. with addition of doxycycline)
  - Screen for other STIs (e.g. HIV, hepatitis, syphilis)
- Prevent spread:
  - Prompt treatment and contact tracing
  - Promote barrier contraception
  - Screen those at risk

Pertussis

CONTENTS

- 'Whooping cough', caused by *Bordetella pertussis*.
- Gram-negative rod, aerobic.

5.1 Epidemiology

- Highly contagious.
- Uncommon in UK children due to immunization.
- In countries without immunization it occurs in epidemics, and most children get it at some stage.

5.2 Basis of infection

- Respiratory droplet transmission.
- Adheres to ciliated epithelium in upper respiratory tract.
- Produces exotoxins that cause death of ciliated epithelial cells.

5.3 Clinical features

- Incubation period 5–14 days.
- Initially presents with 'catarrhal phase':
  - Symptoms of URTI
  - Rhinorrhoea, conjunctivitis, malaise, mild fever, then progresses to dry, non-productive cough
  - Lasts 1–2 weeks
- Next develops into the 'paroxysmal phase':
  - Cough becomes increasingly severe
  - Spasms of coughing followed by a 'whoop' as patient inspires rapidly
  - May become cyanotic during coughing
  - Copious amounts of mucus may be produced

- ■ Vomiting and exhaustion also feature
- ■ Lasts 3–4 weeks
- Finally the 'convalescent phase':
  - ■ Takes additional 3–4 weeks

5.3.1 Complications

- Secondary infections including pneumonia, bronchiectasis, otitis media.
- Encephalopathy, seizures.

5.4 Basis of diagnosis

- Initially a clinical diagnosis (characteristic cough 'whoop').
- Suspect if catarrhal symptoms 1–3 weeks post exposure to pertussis.
- Nasopharyngeal swabs on special culture medium must be taken for microscopy and culture: selective agar yields positive result in 3–6 days.
- More rapid result via direct fluorescent antibody test on nasopharyngeal smears.
- Serologic tests for antibodies.

5.5 Medical management

- If caught early during catarrhal stage give erythromycin to reduce duration and severity of disease and minimize spread of infection.
- Once coughing phase has started, antibiotics have little impact on illness.
- However, antibiotics are often given in first few weeks to patients and contacts to limit spread of infection.
- If erythromycin treatment fails consider trimethoprim and sulfamethoxazole.
- Routine childhood vaccination at 2, 3, and 4 months of age followed by a preschool booster.

Klebsiella, Salmonella, Escherichia coli

CONTENTS

6.1 *Klebsiella*

- *Klebsiella pneumoniae* and *Klebsiella oxytocal*.
- Enterobacteria.
- Gram-negative rods.
- Encapsulated, produce exotoxins.

6.1.1 Epidemiology

- Primarily opportunistic and nosocomial pathogen.
- Colonizes skin, nasopharynx, and GI tract.
- Frequently colonizes hospitalized patients and contaminant in critical care areas and ventilators.
- Associated with antibiotic treatment, indwelling catheters, and immunocompromised patients.

6.1.2 Sites of infection

- Primarily an infection of the respiratory tract.
- *K. pneumoniae* and *K. oxytoca* cause necrotizing lobar pneumonia in the immunocompromised (e.g. alcoholics, diabetics, COPD). May develop bacteraemia and septic shock. High mortality associated with *Klebsiella* pneumonia.
- *Klebsiella* UTIs and URTIs also occur.
- Rhinoscleroma and ozena are rare chronic inflammatory processes involving the nasopharynx.

6.1.3 Medical management

- Widespread antibiotic use has led to the development of highly virulent, multidrug-resistant *Klebsiella*, including some ESBL-producing strains.
- Treat as per sensitivities.
- Empirical treatment for severely ill patients may include cephalosporins, carbapenems, aminoglycosides, and quinolones.

6.2 *Salmonella*

- 2500 different strains, but *Salmonella enterica* is the primary pathogen.
- Gram-negative facultative anaerobe.
- Intracellular parasite, survives in phagocytic cells.

6.2.1 Sources of infection

- *S. typhi* exclusively infects human.
- Other strains are associated with animals and food (e.g. meat, eggs, poultry).
- >95% *Salmonella* infections are food-borne.
- Faecal–oral transmission occurs and may lead to a carrier state.
- Young children and the elderly are particularly susceptible.
- Epidemics occur in crowded institutions.

6.2.2 Clinical features of infection

- Salmonella invades epithelial cells of the small intestine.
- Disease may remain localized in small intestine or become systemic.
- Gastroenteritis (salmonellosis):
  - *S. enteriditis* and *S. typhimurium*
  - Incubation period 12–48 hours
  - Diarrhoea (non-bloody), nausea, vomiting, abdominal pain, fever
  - Self-limiting, lasts 48–72 hours
  - Carriage may persist for more than a month
- Enteric (typhoid) fever:
  - *S. typhi*
  - Severe, life-threatening, systemic illness
  - Characterized by fever and abdominal symptoms
  - Chills, sweats, headache, anorexia, weakness, sore throat, cough, myalgia, diarrhoea, constipation
  - 30% have faint maculopapular rash on trunk (rose spots)
  - Incubation period 5–21 days
  - Lasts 3–4 weeks
  - 15% mortality unless given timely antibiotics and supportive treatment
- Complications:
  - Osteomyelitis and septic arthritis
  - GI haemorrhage
  - *Salmonella* bacteraemia
  - Vascular infections and endocarditis
  - Hepatobiliary and splenic infections

6.2.3 Treatment

- Gastroenteritis in non-immunocompromised: supportive treatment only, no antibiotics required and may prolong carrier state.
- Enteric fever: ceftriaxone, ciprofloxacin.
- Prevent *Salmonella* infection with proper sewage disposal, correct food handling, thorough cooking, and good personal hygiene. Food handlers should not return to work until carrier state excluded.
- Vaccination against typhoid for those at risk.

6.3 *Escherichia coli*

- Gram-negative rod.

6.3.1 Infective sites

- Part of normal flora of colon.
- Different strains of *E. coli* with variable virulence.
- Pili aid adherence to mucosal surfaces.
- Transmission via faecal–oral route from contaminated food/water.
- Intestinal disease—5 main types:
  - Enterotoxigenic: travellers' diarrhoea
  - Enteropathogenic: important in infants in areas of poor sanitation
  - Enterohaemorrhagic: exotoxin-mediated 'haemorrhagic colitis' associated with haemolytic uraemic syndrome in children
  - Enteroinvasive: dysentery-like syndrome
  - Enteroadherent: travellers' diarrhoea and persistent watery diarrhoea in children and HIV
- Extraintestinal disease:
  - Often caused by patients' own flora, which is not pathogenic in their own intestine
  - UTI:
    - *E. coli* is the most common cause of UTIs, especially in women
    - Caused by uropathogenic strains of *E. coli*
    - Virulence factors include P fimbriae (an adherence factor), haemolysin, colicin V, and resistance to the bacteriocidal activity of serum complement
    - *E. coli* is a major cause of neonatal meningitis, and one of the most common causes of neonatal sepsis
  - Nosocomial infections:
    - Postoperative meningitis
    - Bacteraemia
    - Endotoxic shock
    - Pneumonia

6.3.2 Treatment of infection

- Prevention: careful food and water preparation, hand hygiene.
- Symptomatic: fluid and electrolyte maintenance.
- Intestinal disease:
  - Antibiotics may shorten duration of symptoms
  - Resistance is widespread
  - Rifaximin is an appropriate non-absorbable GI-selective oral antibiotic
- Systemic disease:
  - According to sensitivities
  - Ampicillin, cefotaxime, ciprofloxacin, trimethoprim
- Extraintestinal disease:
  - UTIs—according to sensitivities
  - Trimethoprim, ciprofloxacin, cephalosporins, tetracyclines, aminoglycosides
  - Neonatal meningitis—cephalosporins

Gram-negative gastrointestinal disease

CONTENTS

7.1 *Helicobacter pylori*

- Gram-negative curved/spiral rods.

7.1.1 Background to infection

- Common worldwide.
- Transmission person to person.
- Can colonize the stomach, duodenum, and oesophagus.
- Causes non-invasive chronic infections if untreated.
- Survives in mucus layer that coats epithelium resulting in chronic inflammation of mucosa.
- Produces urease, which creates ammonia ions, which elevates pH and prevents attack from stomach acid, favouring bacterial replication.
- Ammonia also potentiates the effects of *H. pylori* cytotoxin in destruction of mucus-producing cells, exposing underlying connective tissue to stomach acid.

7.1.2 Clinical features of infection

- May be asymptomatic (carrier state).
- Presents with superficial gastritis, epigastric discomfort, and sometimes diarrhoea.
- *H. pylori* is closely linked with gastric and duodenal ulcers and is also a risk factor for developing gastric carcinoma and gastric B-cell lymphomas.

7.1.3 Basis of diagnosis

- Urea breath test: oral radiolabelled urea is given to the patient. If *H. pylori* are present, urease will split forming radiolabelled carbon dioxide and NH_3.
- Gastric biopsy by endoscopy: *H. pylori* evident histologically, by culture, or urease test.
- Stool/serum antigen.

7.1.4 Principles of medical management

- Elimination of *H. pylori* is with combination therapy as resistance easily develops.
- 2 antibiotics plus proton pump inhibitor (PPI) (e.g. amoxicillin plus clarithromycin plus omeprazole).

7.2 *Campylobacter*

- Gram-negative curved/spiral rods.

7.2.1 Background to infection

- *Campylobacter* is a commensal of many mammals and birds, which serve as reservoirs for infection.
- Transmitted to humans via faecal–oral route:
  - Direct contact
  - Contaminated meat, milk, water
- *Campylobacter* adhesins aid binding to host cells and mucosal colonization.
- *C. jejuni* is primary human pathogen causing both intestinal and extraintestinal infection.

7.2.2 Clinical features of infection

- Incubation period 1–7 days.
- Intestinal infection:
  - Ulcerative inflammatory lesions throughout bowel
  - Acute gastroenteritis
  - Fever, headache, myalgia, abdominal cramps, diarrhoea (± blood)
  - Lasts several weeks, usually self-limiting, although bacteraemia may occur
  - Major cause of travellers' diarrhoea and pseudoappendicitis
- Complications:
  - Guillain–Barré syndrome
  - Septic abortion
  - Reactive arthritis

7.2.3 Basis of diagnosis

- Isolated from faeces, cultured using selective media.

7.2.4 Principles of management and control

- Symptomatically treat diarrhoea with fluid/electrolyte replacement.
- Limited role for antibiotics:
  - Consider (e.g. ciprofloxacin) if severe symptoms, high fever, bloody diarrhoea, worsening illness, illness more than 1 week's duration.
- Prevention:
  - Thorough cooking of potentially contaminated foods (e.g. poultry)
  - Pasteurization of milk products
  - Clean surfaces used to prepare raw meat

Legionella

CONTENTS

- *Legionella pneumophilia* is the primary pathogen in human disease.
- Gram-negative rod in nature but in clinical material appear cocco-bacillary.
- Aerobic intracellular parasite.

8.1 Background to infection

- Normal habitat soil, warm water, and sources of moist heat (e.g. water-cooling towers, water-distributing systems).
- Chlorine tolerant.
- Most infections transmitted by inhalation of contaminated aerosol or aspiration of water, but may occur from swimming in contaminated water.
- No human-to-human transmissions.
- Primarily causes respiratory tract infections.
- May be sporadic cases or localized outbreaks.
- Inhaled bacteria reach alveoli and are phagocytosed by alveolar macrophages.
- Organisms multiply within phagosome until cell ruptures, releasing multiple bacteria.

8.2 Clinical features of infection

- 2 different presentations:

8.2.1 Legionnaires' disease

- Atypical lobar pneumonia with multisystem involvement.
- Responsible for 1–5% of community-acquired pneumonia in adults.
- Affects 1–5% of those exposed to common source, more often those with some form of immunocompromise/respiratory disorder.
- Incubation period 2–10 days.
- Severity and range of symptoms vary substantially; can be fatal in up to 30%.
- Early symptoms are non-specific, including fever, malaise, myalgia, anorexia, and headache.
- Respiratory infection: productive cough, chest pain, respiratory compromise.

- Multisystem involvement:
  - GI: watery diarrhoea, nausea, vomiting, pancreatitis, peritonitis
  - Neurological symptoms: headache, encephalopathy, altered mental state
  - Cardiac: myocarditis, pericarditis, endocarditis
  - Acute kidney injury

8.2.2 Pontiac fever

- Affects healthy individuals, and ~90% of those exposed to source of *L. pneumophilia*.
- Symptoms similar to influenza.
- Recovery usually within 1 week.
- No specific therapy required.

8.3 Basis of diagnosis

- Definitive diagnosis: culture *Legionella* from sputum/alveolar aspirate, visible colonies form in 3–5 days.
- Urinary antigen test: results available within hours, and positive tests may persist even during administration of antibiotic.
- Serology: immunofluorescent antibodies/ELISA are readily available but require a 4-fold increase in antibody titre, which takes 4–8 weeks. Paired measurements from both the acute and convalescent periods should be obtained.

8.4 Medical management of infection and principles of prevention and public health

- Clarithromycin is commonly used with the addition of rifampicin if symptoms are not settling.
- Macrolides, doxycycline, and fluoroquinolones also generally effective.
- Pontiac fever is treated symptomatically; antibiotics are not required.
- Legionnaires' disease is a notifiable disease.
- Control and prevention of the disease is through identification and treatment of the source of the infection, that is, by treating the contaminated water systems, and good design and maintenance to prevent growth in the first place.
- Gram-negative encapsulated rod, obligate aerobe.

Pseudomonas

CONTENTS

- *Pseudomonas aeruginosa* is the primary pathogen.
- Found in soil, water, plants, and animals.
- Grows in moist environments including hot tubs, wet intravenous tubing, and other water-containing vessels.
- Moist environments within hospitals are a potent source of *Pseudomonas*.
- Hospital reservoirs include disinfectants, respiratory equipment, food, sinks, taps, toilets, showers, and mops.
- Spread occurs from patient to patient on the hands of hospital personnel, by direct patient contact with contaminated reservoirs, and by the ingestion of contaminated foods and water.
- Opportunistic pathogen and major cause of nosocomial infections.
- May colonize healthy humans but rarely infects uncompromised tissues.

9.1 Basis of infection

- Pili facilitate attachment to host tissue.
- The capsule reduces the effectiveness of normal host clearance mechanisms allowing colonization.
- Cytotoxins and damaging proteases promote local invasion and dissemination of infection.
- Virtually any tissue or organ system can be infected; infections may be localized or systemic.

9.2 Clinical features of infection

- Severe hospital-acquired infections—especially in immunocompromised patients and those undergoing chemotherapy or antibiotic therapy.
- Infections:
  - Eye: keratitis, scleral abscess, and endophthalmitis
  - Ear: otitis externa
  - Skin: surgical wound and burn infections, 'hot tub or swimming pool folliculitis' (pustular lesions on any part of the body that was immersed in water)
  - Bone: osteomyelitis (especially vertebral, pelvis, and sternoclavicular joints), septic arthritis

- CNS: meningitis, brain abscesses (especially post trauma/neurosurgery)
- UTI: usually hospital acquired, associated with catheterization
- Pneumonia: in those with COPD, CCF, cystic fibrosis, ventilated, immunocompromised
- Septicaemia: especially in immunocompromised hosts

9.3 Basis of diagnosis

- Culture: *Pseudomonas* can be isolated on a variety of media, including MacConkey agar.

9.4 Principles of treatment

- *Pseudomonas* is often antibiotic resistant, complicating choice of therapy.
- Antibiotic resistance stems from the permeability barrier of the Gram-negative outer membrane. It colonizes surfaces in a biofilm form, which makes the cells impervious to therapeutic concentrations of antibiotics.
- Antibiotic selection depends on clinical presentation and antibiotic sensitivity of isolate.
- Often combination therapy is advised, for example, an aminoglycoside and a broad-spectrum antipseudomonal (penicillin or cephalosporin).

9.5 Implications within hospital setting

- Infection control:
  - Isolation
  - Aseptic techniques
  - Cleaning and monitoring of respirators, catheters, and other instruments

Chlamydia

CONTENTS

- An obligate intracellular parasite.
- 3 species:
  - *Chlamydia trachomatis* causes diseases of genitourinary tract and eye
  - *Chlamydia psittaci* is a respiratory pathogen, transmitted by contact with birds, causes psittacosis
  - *Chlamydia pneumoniae* causes atypical pneumonia

10.1 *Chlamydia trachomatis*

- Incubation period 1–3 weeks.
- Responsible for genital infection and ophthalmia neonatorum.

10.1.1 *Chlamydia* genital infection

- Sexually transmitted.
- Highest incidence in young.
- Often asymptomatic.
- Asymptomatic/untreated act as reservoirs for infection.
- Cervicitis, urethritis, endometritis, salpingitis, pelvic inflammatory disease, epididymitis, proctitis.
- Symptoms:
  - Vaginal, urethral, or rectal discharge (often mucoid)
  - Post-coital or intermenstrual bleeding
  - Abdominal pain
  - Fever
  - Painful, swollen scrotum
- Complications: Reiter syndrome.
- Diagnosis:
  - Endocervical swabs, urethral swabs, or MSU
  - *Chlamydia* can be identified by light microscopy and staining, culture, direct immunofluorescence, and chlamydial antigen detection

- Management:
  - A course of doxycycline, or azithromycin as a stat dose can be given to ensure compliance
  - Children/pregnant/breastfeeding: use erythromycin
  - Often coexists with gonorrhoea so screen and treat for both, and other STIs

10.1.2 Chlamydial ophthalmia neonatorum

- Over 50% of infants born to genitally infected mothers will contract *Chlamydia trachomatis* infection on passage through birth canal.
- Acute purulent conjunctivitis ('inclusion conjunctivitis' as inclusion bodies seen in epithelial cells).
- Presents 5–14 days after birth as a uni/bilateral watery discharge, which becomes copious and purulent.
- Following treatment usually heals without permanent damage to the eye. If untreated can cause blindness.
- 10% of infected infants will develop interstitial pneumonitis. *C. trachomatis* is one of the most common causes of pneumonia in the newborn.
- Conjunctival swabs should be taken.
- Treatment: erythromycin syrup. Topical ocular preparations provide some prophylaxis for newborns but are insufficient for treatment.
- The mother (and partner) must also be assessed and treated.

Herpes simplex and zoster

CONTENTS

- Herpesviridae—enveloped double-stranded DNA virus.
- There are 8 strains of human herpes virus, including:
  - Herpes simplex
  - Varicella zoster
  - Cytomegalovirus
  - Epstein–Barr virus
- All have ability to enter a latent state following primary infection and be reactivated at a later time.

11.1 Herpes simplex

11.1.1 Epidemiology

- Transmission via direct contact with lesions or virus-containing secretions.
- HSV infection is accompanied by viral release into saliva and genital secretions, therefore can be spread via kissing, vertical transmission, and sexual transmission.
- HSV multiply in epithelial cells of mucosal surface, producing vesicles or ulcers containing infectious virus.
- Virus enters sensory neurons at site of infection, establishing lifelong latent infection in the nerve ganglia.
- Various triggers induce reactivation and replication of the latent virus. HSV is then transported down the nerve axon to the nerve endings from which the virus is released, infecting surrounding tissue.
- In immunocompetent patients, herpes simplex remains localized as cytotoxic T lymphocytes recognize HSV-specific antigens on infected cells and kill them prior to progeny virus production.
- By this mechanism, dissemination of herpes simplex infection occurs in people with impaired T-cell immunity, such as in organ transplant recipients and AIDS patients.

11.1.2 Clinical features of infection

- Primary infection: may be subclinical.
- Prodrome: 6 hours of tingling, discomfort, itching (sensory nerve symptoms).
- Active:
  - Small clusters of vesicles/shallow ulcers, erythematous base
  - Vesicles present for a few days then dry, forming a yellowish crust
  - May be associated with systemic symptoms—fever, malaise, tender lymphadenopathy, and myalgia
  - Heals at 8–12 days
- Latent period: after primary infection, HSV remains dormant in nerve ganglia.
- Reactivation:
  - Lesions usually smaller and less severe but in same area
  - Triggers often unknown
  - Recurrent infection may be subclinical but still results in virus shedding and transmission
  - Reactivation is more common and severe in immunocompromised people
- HSV types 1 and 2:
  - HSV 1: mostly oral, eye, CNS
  - HSV 2: usually genital herpes
  - However, lesion location is not necessarily indicative of virus type
- HSV may present as:
  - Herpes labialis (typical cold sore lesion at border of lips)
  - Genital lesions
  - Gingivostomatitis
  - Pharyngotonsillitis
  - Keratoconjunctivitis
  - Herpetic whitlow—small, painful, erythematous lesion of the distal phalanx. Caused by inoculation of HSV through a skin break
- HSV complications:
  - Meningitis, encephalitis
  - Neonatal herpes via vertical transmission through birth canal. Often results in systemic infection involving CNS. High mortality if untreated

11.1.3 Basis of diagnosis

- For characteristic lesions in otherwise healthy patients the diagnosis is usually clinical.
- It is important to identify HSV in encephalitis, keratoconjunctivitis, infection of the immunocompromised, and in prevention of neonatal infection (in which early initiation of therapy is essential).
- Confirm diagnosis with swab, vesicle scraping, CSF.
- Tissue cell culture, immunofluorescence or immunoperoxidase staining, serology, and viral PCR can also be used.

11.1.4 Treatment

- Cannot cure latent infection but can minimize viral shedding and symptoms.
- Aciclovir is drug of choice and can be given topically, orally, or intravenously depending on disease presentation and immune state of host.

11.1.5 Herpes encephalitis

- HSV is the most common cause of viral encephalitis.
- 70% mortality rate if untreated.
- May present with a prodrome of malaise, fever, headache, and nausea. This is followed by acute or subacute onset of an encephalopathy; seizures may occur.

- Lumbar puncture is essential for diagnosis with CSF sent for PCR.
- Intravenous aciclovir should be commenced empirically if viral encephalitis suspected.
- MRI is preferred for imaging and follow-up studies of herpes encephalitis.
- CT classically reveals hypodensity in the temporal lobes; oedema and haemorrhages may occur. Contrast enhancement may be evident after a week.
- EEG is abnormal in most cases.

11.2 Herpes zoster

- Varicella zoster virus.
- Primary infection with varicella zoster causes chicken pox, and reactivation of latent virus causes shingles.
- In contrast to HSV, initial and reactivation disease are quite different.
- Neither is life-threatening to healthy individuals but both can be in immunocompromised patients.

11.2.1 Chicken pox (primary infection)

- Epidemiology:
    - Common in under 10s
    - Seasonal variation: peaks in spring
    - 90% of adults are immune
    - Transmission via respiratory droplets
    - Initial invasion of respiratory mucosa, followed by spread to regional lymph nodes where it replicates
    - Spreads to liver and spleen and is disseminated throughout the body by infected mononuclear leucocytes
    - Endothelial capillary cells and ultimately skin epithelial cells become infected, resulting in typical virus-containing vesicles of chicken pox that appear 14–21 days following exposure
    - Contact with vesicular fluid is not a common mode of transmission
- Clinical features of infection:
    - Incubation period 14–21 days
    - Prodrome (1–2 days): fever, malaise, headache, abdominal pain
    - Rash:
        - Occurs in crops initially on face/head/trunk
        - Itchy erythematous macules initially become papules then vesicles
        - Crust over after about 48 hours
        - Last 5–7 days
        - Infectious 1–2 days prior to rash development and up to 5 days after rash develops
- Complications:
    - Encephalitis
    - VZV pneumonia is a common complication in adults and the immunocompromised and can result in significant morbidity and mortality
    - Congenital varicella syndrome

11.2.2 Shingles

- Epidemiology:
    - After primary infection as chicken pox, VZV remains dormant in sensory nerve roots for life
    - On reactivation the virus replicates and spreads along the sensory ganglion causing the characteristic painful dermatomal rash
    - Most common in the elderly and immunocompromised
    - Infectious until all lesions scabbed over, with non-immune contacts developing chicken pox

- Clinical features of infection:
  - Unilateral painful/hyperaesthetic area in dermatomal distribution
  - Malaise, myalgia, headache, and fever may occur
  - Erythematous macules and papules develop in dermatomal distribution on day 3–5
  - Progress to vesicles, which scab over and fall off in less than 14 days
- Complications:
  - Postherpetic neuralgia—pain in distribution of the rash. Common
  - Trigeminal herpes zoster
  - Ramsay–Hunt syndrome
  - Disseminated infection may occur in the immunocompromised

11.2.3 Basis of diagnosis

- Clinical in immunocompetent.
- In immunocompromised patients, it is important to confirm via cell tissue culture of vesicular fluid, immunofluorescence, or immunoperoxidase staining.

11.2.4 Treatment

- Treatment options are based on the patient's age, immune state, duration of symptoms, and disease presentation.
- For healthy children with chicken pox, treatment is supportive (topical calamine, antipyretics).
- For immunocompetent adults, chicken pox infection tends to be more complicated and therefore oral aciclovir is recommended for those over 12.
- In the immunocompetent with shingles, the main purpose of antiviral treatment is to decrease the duration of symptoms and the likelihood of postherpetic neuralgia. Oral aciclovir may be given but is only effective if initiated within 48 hours of onset.
- Intravenous aciclovir is given to the immunosuppressed and those with complicated/disseminated disease.

11.2.5 Prevention

- Live attenuated vaccination.
- Varicella zoster immunoglobulin can be given to immunosuppressed patients, pregnant women, and neonates with exposure to chicken pox or shingles within 3 days of exposure. Primary maternal chicken pox infection during the first 20 weeks of gestation may cause severe congenital abnormality.

CHAPTER C12

HIV

CONTENTS

- Human immunodeficiency virus.
- Retrovirus. Single-stranded, positive sense, linear RNA. Contains reverse transcriptase.

12.1 Epidemiology

- Transmission:
  - Sexual (present in semen and vaginal secretions)
  - Infected blood/blood products (e.g. IVDUs, haemophiliacs)
  - Vertical (transplacental, passage through birth canal, or breastfeeding)
- Risk factors:
  - Location—sub-Saharan Africa is home to 60% of all people living with HIV
  - In the UK, men who have sex with men remain the group at highest risk of acquiring HIV; however, the number of diagnoses among heterosexuals has risen significantly over the past 15 years
  - Intravenous drug usage
  - Sexual contact with members of the earlier-listed high-risk groups or known HIV-positive patients
  - Blood or blood product transfusion prior to 1985

12.2 Pathogenesis

- Retrovirus.
- HIV binds to CD4 receptors on helper T lymphocytes, monocytes, macrophages, and neural cells.
- CD4 cells migrate to the lymphoid tissue where the virus replicates and then infects new CD4 positive cells.
- As the infection progresses, depletion or impaired function of CD4 cells predisposes to the development of immune dysfunction.
- The host fails to adequately respond to opportunistic infections and normally harmless commensals.
- Cellular immunity is mainly affected, therefore infections tend to be non-bacterial (fungal, viral).

12.3 Clinical features

- Seroconversion—period of high level of virus replication in CD4+ T-helper cells:
  - Occurs several weeks after initial infection
  - May be asymptomatic or may experience fever, fatigue, diffuse maculopapular rash, lymphadenopathy
- Asymptomatic infection—following seroconversion plasma load reduces and plateaus, which is mostly asymptomatic:
  - Persistent generalized lymphadenopathy may occur
- Symptomatic infection/AIDS-related complex:
  - A prodrome to acquired immunodeficiency syndrome (AIDS)
  - Constitutional symptoms—night sweats, generalized lymphadenopathy, diarrhoea, and weight loss
  - Minor opportunistic infections
- AIDS:
  - Defined by CD4 count <200 and acquisition of serious opportunistic infections or AIDS-defining illness
  - Death from opportunistic infections, malignancies, neurological disease, wasting, malnutrition, and multisystem failure

12.3.1 AIDS-defining illness

- Candidiasis of bronchi, trachea, lungs, oesophagus.
- *Mycobacterium tuberculosis*.
- *Pneumocystis* pneumonia.
- Cerebral toxoplasmosis.
- Chronic intestinal cryptosporidiosis.
- Disseminated cytomegalovirus disease/cytomegalovirus retinitis.
- HIV-related encephalopathy.
- Kaposi sarcoma (HHV8).
- Lymphoma.
- HIV wasting syndrome.

12.4 Basis of diagnosis

- Pretest counselling is important to obtain informed consent; however, lengthy pretest counselling is not required and the current consensus is that doctors should be able to obtain informed consent for an HIV test in the same way they do for any other medical investigation. A significant number of HIV infections go undiagnosed and new treatment significantly reduces morbidity and mortality. More lengthy counselling and psychological support will be required following a positive result.
- PCR amplification of viral RNA/DNA is used to detect the virus, and can be quantified to monitor progression of disease/efficacy of treatment.
- For early detection, ELISA can detect the p24 antigen in serum about a week earlier than tests for antibody.
- ELISA can also be used to detect HIV antibody.
- CD4 count can be quantified to monitor progression of disease/efficacy of treatment.

12.5 Basis of management

- Treatment of HIV aims to minimize viral replication, prevent viral resistance, and repair the immune response.
- Antivirals—function either by inhibiting viral reverse transcriptase, thereby preventing establishment of HIV infection, or inhibiting viral protease, which delays production of virus by the host cell:
    - Nucleoside reverse transcriptase inhibitor (e.g. zidovudine)
    - Non-nucleoside reverse transcriptase inhibitors (e.g. nevirapine)
    - Protease inhibitors (e.g. indinavir)
- Combination therapy is used comprising 3 drugs. Adherence to treatment is essential to avoid resistance.
- Prophylaxis against opportunistic infection is important when CD4 count is low.

CHAPTER C13

Hepatitis

CONTENTS

13.1 Hepatitis A

13.1.1 Epidemiology

- Common.
- Virus shed in faeces, therefore predominantly spread via faecal–oral route; blood spread is rare.
- Can be transmitted by eating uncooked shellfish harvested from sewage-contaminated water.
- Common in underdeveloped countries with poor sanitation and in institutions.
- Hepatitis A is most often seen among children, particularly in crowded accommodation. The severity of symptoms following hepatitis A infection directly correlates with age. In children the disease is often mild and subclinical.
- Hepatitis A virus (HAV) enters GI tract where it replicates, and is transmitted via the bloodstream to the liver.
- HAV replicates in hepatocytes causing likely immune-mediated cytopathology and derangement of liver function.
- Virions are secreted into bile and released in the stool.
- Incubation period 3–5 weeks.
- The period of greatest faecal shedding and transmission of HAV is during the prodrome (2–3 weeks after infection). The active virus continues to be faecally shed after the development of jaundice, although amounts fall rapidly.
- HAV may be detected in the blood from ~3–4 weeks following infection, just prior to derangement of LFTs and the icteric phase.

13.1.2 Typical clinical features

- Prognosis generally favourable, development of persistent infection/chronic hepatitis is rare, and the infection itself may be asymptomatic.
- Prodrome (days 14–21):
  - Fever
  - Anorexia
  - Nausea

- Vomiting
- Fatigue
- Myalgia
- Headache
- Icteric phase
  - Bilirubinuria
  - Pale stools
  - Jaundice
  - Abdominal pain
  - Hepatomegaly
  - Arthralgia
  - Diarrhoea
- Relapsing hepatitis A:
  - Rare
  - Most common in the elderly
- After infection, immunity is lifelong.

13.1.3 Basis of diagnosis

- Hepatitis serology—anti-HAV IgM antibodies indicate recent infection, anti-HAV IgG remain detectable lifelong.

13.1.4 Medical management

- Treatment is supportive.
- Most recover in 2 months.
- Advise abstinence from alcohol until LFTs normal.
- Locate primary source and prevent outbreaks.

13.1.5 Prevention

- Locate primary source and prevent outbreaks.
- Good sanitation.
- Avoid faecal contamination of food/water.
- Vaccination for travellers to high-risk areas, those with chronic liver disease, and high-risk workers.
- Close contacts of hepatitis A patients can be given passive immunization with human immunoglobulin.

13.2 Hepatitis B

13.2.1 Epidemiology

- Common, affects almost 300 million people worldwide.
- Endemic in Far East/Asia.
- Leading cause of chronic hepatitis, cirrhosis, and hepatocellular carcinoma.
- Transmission:
  - Infectious HBV is present in all body fluids of an infected individual
  - Therefore transmission commonly occurs via IVDU, needle stick injury, blood/blood product transfusion, sexual intercourse, human bites, and vertical transmission

13.2.2 Pathogenesis

- Hepatitis B virus infects hepatocytes.

- HBV is not directly cytopathic and liver damage is produced by the cellular immune response of the host.
- Cytotoxic T cells react with HBcAg and HBeAg, which are expressed on the surface of infected hepatocytes. This helps limit infection by removing virus-producing cells.
- Humoral anti-HBs antibody appears during the convalescent period when it gives protection against re-infection and may aid in clearing circulating virus.

13.2.3 Acute phase infection

- Hepatitis B surface antigen (HBsAg): a protein on the surface of HBV. Appears 6 weeks to 3 months following an acute infection and disappears if infection cleared. If persistent, it indicates chronic infection.
- Hepatitis B e-antigen (HBeAg): rises early and declines rapidly in acute infection. Persistent HbeAg indicates increased severity and infectivity, and increased risk of developing chronic liver disease.
- HBV DNA: implies viral replication.
- Total hepatitis B core antibody (anti-HBc): the first antibody to appear at the onset of symptoms in acute hepatitis B and persists for life. Anti-HBc indicates previous or ongoing infection with HBV.
- IgM anti-HBc: (high titre) indicates acute infection.
- Hepatitis B e-antibody (Anti-HBe): indicates seroconversion, HBeAg will disappear. Indicates decreased infectivity. A predictor of long-term clearance of HBV in patients undergoing antiviral therapy.
- Hepatitis B surface antibody (anti-HBs): appears late, indicates recovery and immunity from HBV infection. Persists for life.

13.2.4 Acute infection leading to chronic hepatitis B

- HBsAg: persistence indicates chronic infection or carrier state.
- HBeAg: persistence indicates increased severity and infectivity, and increased risk of developing chronic liver disease.
- HBV DNA: implies viral replication.
- IgM anti-HBc: (low titre) indicates chronic infection
- IgG: past exposure to HBV (HBsAg negative)
- Incubation period 1–6 months.

13.2.5 Acute infection

- Pre-icteric phase:
  - 3–7 days
  - Mild fever, malaise, anorexia, myalgia, nausea
- Icteric phase:
  - 1–2 months
  - Jaundice, bilirubinuria, tender hepatomegaly
- Fulminant hepatitis:
  - A minority (1–2%) progress to fulminant hepatitis, which is fatal in 80% cases
  - Characterized by extensive liver necrosis in the first 8 weeks of acute illness, high fever, abdominal pain, renal dysfunction, encephalopathy, coma, and seizures
- Convalescent period:
  - Around 80% undergo a convalescent period following the icteric phase, leading to complete recovery
- In two-thirds of patients primary infection is asymptomatic. These patients may still go on to develop symptomatic chronic liver disease.

13.2.6 Chronic phase

- Following acute infection, 2–10% of adults remain chronically infected in various states:
  - Asymptomatic carrier state (most frequent):
    - Mostly HBsAg and anti-HBe positive
    - Minimal or no infectious virus in blood
    - Asymptomatic, rarely develop liver damage
  - Minimal chronic hepatitis/chronic persistent hepatitis:
    - Mostly asymptomatic
    - More likely to suffer reactivation of disease
    - May progress onto cirrhosis
  - Severe chronic hepatitis/chronic active hepatitis:
    - More frequent exacerbations of acute symptoms
    - Progressive liver damage
    - May go on to develop cirrhosis/hepatocellular carcinoma
    - Chronic fatigue, anorexia, malaise, and anxiety often feature
    - Exacerbations are associated with high viral titres, detectable HBeAg, elevated liver enzymes, and bilirubin
    - The risk of developing cirrhosis is highest in carriers with frequent recurrence of acute disease and those who are HBeAg positive
- Hepatitis D may be acquired as a co-infection with HBV, or as a superinfection in those with existing chronic HBV. It is unable to replicate on its own but becomes activated by the presence of HBV. Leads to a flare-up of acute disease, more rapidly progressive chronic disease, and development of cirrhosis in only a few years.

13.2.7 Basis of diagnosis

- LFTs:
  - Transaminases begin to rise on/before the onset of symptoms.
  - The level of ALT rises sharply and peaks in the low thousands.
  - In cases of acute infection ALT starts to drop and returns to normal around 1–4 months following infection.
  - If ALT remains elevated for more than 6 months this suggests chronic hepatitis B infection.
  - Elevation of ALT greater than AST is usually seen in viral hepatitis.
- Hepatitis serology via immunoassay for detection of viral antigens and antibodies to differentiate between acute and chronic infection (see Table C.13.1):
  - HBsAg appear 1–6 months following infection. If persist longer than 6 months post exposure, indicates carrier state or chronic infection
  - HBeAg appear at 6 weeks to 3 months during acute illness, but persistence indicates chronic infection. Correlates with increased severity and infectivity
  - Anti-HBc appears at around 2 months and persists for life

Table C.13.1 Hepatitis serology

	HBeAg	HBsAg	Anti-HBc	Anti-HBs
Acute	+/−	+	+	−
Resolved	−	−	+	+
Chronic	+/−	+	+	−
Vaccinated	−	−	−	+

- Anti-HBc IgM suggests acute infection
- Anti-HBe appears after anti-HBc and its presence represents decreased infectivity
- Anti-HBs antibodies appear 5 months following infection and imply immunity
- HBV DNA can also be detected, which indicates continual viral replication

13.2.8 Medical management

- Advise abstinence from alcohol.
- Interferon alpha and antiviral therapies including lamivudine.
- Transplant may be required.

13.2.9 Prevention

- Active immunization of at-risk population.
- Passive immunization with human hepatitis B immunoglobulin (e.g. for postexposure prophylaxis).
- To prevent vertical transmission give passive and active immunization at birth.

13.3 Hepatitis C

13.3.1 Epidemiology

- In the UK 0.3–0.7% of the population have HCV; however, there are a large number of undiagnosed cases and true prevalence may be much higher.
- Transmission:
  - Spread via infected blood, vertical transmission; rarely sexually transmitted
  - Risk factors:
    - Intravenous drug use is the largest risk factor
    - Blood/blood product transfusions before 1991
    - Needle stick injuries
    - Haemodialysis
    - Infants born to infected mothers
    - Tattoos
    - Human bites
- HCV replicates in hepatocytes, and probably also lymphocytes and macrophages.
- Destruction of liver cells may be a result of both viral replication and host immune response.

13.3.2 Typical clinical features

- Incubation period 6–9 weeks.
- May be asymptomatic, and many cases are very mild.
- 25% get acute hepatitis:
  - May present with fever, malaise, anorexia, abdominal pain, fatigue, arthralgia, urticaria, pale stools, bilirubinuria, jaundice, or deranged LFTs
  - Acute hepatitis may resolve over the course of months, or may progress on to chronic hepatitis C
- Chronic hepatitis C may cause liver failure, cirrhosis, and hepatocellular carcinoma.

13.3.3 Basis of diagnosis

- Immunoassay—anti-HCV antibody detectable 3–4 months post-infection.
- Viral PCR also possible.

13.3.4 Medical management

- Advise abstinence from alcohol.
- The goals of treatment are to achieve sustained eradication of hepatitis C virus and prevent progression to cirrhosis.
- Treatment of choice is combination interferon alpha and ribavirin.
- Liver transplant may be required.

13.3.5 Indications for transplant

- Liver transplantation is not a cure for hepatitis C, as it essentially recurs universally following transplant.
- End-stage liver disease that has failed medical therapy, including:
  - Decompensated cirrhosis
  - Recurrent variceal haemorrhage
  - Intractable ascites
  - Spontaneous bacterial peritonitis
  - Refractory encephalopathy
  - Fulminant hepatic failure

Measles, mumps, rubella

CONTENTS

14.1 Measles

14.1.1 Epidemiology

- A disease of childhood now rare in the UK as a result of vaccination.
- Transmission is via respiratory droplets.
- Incubation period is 10–18 days.
- Measles is extremely infectious and patients are infective from 1–2 days before initial symptoms until 5 days after rash appears.
- Infection is followed by lifelong immunity.

14.1.2 Usual clinical features

- Early (prodrome) lasts 2–4 days:
  - High fever
  - Conjunctivitis
  - Non-productive cough
  - Coryza
  - Diarrhoea
  - Koplik spots—small white spots on red buccal mucosa of mouth and throat
- Rash:
  - Generalized maculopapular rash appears ~10–14 days after infection, beginning at head and neck and spreading to the trunk and finally limbs
  - Fades after 3–4 days
- Complications:
  - Secondary bacterial infections including bronchopneumonia, otitis media
  - Acute demyelinating encephalitis—an autoimmune disease that complicates 1 in 1000 cases of measles. Usually occurs within 2 weeks of onset of rash. Presents as seizures, fever, irritability, headache, and altered conscious level. Treatment is supportive
  - Subacute sclerosing panencephalitis—commoner in boys. Onset is usually 5–10 years following measles, with disturbance in intellect, personality, behavioural disorders, and worsening schoolwork. This is followed by seizures, evidence of pyramidal and extrapyramidal disease, decerebrate rigidity, and death. This condition is untreatable
  - Transient hepatitis

14.2 Mumps

14.2.1 Epidemiology

- Previously a common childhood infection and pre-vaccine was the most common cause of viral encephalitis.
- Transmission via respiratory droplets.
- Incubation 14–21 days.
- Infective from 3 days prior to salivary swelling and up to 1 week following.
- Lifelong immunity is the rule following mumps but re-infection does occur.

14.2.2 Usual clinical features

- May be subclinical.
- Initially prodromal phase characterized by high fever, malaise, myalgia, and headache.
- Infection and swelling of the salivary glands then occurs, mainly the parotid (parotitis), but also sometimes the submandibular glands. May be unilateral or bilateral and is usually tender.
- Complications:
  - Meningo-encephalitis; may occur in the absence of parotitis
  - Epididymo-orchitis—usually presents 4–5 days following parotitis but may occur in isolation. Most common in adolescent male mumps infection. May cause sterility
  - Pancreatitis
  - Mumps arthritis

14.3 Rubella

14.3.1 Epidemiology

- Prior to vaccination programme epidemics occurred in spring/early summer every 6–9 years; however, rubella is now rare in the UK.
- Transmission: respiratory droplet.
- Incubation period 14–21 days.
- Infective from 1 week before to 5 days after onset of rash.
- Natural infection is followed by protection from further infection. If re-infection does occur it is often subclinical.

14.3.2 Clinical features

- Usually mild, may even be subclinical.
- Prodrome:
  - Fever
  - Headache
  - Conjunctivitis
  - Anorexia
  - Rhinorrhoea
- Rash:
  - Generalized pink maculopapular rash usually lasts 3 days
  - Initially on face/head, spreading to trunk and extremities
- Occipital, cervical, and postauricular lymphadenopathy is characteristic.

- Complications:
  - Main morbidity is due to congenital rubella
  - Other complications are rare:
    - Arthropathies
    - Thrombocytopenia
    - Rubella encephalopathy
    - Orchitis

14.3.3 Congenital rubella

- Main morbidity of rubella is caused by congenital infection.
- Rubella is teratogenic and infection in pregnancy causes birth defects including congenital heart disease, sensorineural deafness, mental retardation, motor dysfunction, cataracts, retinopathy, glaucoma, hepatitis, and impaired fetal growth.
  - 1st trimester: infection incurs the highest risk of defects to the baby (~70%) and may also cause miscarriage.
  - 2nd trimester: infection is less problematic; most commonly only sensorineural deafness or occasionally retinopathy occur.
  - 3rd trimester: infection carries a very low risk of birth defects.
- Postexposure immunoglobulin does not prevent infection but may reduce viraemia and severity of infection:
  - It is therefore given to pregnant women who come into contact with rubella.
  - Live vaccine cannot be given in pregnancy.

14.4 MMR

- Combined injection of live attenuated measles, mumps, and rubella.
- Given at 13 months when maternal immunity has disappeared, with a preschool booster.
- Malaise, fever, and rash are common ~1 week after immunization, typically lasting 2–3 days.

CHAPTER C15

Respiratory viruses

CONTENTS

15.1 Rhinovirus

15.1.1 Epidemiology

- There are more than 100 different serotypes of rhinovirus.
- Rhinovirus is chiefly limited to upper respiratory tract infections and is the major cause of the common cold.
- Transmission:
  - Primarily by direct contact
  - Respiratory droplets
- Incubation period is 12–72 hours.
- Virus shedding peaks at 48 hours but can last up to 3 weeks.

15.1.2 Usual clinical features

- Sore throat, nasal congestion, sneezing, headache, and cough are common features. Fever and malaise are unusual.
- Symptoms last 7–14 days, viral shedding persists past symptom resolution.
- Infection results in sinusitis, otitis media, and may exacerbate asthma/COPD.

15.1.3 Basis of diagnosis

- Diagnosis is primarily clinical.
- Rhinovirus can be detected by PCR and viral culture.

15.1.4 Basis of immunity

- Serotype-specific antibodies are found 7–21 days after rhinovirus infection in most patients.
- These antibodies persist for years, providing long-lasting immunity to that serotype.
- However, because of the vast range of serotypes, adults experience the common cold on average 2–4 times per year, each caused by a different serotype.

15.1.5 Management

- Rhinovirus infections are predominantly mild and self-limiting, therefore symptomatic relief and prevention of spread are the main aims.

15.2 Influenza

15.2.1 Epidemiology

- Respiratory tract infection.
- Spread by respiratory droplets.
- Viral shedding occurs between 0 and 24 hours of infection and continues for 5–10 days.
- Classification:
  - 3 basic subtypes of influenza, A, B, and C, classified according to inner antigen proteins
  - Type A is further divided into subtypes H and N depending on surface antigens
  - In humans only subtypes H1, H2, and H3, and N1 and N2 are found
- Over years, marked variation in antigenic properties has occurred as a result of the following:
  - Antigenic drift—minor antigenic changes in H and N surface antigens occur each year due to random mutations in viral RNA and small amino acid substitutions in H/N
  - Antigenic shift—only occurs in type A influenza. A 'reassortment' of viral RNA segments causes a more dramatic change in antigenic properties of H/N proteins, and a complete change in subtype occurs approximately every 10–20 years:
    - If a cell is infected with 2 distinct influenza viruses, the genomic RNA of both parental viruses is replicated and progeny viruses are assembled that contain segments from both parents, creating a new and different virus
    - Where humans live in close proximity to farm animals, new viral subtypes are more likely to develop as reassortment can occur between influenza A viruses from different animal/bird species
- Because of antigenic shift, new types of virus appear that have not been in circulation for many years, therefore many people are immunologically unprotected and previous vaccines are not effective.
- It is antigenic shift that results in major influenza epidemics/pandemics.
- Influenza epidemics typically occur in winter months and severity varies depending on the subtype involved.

15.2.2 Usual clinical features

- Incubation period is 18–72 hours.
- Acute onset.
- High fever, sore throat, myalgia (caused by circulating cytokines), headache, rhinitis, drowsiness, fatigue, cough, diarrhoea.
- Lasts 4–5 days followed by gradual recovery.
- Complications occur in the very young, elderly, immunodeficient, those with chronic cardiac or pulmonary disease, and diabetics, and include:
  - Viral pneumonia
  - Secondary bacterial pneumonia (especially *S. aureus*)
  - Acute bronchitis
  - Febrile convulsions
  - Myositis/myocarditis
  - GBS
  - Encephalitis

15.2.3 Basis of diagnosis

- Diagnosis is essentially clinical, as in most cases it is not necessary to make a specific lab diagnosis.
- Diagnosis can be made from direct viral culture of respiratory tract secretions, PCR, immunofluorescence of respiratory tract secretions, and acute and convalescent serology 10–14 days apart.

15.2.4 Principles of management

- Most often supportive management only is required.
- Antiviral therapy is available, which shortens duration of illness by 2 days and reduces severity. This may lead to resistance and is not routinely given.
- Vaccination:
  - Inactivated influenza virus
  - Recommended for high-risk groups, including patients over 65, patients with COPD, asthma, chronic cardiac disease, chronic renal failure, diabetes, chronic liver disease, cerebrovascular disease, and immunosuppression, and transplant recipients
  - Must contain the specific subtypes of influenza virus that are in circulation at the time
  - Usually contains the principal strains recovered during the previous year

15.3 Parainfluenza

- Group of human parainfluenza viruses (HPIV).
- Primarily affect young children causing upper and lower respiratory tract infections:
  - Common cold (HPIV1, HPIV3, HPIV4)
  - Croup (HPIV1, HPIV2, HPIV3)
  - Bronchiolitis (HPIV1, HPIV3)
  - Pneumonia
- Each HPIV has differing seasonal variation, accounting, for example, for the epidemics of croup in spring and autumn.
- Re-infection can occur throughout life; elderly and immunocompromised are at most risk of complications.
- Transmission is via direct person-to-person contact with secretions, or respiratory droplet spread.
- Incubation period is generally 2–6 days.
- Diagnosis is essentially clinical.
- Virus can be isolated from nasal secretions but this is rarely required.
- Management mostly consists of supportive care.
- Antivirals are of uncertain benefit.

15.4 Respiratory syncytial virus (RSV)

- The leading cause of lower respiratory tract infections in infants and young children.
- Most common cause of bronchiolitis in infants; causes viral pneumonia in young children.
- Transmitted by respiratory droplets or contaminated hands carrying the virus to nose or mouth.
- Typically presents with cough, coryza, wheeze, fever, and reduced oral intake.
- May develop respiratory distress and cyanosis in advanced disease, or apnoea in young children.
- Frequently associated with otitis media (viral/bacterial).

- Symptoms last 7–10 days.
- Over the age of 3 tends to be limited to the upper respiratory tract but can cause severe bronchiolitis with pneumonia in the elderly and organ transplant recipients.
- Repeated infections are common.
- Lab identification is usually not required if the patient is well. Serum antibody titre or viral antigen can be demonstrated in respiratory secretions.

15.4.1 Treatment

- Mainstay is supportive, ensuring adequate oral intake etc.
- Bronchodilators have been used but there is no evidence to demonstrate their efficacy.
- Ribavirin (aerosol) is a broad-spectrum antiviral agent used in the severely ill.

Gastrointestinal viruses

CONTENTS

16.1 Rotavirus

16.1.1 Epidemiology
- Causes severe gastroenteritis, especially in children and infants.
- Responsible for 50% of cases of severe diarrhoea in children under 2 years.
- Seasonal variation in incidence, peaking in winter months.
- Faecal–oral transmission from contaminated food, water, and surfaces.
- Rotavirus survives for extended periods on surfaces.

16.1.2 Pathological basis
- Following ingestion, rotavirus primarily infects and multiplies within enterocytes. The virus destroys enterocytes and damaged cells are sloughed off, releasing large numbers of viral particles into the stool.
- Destruction of enterocytes of the small intestine leads to malabsorption by:
  - Loss of digestive enzymes
  - Shortening and atrophy of the villi, thereby decreasing the surface area of the small intestine
- The malabsorptive state creates a hyperosmotic effect leading to excessive fluid loss via diarrhoea. A secretory component causes increased motility further exacerbating the diarrhoea.
- Rotavirus is shed in the stool from before the onset of symptoms and persists for up to 10 days after symptom appearance.
- Incubation period 1–7 days (usually 48 hours or less).
- Infection may be subclinical but if symptomatic classically lasts 3–8 days and presents with non-bloody diarrhoea, vomiting, fever, malaise, dehydration, and loss of electrolytes.
- Fluid stool loss may be dramatic and death from dehydration is not uncommon, particularly in developing countries where medical facilities are lacking and unable to rehydrate/replace electrolyte loss.

16.1.3 Diagnosis

- Identification of virus in stool is primarily via nucleic acid antigen test (NAAT).

16.1.4 Principles of management

- Fluid/electrolyte replacement.
- No specific antiviral therapy is used.

16.2 Norovirus

16.2.1 Epidemiology

- Commonest cause of gastroenteritis in England and Wales.
- Highly contagious and a major cause of epidemic gastroenteritis, especially in institutions such as hospitals, schools, military barracks, and prisons.
- Norovirus is shed in stool and therefore transmission is via the faecal–oral route: ingestion of contaminated food/water or contact with an infected patient.
- Norovirus can also be spread by particles aerosolized by vomiting.

16.2.2 Pathological basis

- Norovirus infects small bowel epithelium, which serves as the host for viral replication.
- Damage occurs to microvilli in small intestine causing malabsorption.
- Norovirus also causes delayed gastric emptying resulting in vomiting.

16.2.3 Typical clinical features

- Self-limiting infection lasting 12–60 hours.
- Fever, nausea, vomiting (often projectile), watery diarrhoea, abdominal cramps.

16.2.4 Diagnosis and management

- Stool samples are essential in outbreaks to identify virus and control infection.
- Treatment is supportive.
- Prevention:
  - Isolation is essential
  - In hospital settings it is often necessary to close affected wards to limit the outbreak
  - Particular attention to handwashing, food hygiene, and cleaning of hard surfaces with bleach will also prevent spread

Yeasts and fungi

CONTENTS

17.1 *Candida*

- *Candida* occurs as part of the normal flora of the mouth, skin, vagina, and GI tract.
- Opportunistic infection, frequently presenting in association with immunocompromise and antibiotic use.
- The use of broad-spectrum antibiotics eliminates competing bacterial flora allowing the yeast to overgrow.
- Various manifestations depending on site.

17.1.1 Localized

- Genital:
  - White plaques on mucous membranes accompanied by a white discharge
  - Dyspareunia, dysuria, and burning vulvovaginitis occur
- Oral:
  - Raised white plaques on oral mucosa, tongue, and gums, which may become confluent and ulcerated and spread to throat.
  - May be associated with angular stomatitis
  - In immunocompromised patients, progresses to oesophageal candidiasis
- Intertrigo.
- Nappy candidiasis.
- Chronic paronychia.

17.1.2 Systemic candidiasis

- Occurs in immunosuppressed/debilitated (i.e. HIV, malignancy, chemotherapy, systemic corticosteroids, broad spectrum antibiotic use).
- High mortality rates.
- Candidaemia may be a complication of line infection. Usually responds to line removal and antifungal agents.
- *Candida* endocarditis.
- *Candida* endophthalmitis.
- Renal candidiasis.

- *Candida* meningitis.
- *Candida* peritonitis.
- *Candida* pneumonia.
- Hepatosplenic candidiasis.

17.1.3 Diagnosis

- Localized infections can often be diagnosed clinically.
- Swabs of lesions may be sent for microscopy and culture.
- Laboratory identification of candidal infection is limited and it is necessary to correlate results to clinical features.
- Blood cultures are only positive in 50–60% of cases of disseminated infection, therefore systemic candidiasis should be suspected and treated empirically in patients with persistent leucocytosis/neutropenia or other risk factors and who remain febrile despite broad-spectrum antibiotic therapy.
- A positive culture from a sterile site (blood, CSF) is always significant.
- A positive culture from GI or respiratory tract may represent colonization rather than active infection.
- In disseminated disease, positive cultures should be sent for susceptibility testing.

17.1.4 Management

- Depending on site and immune status of host:
  - Oral candidiasis: nystatin oral suspension, amphotericin lozenge, miconazole gel
  - Genital candidiasis: topical clotrimazole, oral fluconazole
  - Intertrigo: clotrimazole cream ± mild topical steroid
  - Oral/intravenous antifungals in systemic disease/immunocompromise: ketoconazole, fluconazole, itraconazole, amphotericin B, caspofungin

17.2 Cryptococcus

- Opportunistic mycosis.
- Severe/extrapulmonary infection with a high mortality is usually a result of prior immunocompromise (T-cell compromise being the underlying pathological factor):
  - Transplant recipients
  - AIDS patients
  - Lymphoma
  - Leukaemia
  - Sarcoidosis

17.2.1 Typical features

- Cryptococcosis caused by *Cryptococcus neoformans* found in soil containing bird (especially pigeon) droppings.
- Associated with pigeon fanciers.
- Pulmonary cryptococcosis ('pigeon fanciers' lung') disease spectrum ranges from mild subclinical lung infection to cavitations with pleural effusions and ARDS:
  - Symptoms include cough, dyspnoea, malaise, fever, and pleuritic pain
- In immunocompromised patients, infection often disseminates to CNS causing subacute/ chronic cryptococcal meningitis/meningoencephalitis:
  - Varying clinical presentation; most common symptoms are headache, altered mental status, personality changes, confusion, and coma
  - Classical features of meningism are less common

17.2.2 Basis of therapy

- Depends on disease presentation and immune condition of patient.
- Pulmonary cryptococcosis with normal immunity requires no treatment.
- Antifungals: amphotericin B, flucytosine, and fluconazole are agents used in disseminated infection/immunocompromise

17.3 Dermatophytes

- Dermatophytoses are cutaneous mycoses caused by different organisms including trichophyton, epidermophyton, and microsporum.
- Use keratin as source of nutrition and therefore affect skin, hair, and nails.
- Dermatophytoses are usually identified according to the affected tissue with the prefix 'tinea'.

17.3.1 Basis of transmission

- Most human infections are transmitted from infected skin scales. Requires close personal contact.

17.3.2 Typical features

- Dermatophytoses classically present with patches of itching, scaling skin that can become inflamed and weep.
- Most commonly encountered diseases:
  - Tinea corporis (ringworm) most often occurs on trunk/limbs:
    - Single/multiple plaques, scaling, erythema at edges
    - Lesions enlarge slowly and clear centrally creating a ring
  - Tinea pedis (athlete's foot) infects initially between the toes but can spread to nails:
    - Itchy maceration between toes
    - Risk factors include swimming, occlusive footwear, hot weather
    - Can develop secondary bacterial infection
  - Tinea capitis (scalp ringworm):
    - Defined, inflamed scaly areas, with broken hair shafts
    - Severity ranges from small patches to entire scalp with extensive alopecia

17.3.3 Basis of diagnosis

- Skin scrapings, hair or nail clippings sent for microscopy and culture.

17.3.4 Principles of management

- Topical application of antifungal agents is the first line:
  - Nail: if limited, distal disease initially, try a nail lacquer (e.g. amorolfine)
  - Skin: clotrimazole or imidazole cream/spray/powder, terbinafine cream
  - Tinea capitis: ketoconazole shampoo, terbinafine cream
- Systemic therapy is usually reserved for onychomycosis, tinea capitis, and when topical treatment has failed or disease is extensive: oral griseofulvin, itraconazole, terbinafine.

Worms

CONTENTS

18.1 Threadworm

- Also known as pinworm or 'enterobiasis', caused by *Enterobius vernicularis*.
- Common, especially in children.

18.1.1 Typical clinical features

- Humans are the only host.
- Transmission is via ingestion of eggs.
- Threadworm larvae hatch in the small intestine and inhabit the colon.
- Leave the bowel at night to lay eggs in perineum.
- Eggs are coated in an irritant mucus that causes pruritus and scratching.
- Eggs are thereby transferred to the hands and mouth, transmitting infection.
- The principal presenting feature is perianal itching and disturbed sleep may be an issue.
- Silvery, white worms may be visible in stool or perianal region.
- Diagnosis requires identification of worms or perianal eggs.

18.1.2 Principles of management

- Mebendazole can be bought over the counter and kills worms.
- Combination piperazine and senna is available for those under 2 years.
- Repeat treatment in 6 weeks is advised in case of re-infection.
- Treat whole household as asymptomatic infection is common and transmission and re-infection may occur, and advise re: personal hygiene.

18.2 Tapeworm (pork and beef)

18.2.1 Epidemiology

- Ribbon-like, segmented worms, primarily intestinal parasites.
- Various species including *Taenia saginata* (beef tapeworm) and *Taenia solim* (pork tapeworm).
- Transmitted to humans in undercooked beef/pork.
- Highest incidence in developing countries.

18.2.2 Basis of infection

- Lifecycle of tapeworm:
  - Eggs are excreted to the environment by the primary host
  - The eggs are ingested by an intermediate host in which they hatch
  - The larvae enter the tissues of the intermediate host and form cysts
  - The primary host ingests the cysts in the flesh of the intermediate host
  - The cysts release tapeworm larvae, which attach onto the intestine with suckers
  - Tapeworms are composed of many segments (proglottids), which generate fertilized eggs
  - Proglottids at the end of the chain with mature eggs break off and pass out of the body in stool
- When humans are the primary hosts, the adult tapeworm is limited to the intestinal tract.
- When humans are the intermediate hosts, the larvae infect the tissues, migrating through the different organ systems.
- *Taenia saginata* (beef tapeworm):
  - Can grow up to 25m
  - Humans only serve as primary hosts, ingesting the cysts in undercooked beef, therefore infection is limited to intestines
- *Taenia solium* (pork tapeworm):
  - Can grow up to 7m
  - Humans are both primary and intermediate hosts
  - Ingestion of larvae from undercooked pork causes intestinal infestation
  - Ingestion of eggs results in the development of larvae, which form cysts in the brain and other tissues
- Tapeworms sequester host's nutrients, excrete toxic waste, and can cause mechanical blockage of the intestine.

18.2.3 Typical clinical features

- Often asymptomatic: tapeworms or proglottids may be discovered by patients during defecation or on toilet paper or underwear.
- 'Taeniasis': intestinal infection caused by both *T. solium* and *T. saginata*. Presents as anal itching, nausea, abdominal pain, anorexia, weight loss, or malaise.
- 'Cysticerosis': extraintestinal infection due to cysts in *T. solium*:
  - Cysts mainly occur in the CNS and skeletal muscles, causing local inflammatory responses and mass effects
  - If neurocysticercosis develops, seizures often present

18.2.4 Basis of diagnosis

- 2–3 independent stool samples are required for examination for ova and parasites, as proglottids are released irregularly into the stool and may be missed on a single sample.
- CT head should be performed for the diagnosis and monitoring of neurocysticercosis.

18.2.5 Principles of management

- Niclosamide or praziquantel, depending on clinical manifestation.
- Disease may be widespread and complicated therefore specialist input is required.

18.3 Roundworm

- Roundworm—*Ascaris lumbricoides*—causes 'ascariasis'.
- Over 1 billion humans are infected worldwide.
- Humans sole host.
- Transmission: ingestion of food contaminated by soil containing eggs.
- Eggs may occur in municipal domestic sewage or on unwashed fruit and vegetables, especially if grown in or near soil fertilized with sewage.
- It is prevalent in deprived areas where there is a combination of poor sanitation and malnutrition.
- Larvae initially enter the intestine, then penetrate the tissues and migrate throughout the body via blood and the lymphatics, commonly to the lungs. The larvae enter alveoli and ascend to the throat, then re-enter the GI tract where they may grow up to 30cm.
- Disease presentation and symptom severity is dependent on the developmental stage of the *Ascaris*, the site of the parasite, and the number of mature worms present:
  - Pneumonitis from larval migration into the lungs
  - Conjunctivitis, seizures, and rash from larval migration elsewhere
  - Intestinal worms cause abdominal pain, colic, nausea, vomiting, anorexia, anal itching, diarrhoea, weight loss, and malabsorption
  - Mature worms may cause GI obstruction, perforation, appendicitis, liver abscess, and respiratory tract obstruction
- Diagnosis: typically eggs in stool, although worms may also be seen.
- Treatment: imidazole therapy.

18.4 Hookworm

- Caused by *Ancylostoma duodenale* and *Necator americanus*.
- Lives in intestine of host (e.g. dog, cat, human). Eggs excreted by host onto soil and thrive in warm earth with heavy rainfall. Larvae hatch and penetrate skin.
- Attaches to intestinal mucosa causing prolonged infection; may live for up to 15 years.
- Presentation: most people are asymptomatic; may cause abdominal pain, diarrhoea, anorexia, chronic GI blood loss, and anaemia.
- Diagnosis: eggs in stool (although not present during first 5–7 weeks).
- Treatment: imidazole therapy.

Malaria

CONTENTS

19.1 Epidemiology

- Protozoal disease.
- *Plasmodium* spp.:
  - *P. falciparum* (15%)
  - *P. vivax* (80%)
  - *P. ovale*
  - *P. malariae*
- High-risk areas: Central/South America, SE Asia, sub-Saharan Africa.
- Transmission:
  - Vector is female *Anopheles* mosquito
  - Mosquito bite injects plasmodium sporozoites into the bloodstream, which migrate to liver and form merozoites
  - Merozoites are released and invade red blood cells
  - Using haemoglobin as a nutrient they multiply within the erythrocyte
  - Infected red cells rupture, releasing *Plasmodium* merozoites to invade other erythrocytes
  - Rupture of thousands of erythrocytes simultaneously causes massive release of toxic substances and sudden onset of high fever

19.1.1 Falciparum malaria

- Caused by *Plasmodium falciparum*.
- Incubation 7–14 days, occasionally longer.
- Most dangerous plasmodial species because it invades all ages of erythrocytes and can adhere to endothelial walls causing vascular obstruction.
- Rapidly fulminating with high fever and hypotension.
- Can be fatal in less than 24 hours if treatment is not prompt.
- Complications:
  - 'Black water fever': massive intravascular red cell haemolysis results in high fevers and haemoglobinuria. Associated with renal failure
  - Cerebral malaria, coma
  - Severe anaemia

- Pulmonary oedema
- Splenic rupture
- DIC

19.1.2 Benign malaria

- Caused by *Plasmodium vivax, ovale*, and *malariae*.
- Low mortality as it invades only young or old erythrocytes.
- Incubation 12–40 days, occasionally up to 18 months.
- Relapse may occur weeks to years after initial infection as parasites lay dormant in liver or blood.

19.2 Usual clinical features

- Consider in any traveller with fever within 6 months of return from high-risk area.
- Varying symptoms.
- Headache, malaise, myalgia, arthralgia, anorexia, cyclical high fevers, rigors, sweats (classically every 48–72 hours).
- May be anaemia, jaundice, hepatosplenomegaly.

19.3 Basis of diagnosis

- Serial blood films are required—3 thick and thin smears should be obtained 12–24 hours apart to allow detection of malaria parasite within red blood cells.
- The highest yield of peripheral parasites occurs during or soon after a fever spike; however, smears should not be delayed while awaiting fever spikes:
  - Thick smears are more sensitive but less specific than thin smears. This is a quantitative test as the parasitaemia is calculated based on the number of infected RBCs
  - Thin smears allow identification of *Plasmodium* spp. responsible for the infection, which is essential to plan treatment
- *P. falciparum* infection may not be detected on thick and thin films as the parasite can be sequestered out of the peripheral blood in late-stage forms. If no alternative diagnosis is found in an at-risk patient with possible cerebral malaria, initiate therapy for presumptive malaria and continue to obtain additional blood smears to confirm the diagnosis.

19.4 Therapy

- Refer to infectious diseases for specialist advice as *P. falciparum* malaria can be rapidly fatal if inadequately treated.
- Treatment depends on stage of infection—drugs include primaquine, chloroquine, quinine, mefloquine, and pyrimethamine.

PHYSIOLOGY

Basic cellular physiology

CONTENTS

1.1 Homeostasis

- This is 'the property of a system that regulates its internal environment and tends to maintain a stable, constant condition' as described by Claude Bernard in 1865.
- This concept is essential for survival due to the fact that our external environment is constantly changing and yet we need to maintain our internal environment between fine parameters so that cellular structure and function isn't damaged.
- All homeostatic control mechanisms require at least 3 components for the variable being regulated:
  - A sensory system that monitors and responds to changes in the environment:
    - A **receptor** is therefore required that receives the signal from the environment and relays this information to a **comparator**
  - The **comparator** has a 'set point' for what is normal and determines an appropriate response to the stimulus:
    - A signal is then sent to a '**control centre**'
    - In most homeostatic mechanisms the comparator and control centre is the brain
  - A signal is then sent via an effector mechanism, which in humans can be a muscle contraction, hormone release, or a variety of other mechanisms:
    - A change then occurs to correct the deviation by either *increasing it* with **positive feedback** or *reducing it* with **negative feedback**
- The 'set point' mentioned is regarded as the normal range that the body or control centre will allow deviation from (e.g. an internal temperature of 36.8°C ± 0.7°C before a change needs to occur)
- The change that occurs following signal of a change in conditions is usually via either **negative** or **positive feedback** mechanisms. These processes help to accurately maintain the 'set point'. However, they do have disadvantages:

- Negative feedback control works well for slower processes within the body (e.g. maintenance of body posture). However, when fast, complex feedback is required, the negative feedback is too slow, which causes a time lag between the real-time stimulus and reaction required:
  - For this reason there are **feed forward** controls that involve processing in the brain based on information from events that have occurred previously (i.e. *learnt behaviours* such as catching a fast ball)
- Positive feedback controls are designed to accelerate or enhance the action created by a stimulus received. This acts to increase the 'set point' to the higher end of the normal range and if not controlled can go past the point of normal (e.g. a fever) as a response to infection, can cause shivering, which further increases body temperature:
  - For this reason, positive feedback mechanisms are less common in the body due to risks of uncontrolled acceleration
- The main reason why homeostasis is so important in living organisms is the *denaturation* of **proteins**. The main factors that affect this in the body are **temperature** and **pH**
- If the normal ranges of these variables are affected then the structure of proteins begins to be affected
- Proteins can be 'unfolded' making them inactive if the pH and temperature are outside of the normal ranges
- As proteins are essential for cell structure, metabolic processes, energy production, enzymatic activity, cell signalling, and transport, they are essential for life and consequently homeostatic mechanisms evolve around protein structure maintenance

1.2 Compartments and fluid spaces in health

1.2.1 Osmosis

- Describes the diffusion of water across a semipermeable membrane down a concentration gradient (i.e. from low solute concentration to high solute concentration) until there is equilibrium on either side of the membrane.
- The *osmotic pressure* is the force required to prevent the movement of water down the concentration gradient (i.e. the force generated by the movement of water by osmosis).
- Osmosis is only influenced by solutes that are unable to cross the semipermeable membrane.
- This is the main driving force of fluid shifts in humans, as approximately 60% of the body is water; it plays an essential role in the homeostasis of cells and the transport of substances.

1.2.2 Tonicity

- Tonicity is a measure of the osmotic pressure of 2 solutions separated by a semipermeable membrane.
- There are therefore 3 types of tonicity that a solution can have in relation to another:
  - **Isotonic**: an equal distribution of solute either side of the membrane (iso = same)
  - **Hypertonic**: a higher concentration of *impermeable* solute than the solution on the other side of the membrane
  - **Hypotonic**: a lower concentration of *impermeable* solute than the solution on the other side of the membrane

- For human cells (eukaryotic cells) the shift of fluid into or out of the cell depends on the solution surrounding it:
  - If immersed into **isotonic fluid**—there will be *no net gain or loss* from the cell as the solute content in the surrounding fluid is the *same*
  - If immersed into **hypertonic fluid**—there will be a *net loss* of fluid **from** the cell due to osmosis (movement of water from a low to high solute concentration):
    - The cell becomes small and wrinkled, known as *crenation*
  - If immersed into **hypotonic fluid**—there will be a *net gain* of fluid **into** the cell due to osmosis and the cell becomes swollen and can eventually rupture, known as *cytolysis*

1.2.3 Fluid compartments

- As already mentioned, the human body (average weight 70kg) is composed of approximately 60% water (42L).
- Fluid in the body can be divided into 2 groups:
  - **Intracellular** (ICF) (60% total body water—28L)
  - **Extracellular** (ECF) (40% total body water—14L). This compartment can be divided into:
    - Interstitial fluid (60% extracellular volume—10.5L)
    - Intravascular fluid (plasma) (40% extracellular volume—3.5L)
  - As seen earlier in this list, the fluid compartments can *generally* be thought of in principles of two-thirds
  - The ICF and ECF differ in their concentrations of cations as seen in Table D.1.1
- As demonstrated in Table D.1.1, there is a large difference in concentration of electrolytes within the compartments of the body. This difference in concentrations is due mainly to the Na^+/K^+ ATPase channel, which ensures a difference in these cations across the cell membranes via active transport.
- The other electrolytes are therefore transported mostly as a consequence of the electrochemical gradient created by this transporter.
- The movement of small anions such as Cl^- is slightly different to that of small cations such as K^+ or Na^+. This is due to the differences that occur when these charged ions are close to a semipermeable membrane, known as the **Gibbs–Donnan equilibrium**:
  - For example, in plasma fluid some small cations are attracted to large plasma proteins as these tend to have a negative charge
  - This means that small anions will cross membranes more readily than small cations, as the cations are 'pulled back' into the plasma by the negative proteins

Table D.1.1 Cation and anion concentrations in body fluids

	ECF concentration (mEq/kg H_2O)	ICF concentration (mEq/kg H_2O)
Cation:		
Na^+	145	10
K^+	4	159
Ca^{2+}	3	1
Mg^{2+}	2	40
Anion:		
Cl^-	117	3
HCO^-	28	7

1.3 Key aspects of cell structure and function

1.3.1 Organelle function

See Figure D.1.1.

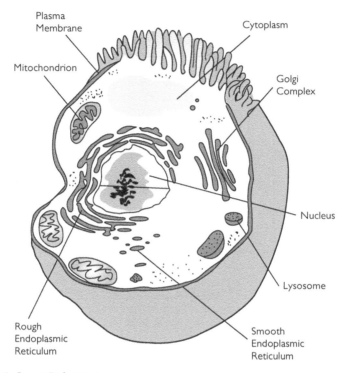

Figure D.1.1 Organelle function

Mitochondria

- Energy producers for cells.
- Location of aerobic respiration pathway → 36 ATP molecules produced from 1 molecule of glucose.
- Cylindrical structures 0.5–1.0μm in diameter:
  - Outer membrane smooth and unfolded
  - Inner membrane has numerous infoldings known as *cristae*
- Membranes divide structure into 2 areas:
  - The narrow intermembrane space
  - Large matrix
- Matrix contains many enzymes responsible for reactions such as the **Krebs cycle**, **citric acid cycle**, and **tricarboxylic acid cycle**.
- Hepatocytes are rich in mitochondria for energy production and other metabolic processes.

Nucleus

- Production centre of **DNA** and **RNA**, and control of cellular functions.

- Regulates gene expression.
- Composed of:
  - Nuclear envelope:
    - Contains *nuclear pores* for selective movement of proteins and RNA
    - Outer membrane continuous with endoplasmic reticulum (ER) and attached to ribosomes for protein synthesis
    - Inner membrane provides a structure for chromosomes
  - Chromatin:
    - Made up of DNA + histones + other nuclear proteins
  - Nucleolus:
    - Site of rRNA transcription
    - Regulates cell cycle

Endoplasmic reticulum (ER)

- 2 distinct types: rough ER and smooth ER.
- Rough ER:
  - Ribosomes bound to outer surface (therefore rough)
  - Amino acids are combined to form polypeptides at the ribosomes and undergo further folding in protein synthesis inside the ER
- Smooth ER:
  - Synthesis of triglycerides, phospholipids, and steroids
  - These form complexes with proteins in the ER lumen to form **lipoproteins**
  - Therefore has important role of cellular membrane formation
- Once proteins and/or lipids are formed, they leave the ER and become a *transition vesicle* that moves to the Golgi apparatus.

Golgi apparatus

- Modification of structures produced by the ER:
  - Structures (proteins and/or lipids) are modified and packaged into *vesicles*
- The Golgi is made up of *stacks*:
  - The *cis* or ER-facing part of the stacks receives the transition vesicle from the ER and then modifies the structures produced
  - The *trans* or cell membrane-facing part of the stacks releases vesicles towards the cell membrane for release

Lysosomes

- Have the ability to break down any macromolecule in the body
- Contain around 50 different digestive enzymes
- *Primary lysosomes*: contain digestive enzymes made from the Golgi apparatus
- *Secondary lysosomes*: contain both enzymes and substrates, the largest being digestive vacuoles that break down foreign substances (e.g. bacteria). This process is known as **phagocytosis**, i.e. the ingestion of foreign substances.
- When the lysosome breaks down its own cellular organelle, this is known as **autophagy** and can be a normal process of cellular 'housekeeping'.

1.3.2 Cell membrane structure

- Consists of lipids and protein—forms a *lipid bilayer*.
- Contents of cell membrane are cell specific, for example:
  - Nerve cell membranes contain a majority of lipid to preserve nerve conduction signals
  - Kidney cells may contain protein-rich cell membranes for cellular transport

- Lipids:
  - Are phospholipids, cholesterol, or glycolipids
  - Contain a hydrophilic and a hydrophobic end
  - Therefore form bilayer structures (hydrophobic ends face in towards each other and hydrophilic heads face outwards)
- Carbohydrates are present on cell surface membrane:
  - For cellular recognition
  - Also receptors for specific extracellular messages
- Proteins:
  - Act as transport channels (see Chapter D1, Section 1.3.3: Cell membrane transport) and hormone receptors
  - Largest number of membrane receptors are linked to **G-proteins**
  - G-proteins help to transfer the signal from outside the cell to stimulate processes within the cell via the receptor protein
- G-proteins:
  - When inactivated are composed of 3 subunits (α, β, and γ) linked to the cell receptor
  - When the receptor is activated, GDP is replaced by GTP causing the subunits to divide to make the α subunit separate from β and γ
  - The α subunit moves through the cell membrane and stimulates or inhibits another cell membrane protein, which could be an enzyme for intracellular signals or a cell ion channel
  - Different cell receptors are associated with different G-proteins and therefore have different mechanisms of action within the cell

1.3.3 Cell membrane transport

- 3 types of cellular transport:
  - Passive transport
  - Facilitated diffusion
  - Active transport:
    - The most common example of active transport within a cell membrane is the **Na$^+$/K$^+$ ATPase pump**
- Na$^+$/K$^+$ ATPase pump:
  - Found in the basolateral membrane of nearly all cells of the body
  - Uses energy derived from adenosine triphosphate (ATP)
  - For 1 molecule of ATP:
    - 3 Na$^+$ molecules pumped *out of* the cell
    - 2 K$^+$ molecules pumped *into* the cell
  - Energy from ATP is used to transport Na$^+$ and K$^+$ against a concentration gradient:
    - Maintains electrochemical gradient across cell membrane
  - Energy from this channel can help to facilitate movement of other substances (facilitated diffusion)
- Other protein channels help to facilitate substance transport:
  - Channel interacts with molecules (e.g. K$^+$ and Na$^+$) and assists in movement of molecule
  - Channels open and close once stimulated, therefore act like a gate
  - Stimulation can be electrical (voltage-gated) or molecular (ligand-gated)
  - Transport is much greater than simple diffusion
  - Channels are specific to the molecules transported and can be 'saturated' once the transport molecule reaches a certain concentration
  - Channels can be competitively and non-competitively inhibited

1.4 Vessel fluid dynamics

1.4.1 Permeability

- Cell membranes are composed mainly of lipid and protein. They contain channels for the movement of specific molecules, ions, or substances. This is so that the cell can regulate its own contents.
- For this reason the cell membrane must be *selectively permeable*, i.e. it allows the diffusion of certain molecules (e.g. non-polar molecules) and not others (e.g. ions and polar molecules).
- The permeability of a cell membrane will depend on certain characteristics:
  - Cell membrane thickness
  - Lipid solubility of substance
- These 2 factors govern the *permeability coefficient* of the cell membrane.
- Given a constant permeability coefficient for a non-polar substance, the major factor defining the diffusion rate of the substance will be the *concentration gradient* across the cell membrane.
- However, if the molecule has a charge (e.g. an ion such as Na^+ or K^+) then the movement of the substance across the cell membrane is governed by the *electrochemical gradient*.
- Due to the action of the **Na^+/K^+ ATPase pump,** as mentioned earlier, a typical cell has a resting membrane potential of -70 millivolts (mV):
  - This enables the entry of positively charged ions, which are at a lower concentration within the cell, for example, Na^+
  - For this reason Na^+ entry into the cells can be a passive process, as this ion can move down both a concentration and an electrical gradient

1.4.2 Tube flow

- The movement of a fluid through a vessel (flow, F) is determined by the following in Poiseuille's law:
  - The radius of the vessel (r)
  - The viscosity of the fluid (η)
  - The length of the vessel (L)
  - The pressure difference across the vessel ($P_1 - P_2$)
- Flow $= \dfrac{(P_1 - P_2) \times \pi r^4}{8\eta L}$:
  - So as the length or viscosity increases, the flow decreases
  - As radius increases the flow increases to the power of 4, meaning that a change in the vessel radius has a more significant impact on flow than the other factors
  - Therefore if the length of the vessel, viscosity of the fluid, and pressure across the vessel were constant, the major determinant of flow would be the diameter of the vessel:
    - For example, if the radius of an arteriole is halved then the resistance increases by 16 times
- In humans, where the viscosity of blood and length of blood vessels aren't changed dramatically in normal situations, blood flow is therefore determined by 2 major factors:
  - Blood pressure
  - Blood vessel diameter
- Normally blood flows smoothly through vessels in the body. This smooth flow of fluid or blood is known as **laminar flow**:
  - Flow of fluid is in layers within a vessel
  - Flow is unidirectional for all fluid layers

- Fluid at the surface of the vessel walls travels slowest
- Fluid at the centre of the vessel travels fastest
- Flow is therefore proportional to pressure
- Most flow in blood vessels occurs this way
- However, there are situations in the body when **turbulent flow** occurs, and the fluid flow is therefore disrupted and disorganized:
  - Velocity of flow is too great and fluid no longer flows in layers
  - Flow is chaotic and multidirectional
  - Flow of fluid travels at different speeds within the vessel
  - Flow is inversely proportional to pressure
  - Can occur where vessel diameter is large and flow is fast (e.g. aorta)
  - Also occurs at stenoses of vessels or across valves
  - Turbulent flow creates audible sounds and therefore creates 'murmurs'

1.4.3 Wall tension

- Blood flow through a vessel creates a tension on the vessel wall—this is in accordance with the law of *Laplace* where $T = \pi r \times p \times \mu$:
  - T = tension of the vessel wall
  - p = pressure across the vessel wall
  - r = vessel radius
  - μ = thickness of the vessel wall
- Therefore, for a constant blood pressure, increasing the radius of the vessel leads to an increase in wall tension.
- In order to cope with this tension, arteries tend to have thicker vessel walls and can withstand the higher blood pressures compared to veins, therefore enabling the high blood velocities through this system.
- Capillaries have a small vessel radius and low wall tension and therefore are able to have thin vessel walls.
- Clinically, damage to the vascular system (e.g. atherosclerosis) can lead to malformations in the vessel walls such as aneurysms:
  - As the vessel becomes weakened by the atherosclerotic lesions it becomes more distensible
  - As the radius of the vessel increases and the thickness of the wall decreases the tension on the vessel wall increases and can eventually lead to a rupture
  - In the arterial system, blood loss through a rupture can be catastrophic due to the high pressures; therefore a ruptured aortic aneurysm can be fatal

1.5 Blood and blood flow

- The normal total volume of blood is around 5.5L (normal range 60–80mL/kg) and is mainly composed of:
  - Red blood cells (RBCs):
    - Measured by **haemoglobin (Hb) level**: 13.5–17.7g/dL for males and 11.5–16.5g/dL for females
  - White blood cells (WBCs):
    - Normal range = $4–11 \times 10^9/L$
  - Platelets:
    - Normal range = $150–400 \times 10^9/L$
- When centrifuged, the blood forms into 2 main parts—RBCs and plasma. The ratio of these 2 parts gives the **haematocrit** ratio, i.e. ratio of RBCs to plasma:
  - Normal haematocrit:

- For males = 47% (±5%)
- For females = 42% (±5%)

1.5.1 Red blood cells (RBCs)

- Approximately one-third of a RBC or 'erythrocyte' is made of Hb. This gives these cells the capacity to transport oxygen and carbon dioxide, as these gases combine with Hb readily.
- Approximately 98% of oxygen is transported with Hb:
  - Each gram of Hb can combine with 1.34mL of O_2
  - Therefore a normal adult with an Hb of 15g/dL can carry approximately 20mL of O_2 per dL
- Production of RBCs is in the red marrow of large bones such as the humerus, femur, ribs, sternum, etc.
- Substances that are required to make RBCs include:
  - Amino acids
  - Iron
  - Copper
  - Vitamin B2 and B12
  - Pyridoxine
  - Folic acid
- The kidneys produce **erythropoietin** when levels of oxygen in the blood are low:
  - This hormone travels in the blood to the bone marrow where it stimulates erythropoiesis—RBC production
  - This increases the oxygen-carrying capacity of the blood meaning it can supply more oxygen to tissues
- The average RBC circulates for approximately 120 days before being removed from the blood by macrophages in the spleen, liver, and bone marrow:
  - Once consumed by macrophages the RBCs are broken down into their components. The haem component is separated into iron and biliverdin. Biliverdin is then reduced to **bilirubin**
  - Bilirubin travels in the plasma, attached to albumin, to the liver where bile salts are produced and excreted into the small intestine

1.5.2 White blood cells (WBCs)

- WBCs or leucocytes can be differentiated into different types—granular and agranular leucocytes:
  - Granulocytes include neutrophils/eosinophils/basophils
  - Agranulocytes include monocytes and lymphocytes
- Each type of WBC has a specific role but collectively they are an important part of the immune system of the body, providing defence against foreign substances.
- WBCs attack other substances with a variety of different mechanisms, such as:
  - Phagocytosis
  - Antibody release
  - Neutralization of toxins
  - Chemical messenger release
  - Enzyme production
- WBC production or **leucopoiesis** occurs in the bone marrow:
  - Here the different types of cells are created, each undergoing different forms of maturation
  - However, potential T lymphocytes mature in the thymus and spleen and potential B lymphocytes mature in the lymphoid tissue of the intestines, spleen, and bone marrow
- When an infection happens then **leucocytosis** occurs, leading to an increase in circulating WBCs to combat the foreign substance that has entered the body.

1.5.3 Plasma

- Plasma is the substance in which blood cells and platelets are contained. (Serum is the same but without clotting factors.)
- The majority of plasma is water (93%), and the rest is composed of protein, organic (e.g. glucose) and non-organic solutes (e.g. Na^+), dissolved gases, waste products (e.g. urea), and amino acids.
- The main proteins found in plasma are **albumin**, **globulins**, and **fibrinogen**. The majority is albumin (60% of plasma protein).
- Albumin:
  - Transports substances within the circulation, for example:
    - Bilirubin
    - Hormones
    - Fatty acids
    - Drugs (e.g. warfarin, digoxin, NSAIDs, midazolam, thiopental)
    - Ions (e.g. calcium)
- Also responsible for acid–base balance due to albumin's negative polarity.
- Provides an oncotic pressure proportional to the size of the molecule:
  - Oncotic pressure (also known as colloid osmotic pressure) is the force created by large molecular weight substances that oppose a force on fluid movement across a capillary wall
  - The oncotic pressure pulls fluid into the vessel due to the difference in osmotic pressure; hydrostatic pressure acts in reverse to force fluid out
  - Therefore albumin plays an important role in fluid balance

1.5.4 Platelets

- A platelet is actually a fragment of a megakaryocyte. They are not produced by mitotic division and are therefore not cells.
- Platelets are small 'packages' containing:
  - Granules
  - Microfilaments
  - Vesicles
  - Microtubules
  - Mitochondria
- The platelet's main role is in haemostasis:
  - When blood vessel damage occurs, platelets stick to the area affected and clump together
  - Here the platelets initiate a cascade of events that leads to vasoconstriction of the blood vessel and formation of a blood clot or 'thrombus'
  - This ultimately leads to reduced haemorrhage and repair of the vessel
- The process of events that occurs with blood vessel injury can be briefly summarized as follows:
  - Damage to the endothelium of the blood vessel leads to release of ADP
  - Platelets are attracted to this site of injury due to this release of ADP, and clump together
  - Platelets then react with the exposed collagen from the blood vessel wall and become activated
  - Activated platelets:
    - Become more 'sticky'
    - Attract more platelets
    - Release chemicals such as ADP, serotonin, and thromboxane A2
    - These chemicals increase the activation of platelets
    - Thromboxane A2 causes vasoconstriction

- Anchor into the collagen to form attachments for the blood clot
- Stimulate a coagulation cascade
- The coagulation cascade occurs in 2 different pathways:
  - Intrinsic
  - Extrinsic
- This involves the formation and stimulation of clotting factors, which lead to the activation of **prothrombin clotting factor**.
- Prothrombin clotting factor initiates the conversion of prothrombin to **thrombin**.
- The enzyme thrombin then converts fibrinogen to **fibrin**:
  - Fibrin is an insoluble protein that forms a network of filaments, which traps blood contents to form a blood clot
- Once a blood clot has stabilized and blood vessel repair has taken place, the clot needs to be resolved:
  - This occurs by the activation of **plasmin**. This breaks down the fibrin links caused by the coagulation cascade (*fibrinolysis*)
  - The activation of plasmin can be stimulated by:
    - Cytofibrokinase (tissue enzyme)
    - Staphylokinase and streptokinase (bacterial enzyme)
    - Plasma kinase (clotting factor enzyme)
    - Tissue plasminogen activator (TPA—produced from endothelial cells)

1.6 Basis of the neurological action potential

- In order for messages to be transmitted throughout the body a signal needs to be generated from one cell to another.
- Most 'excitable cells' in the body rely on this signal to function and include:
  - Nerve cells (neurons)
  - Muscle cells:
    - Skeletal
    - Smooth muscle
  - Cardiac cells
- These cells share 2 main properties:
  - Excitability from a signal
  - Conductivity of the signal

1.6.1 Excitability

- All cells of the human body have an electrical chemical difference across the cell membrane, mostly due to the Na^+/K^+ ATPase, and also due to facilitated diffusion of K^+ out of the cells.
- This difference across the cell membrane is known as the resting membrane potential.
- In neurons this resting membrane potential is approximately −70mV:
  - That is, the inside of the cell is more negative than the outside of the membrane, due to the difference in concentration of K^+, Na^+, and Cl^- in the cell
- In general terms, cells contain high concentrations of K^+ and low concentrations of Na^+, which creates the potential difference across the cell membrane.

1.6.2 Action potentials

- An action potential is the term given to the propagation of a signal along a cell, where a rapid change in membrane potential occurs causing the stimulation of the cellular components and leading to either conduction of the signal or the stimulation of the cellular function (e.g. muscle contraction).

- The stimulation that causes an action potential in excitable cells varies depending on the cellular function. However, the stimulus can be differentiated into 2 main types:
  - Mechanical stimulation (e.g. stretch, of Na^+ channels)
  - Chemical or neurotransmitter stimulation (e.g. acetylcholine (Ach), Na^+ channels)
- Every type of signal has the same consequence in that Na^+ channels are activated:
  - The activation of Na^+ channels causes an influx of Na^+ into the cells
  - If this influx of Na^+ manages to create enough positive charge in the cell so that the membrane **threshold** is breached then **depolarization** of the cell occurs
- In humans, the membrane threshold is −50mV, so when enough Na^+ enters the cell to move the membrane potential from −70mV to −50mV and above, the cell very rapidly allows more entry of Na^+ into the cell and the cell voltage jumps to +30mV:
  - This is known as **depolarization** and creates the **action potential** (see Figure D.1.2)
  - This signal and depolarization that occurs is *all or none*, i.e. either the cell depolarizes or it doesn't:
    - A strong signal will produce the same effect as a weak signal as long as the threshold is breached
    - The strength of the signal comes from the frequency of depolarization
- In order for the cell to return to its resting membrane potential (i.e. −70mV) there is an outflow of K^+. This is known as **repolarization**.
- During this period the cell is not capable of depolarizing again and the period is known as the **refractory period**.
- There are 2 types of refractory periods, *absolute* and *relative*:
  - Absolute refractory period:
    - Na^+ channels are completely inactive and no matter what the strength of the stimulus is, the cell is unable to depolarize
  - Relative refractory period:
    - Some of the Na^+ channels are now reset and can be reactivated, but the signal strength must be much greater than before in order to create an action potential

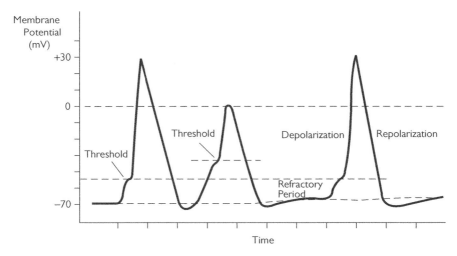

Figure D.1.2 Action potentials

1.7 Conduction of the generated action potential

- The movement of the signal down a neuron or axon relies on the efficient conduction of the action potential. This is made possible by:
  - The speed at which the action potential travels down an axon is directly proportional to the diameter of the axon. This is due to the reduced resistance to the flow of ions along this axon
  - The **myelin sheath** that surrounds the axon:
    - This myelin sheath provides 'insulation' for that part of the axon
    - Where the sheath ends, the axon is exposed to extracellular fluid; these areas are known as nodes of Ranvier
    - Therefore depolarization of lipid-covered areas does not occur, as movement of Na^+ cannot happen due to the presence of myelin
    - However, depolarization does occur at the exposed axon areas (i.e. the nodes of Ranvier)
    - The depolarization at each node is enough to transmit the signal to the next node and thus the signal is transmitted in a unidirectional flow down the axon
    - This is known as *saltatory conduction* and ensures that the signal is conducted and not lost to the surroundings of the axon, maintaining the energy of the signal
    - The speed at which the signal travels is directly proportional to the distance between the nodes of Ranvier
- Therefore propagation of a signal down an axon is directly proportional to:
  - The diameter of the axon
  - The distance between the nodes of Ranvier

1.8 Outline of the function of the sympathetic and parasympathetic nervous systems

- As the name implies, the autonomic nervous system (ANS) controls functions of the body essential for life without conscious thought.
- The ANS is divided into 2 separate parts that have opposite functions to one another. These are:
  - The **sympathetic nervous system**
  - The **parasympathetic nervous system**
- Homeostasis within the body relies on the fine balance between the actions of these 2 systems:
  - This occurs by the transmission of sensory information from different body systems or organs to the ANS, which then relays the information via either excitatory or inhibitory pathways via either the parasympathetic or sympathetic system
  - In this way the ANS is able to sense changes that are occurring both internally and externally and adapt the body systems in an attempt to maintain constant homeostasis within the body
  - As mentioned previously, the changes that occur are via the nervous system, which produces a neurochemical signal to create changes at the desired target organ or body system. This signal occurs at the *postganglionic synapse*
  - At the end of the postganglionic nerves are *terminal boutons*, which make synaptic connections to the *effector* (or target) cells. The boutons contain numerous vesicles, each containing chemicals required for the transmission of the signal to the target cell (e.g. Ach)

- When an action potential arrives at a bouton the *presynaptic membrane* is depolarized and voltage-sensitive Ca^{2+} channels are activated. There is a sudden **influx** of Ca^{2+} into the terminal bouton:
  - This Ca^{2+} influx causes the vesicles, containing neurotransmitter substances, to bind to the presynaptic membrane and release the chemical into the synaptic cleft
  - These chemicals then move across the synaptic cleft to bind to specific receptors on the *postsynaptic* membrane, which causes a specific effect on this area of the cell (e.g. ion channel opening)

1.8.1 Excitatory vs inhibitory

- The effect that a neurotransmitter has on the target cell depends on whether the synapse is excitatory or inhibitory.
- At an excitatory synapse the action of the neurotransmitter tends to cause an increase in the opening of Na^+ channels, thus increasing the likelihood that the postsynaptic membrane will depolarize. The magnitude of the effect is dependent on the amount of neurotransmitter released:
  - This may then lead to an action potential being generated in the cell. This is known as an **excitatory postsynaptic potential** (EPSP)
- At an inhibitory synapse, a neurotransmitter is released that decreases the chance of an action potential occurring. The neurotransmitter that is released causes ion channels to be either opened or closed at the postsynaptic membrane:
  - This leads to the membrane potential becoming more negative, and therefore more difficult to depolarize. In this state, it is said that the postsynaptic membrane is in 'transient hyperpolarization'. This is known as **inhibitory postsynaptic potential** (IPSP)
- At some synapses there is a balance between EPSPs and IPSPs. Therefore the overall action produced depends upon where the majority of the signal comes from:
  - This principle is known as **summation** as the effects of EPSPs and IPSPs cancel each other out

1.8.2 Termination of signal

- Once the neurotransmitter has crossed the synaptic cleft and bound to the postsynaptic membrane to cause an effect, it is then removed from the cleft so that the process can occur again:
  - This reuptake of neurotransmitter occurs at the presynaptic membrane
  - The mechanism of reuptake is specific to the neurotransmitter involved
- Examples of this reuptake process include Ach and norepinephrine (NE):
  - Ach is composed of acetate and choline:
    - When this neurotransmitter is released into a synaptic cleft it binds to receptors in the postsynaptic membrane and is broken down by *acetylcholinesterase* into its 2 original forms
    - The enzyme acetylcholinesterase is found on the postsynaptic membrane and therefore ensures that the signal is terminated, as acetate and choline are inactive molecules. Acetate and choline are reabsorbed by the presynaptic membrane and are used to synthesize more Ach
  - NE reuptake occurs by a slightly different mechanism:
    - Once NE has been released into the synaptic cleft it is rapidly pumped back into the terminal bouton
    - *Monoamine oxidase* (MAO) then acts to break down NE into inactive parts, which are then released back into the bouton or into circulation. MAO is also responsible for breakdown of serotonin, dopamine, epinephrine, and phenylethylamine

- *Catechol-O-methyltransferase* (COMT) is present in the postsynaptic membrane and inactivates the active NE. COMT is also responsible for dopamine and epinephrine breakdown
- These reuptake mechanisms ensure that the signal is recycled back to the presynapse for further release and that there is only a short-lived propagation of a signal across the synaptic cleft.

1.8.3 Sympathetic and parasympathetic effects on the body

- At the extremes of stimulation they have opposite effects, i.e. the sympathetic response is known as the 'fight or flight' and the parasympathetic system is known as the 'rest and digest' response.
- However, in normal situations within the body there is a balance between both systems to maintain homeostasis (see Table D.1.2).

Table D.1.2 Autonomic nervous system and systemic effects

Organ system	Sympathetic effect	Parasympathetic effect
Eye	Dilation of pupil; focusing for distance vision	Constriction of pupil; focusing for near vision
Skin:		
Sweat glands	Increases secretion	None (not innervated)
Arrector pili muscles	Contraction and erection of hairs	None (not innervated)
Tear glands	None (not innervated)	Increases secretion
Cardiovascular system:		
Blood vessels	Vasoconstriction and vasodilation	None (not innervated)
Heart	Increases heart rate and contractility	Decreases heart rate and contractility
Adrenal glands	Secretion of epinephrine and norepinephrine by adrenal medullae	None (not innervated)
Respiratory system:		
Airways	Increases diameter to improve airflow	Decreases diameter to reduce airflow
Secretions	Decreases airway secretions	Increases airway secretions
Respiratory rate	Increases rate	Decreases rate
Digestive system:		
Level of activity	Decreases activity—especially by reducing blood supply	Increases activity—improved blood supply
Liver	Glycogen breakdown and glucose synthesis and release	Glycogen synthesis
Skeletal muscles	Increases force of contraction and glycogen breakdown	None (not innervated)
Urinary system:		
Kidneys	Decreases urine production	Increases urine production
Urinary bladder	Constricts sphincter and relaxes urinary bladder	Contracts bladder and relaxes sphincter
Reproductive system	Increases glandular secretions and ejaculation in males	Arousal of genitalia

1.9 Muscle physiology

1.9.1 Types of muscle

- Muscle can be classified into categories. Using a functional classification the muscles are divided into 3 groups:
  - Skeletal
  - Cardiac
  - Visceral (also known as smooth muscle due to its structural difference from the others, which are striated muscle)
- Skeletal muscle:
  - Large muscle groups
  - Striated muscle
  - Voluntary control
  - Used for movement and posture
  - Most skeletal muscles have a point of origin and point of insertion at the skeleton
  - These points are anchored by tendons
  - Provide short bursts of contraction followed by relaxation
- Cardiac muscle:
  - Found only in the heart
  - Similar structure to skeletal muscle
  - Involuntary control
  - Muscle fibres connect at branching, irregular angles called intercalated discs, which allow neighbouring muscle activation; therefore the heart muscle can be activated regularly from one point
  - Provide repeated contractions that alter in rate and force
- Smooth muscle:
  - Found in the splanchnic organs (e.g. the organs of the GI tract and also found in bronchi, uterus, urethra, bladder, blood vessels, and the arrector pili in the skin)
  - Involuntary control
  - Contractions are long and sustained compared to those of striated muscle
  - Responsible for the 'tone' of blood vessels

1.9.2 Skeletal muscle

- Skeletal muscle bulk is composed of many different muscle cells, or muscle fibres, which are contained within connective tissue known as endomysium.
- This group of muscle cells, arranged in longitudinal formation, is known as a fascicle. These are bundled together within another type of connective tissue, called perimysium, to form fasciculi:
  - Multiple bundles of fasciculi form the bulk of the skeletal muscle and are surrounded by epimysium
- A muscle fibre is composed of multiple **myofibrils**, which are separated by a cell membrane called the *sarcolemma*.
- This cell membrane not only forms a covering for the myofibrils but also contains extensions that pass into the muscle cells, known as **transverse tubules** (T-tubular).
- These T-tubules connect up with another membrane known as the **sarcoplasmic reticulum** and so a connection is made from the outside of the cell to the inside:
  - This connection network is thought to help conduct signals for contraction and relaxation of the muscle

- The myofibrils are made up of the active components of the muscle:
  - **Thick** filaments (made of *myosin*)
  - **Thin** filaments (made of *actin*)
- During the process of contraction the thick and thin filaments overlap and pull against each other. This reduces the length of the myofibril unit and consequently, with enough stimulation, the muscle length.
- The overlap that occurs between the thick and thin filaments is due to the heads of myosin of the thick filaments. These form *cross-bridges* with sites on the thin filaments. When the units are stimulated the myosin heads 'pull' the thin filaments inwards—similar to a rowing motion—and the unit shortens.
  - The degree of shortening depends on the degree of overlap that occurs between the thin and thick filaments
- The stimulation that is required for the thin and thick filaments to become activated originates from an action potential from a motor neuron, causing the release of Ach at the neuromuscular junction. The following actions then occur:
  - Ach binds to **nicotinic** receptors, which causes opening of an ion channel
  - An action potential is generated across the myocyte membrane, which travels down the T-tubules reaching the sarcoplasmic reticulum
  - This signal reaches the muscle cell and causes the release of Ca^{2+} into the cells from the sarcoplasmic reticulum
  - Ca^{2+} binds to troponin-C on actin filaments, which causes the removal of tropomyosin from the binding sites of the myosin heads, therefore allowing the cross-bridges to be formed
  - The myosin is then able to pull the actin filaments towards the centre of the muscle unit, shortening its length
  - This is powered by ATP hydrolysis at the myosin head
  - Ca^{2+} is then actively removed from the cytoplasm, allowing tropomyosin back into position, so blocking the actin sites, and the muscle returns to a resting state
- This process is known as **excitation–contraction coupling**, as an *electrical* signal is transformed into a *mechanical* action.
- The nerve stimulation that arrives at the muscle can arrive in different forms. This means that muscle contraction isn't uniform and can *differ in strength and rate of contraction*:
  - This is important functionally, so that the movement of the skeleton with muscle contraction can adapt to the situation (e.g. picking up a pen vs picking up a heavy bag)
- This concept of change in muscle contraction can be described with 2 types of nerve stimulation:
  - Temporal (frequency) summation:
    - When a nerve impulse arrives at a muscle unit it may not pass the threshold for contraction of that unit, or it may only cause a transient 'twitch' due to only one brief action potential arriving at the muscle cell
    - However, if the rate at which the nerve signal arrives at the muscle cell increases, this *increases* the **force** generated by that muscle unit
    - This is due to the repeated stimulation of the muscle cell causing repeated release of Ca^{2+} from the cell, thus reducing the absolute or relative refractory period. This enables repeated stimulation and a 'summation' of signals, increasing contraction
  - Spatial (multiple fibre) summation:
    - The other mechanism whereby muscle contraction increases in strength is with the recruitment of more muscle cells. This is done by increasing the number and size of contractile units stimulated

- When a weak signal arrives from the nervous system the smaller and weaker muscle cells contract but the larger units are not stimulated. As the nerve impulse increases in size then larger muscle cells are stimulated and so the force of contraction is increased
- As more motor nerves are stimulated more muscle units will be recruited in contraction and consequently more muscle contraction occurs

1.9.3 Cardiac muscle

- This type of muscle is very similar to skeletal muscle; however, there are differences that allow for repeated frequent contractions, changes in contractile force, differences in relaxation, and differences in the rate of contraction.
- In cardiac muscle the mechanism for electrical-contraction coupling is different prior to the above-mentioned mechanisms occurring:
  - This difference is due to calcium-induced calcium release. This occurs when the action potential causes Ca^{2+} release from the ER, which in turn causes further release of Ca^{2+} into the cytoplasm
- The mechanism by which contraction occurs with the heart is as follows:
  - **Pacemaker cells** in the sinoatrial node or atrioventricular node produce an action potential, which is conducted through the cardiac myocytes via **gap junctions**. This allows for electrical coupling between cardiac myocytes, which enables the electrical signal to spread across the myocardium causing the unique contraction method of the atria then the ventricles. This ensures the correct blood flow direction
  - The action potential then causes the release of Ca^{2+} into the cytoplasm of the cardiac myocytes. This causes further Ca^{2+} release from the ER
  - Muscle contractions then occur using a similar mechanism to skeletal muscle
  - Ca^{2+} is actively removed from the cytoplasm with the use of ATP and a Na^+/Ca^{2+} exchanger
  - The reduction in Ca^{2+} allows for the relaxation of the actin and myosin filaments

1.9.4 Frank–Starling mechanism

- The heart has an important functional property that ensures that cardiac output is matched to venous return (i.e. what comes in also goes out):
  - If the venous return to the heart increases, more blood will enter the ventricle. This causes increased stretch of the cardiac muscle cells, that is, the load on the myocytes before contraction increases—this is known as the preload
  - The stretching of the myocytes increases the affinity of troponin C with calcium, causing a greater number of cross-bridges with actin and myosin, leading to an increase in contractile force
- So the stretch of a muscle cell depends on the volume of blood within the ventricle before contraction (i.e. at diastole). Therefore preload is dependent on the *end diastolic volume*, which is directly proportional to the stretch of the cardiac myocyte.
- The stretch of the muscle unit is then directly proportional to the force of contraction, ensuring increased cardiac output with increased venous return.
- This is known as the **Frank–Starling law of the heart**.

CHAPTER D2

Respiratory physiology

CONTENTS

2.1 Lung volumes and pressures

2.1.1 Terminology

- There are 2 different terms applied to lung physiology:
  - *Capacity*:
    - This is used when a volume is made up of 2 or more smaller volumes, for example, FRC = ERV + RV
  - *Volume*:
    - The total amount of air contained in the defined lung physiology
- As seen in Table D.2.1 and Figure D.2.1, in the lungs there is a *residual volume* (RV).
- This is the difference between *vital capacity* (VC) and *total lung capacity* (TLC).
- Only VC can be measured on spirometry as TLC cannot directly be measured:
  - This is because it is not possible to fully exhale all of the air from the lungs, as some will remain (known as the RV)
  - This RV ensures that the airways stay open. If all the air was expelled and the airways closed and collapsed it would be more difficult to re-inflate them. (See Chapter D2, Section 2.3: Lung compliance)
- Another important part of ventilation is the *tidal volume* (V_T):
  - This is the volume of air expired when at rest, i.e. with normal ventilation
  - This is the air movement out of the lungs from the alveoli to the mouth
  - However, only part of this volume will be involved in ventilation of the alveoli
  - This is due to some of the V_T travelling in areas of the lung *not* involved in ventilation, i.e. the trachea, bronchi, and bronchioles. This is termed *dead space volume* (V_D) or the *anatomical dead space*
- The volume of air that is involved in ventilation is referred to as the *alveolar volume* (V_A):
  - Therefore $V_T = V_A + V_D$
  - The ratio of $V_D{:}V_T$ is 0.20–0.35. This means that 20–35% of air entering the lungs isn't involved in gas exchange at the alveolus

Table D.2.1 Definitions of terminology

Term	Value (for an average 70kg male) (L)	Definition
Tidal volume (V_T)	0.5	Volume of air leaving lungs per breath at rest
Vital capacity (VC)	4.8	Volume of air exhaled after maximal inspiration = IRV + V_T + ERV
Residual volume (RV)	1.2	Volume of air remaining in the lungs after maximal expiration
Functional residual capacity (FRC)	2.4	Volume of air remaining in lungs after expiration at rest = ERV + RV
Total lung capacity (TLC)	6.0	Total volume of air in lungs after maximal inspiration = VC + RV
Expiratory reserve volume (ERV)	1.2	Maximal volume of air exhaled after normal expiration
Inspiratory reserve volume (IRV)	3.1	Maximal volume of air inhaled after normal inspiration
Inspiratory capacity (IC)	3.6	Maximal volume of air inspired after normal expiration = IRV + V_T

- NB The V_D value *always* stays the same (i.e. it is fixed) as the anatomical volume will always be the same for each individual.
- Therefore if the V_T is reduced then the gas exchange at the alveolus will be reduced even further
- For example, V_T = 500mL (with ratio of 0.30 of V_D = 150mL) then V_A = 350mL
- If V_T = 300mL (with same volume of V_D as at rest, i.e. 150mL) then V_A = 200mL

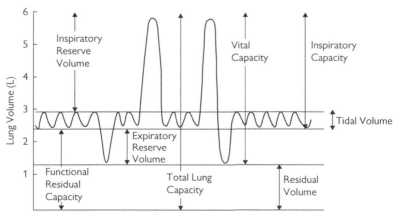

Figure D.2.1 Lung volumes and capacities

2.2 Lung epithelium

- As already mentioned, the lungs can be divided into 2 physiologically separate parts: those involved in gas exchange (V_A) and those areas that aren't (V_D).
- The parts of the airway system not involved with gas transfer have 3 major functions:
  - To conduct air evenly to all possible parts of the lung
  - To warm and humidify air, thus protecting areas lower down (alveoli) from damage
  - To detect and remove foreign substances from the air (e.g. bacteria, dust, toxins, etc.), again protecting airways structures further down in the lungs
- Defence against damaging foreign bodies is provided by ciliated columnar epithelial cells, which line the lumen of airways.
- The cilia beat together in a 'metachronal rhythm' so that there is synchronicity between the cells, ensuring efficient expulsion of material. An analogy of this would be a 'Mexican wave' effect, so that any foreign material that is trapped in the cilia is moved *upwards* towards the mouth, where it is coughed up or swallowed in phlegm.
- The process of moving substances is aided by the formation of mucus that coats the cilia. This also adds to the trapping effect of foreign material, for example, bacteria will be caught by the 'sticky' mucus *and* the fine cilia hairs:
  - This process is known as **mucociliary transport**
- The mucus involved in this system also has antipathogenic properties due to infiltration of inflammatory cells:
  - These inflammatory cells release proteases such as elastase to break down microorganisms trapped in the mucus
  - However, much of the lung is made up of elastin, therefore if left uncontrolled the lung would also be broken down by these proteases
  - For this reason a substance known as *alpha-1 antitrypsin* is found in the alveoli, which inhibits the proteases after their action in the mucus
- In some clinical circumstances there can be disruption of mucociliary transport. This can be due to:
  - Increased production of mucus:
    - For example, cystic fibrosis—a deficiency in a chloride channel that operates at the apical membranes throughout the body. One major effect clinically is the production of viscous mucus within the lung
    - This is thought to be due to a lack of the movement of water into the airways that normally occurs in healthy patients. This lack of water movement is a consequence of the cells' inability to transport Cl^-, due to the channel defect
    - Within this viscous, dehydrated mucus, more bacteria are trapped in the airways, as the mucociliary transport system is unable to move this concentrated mucus
  - Decreased movement of cilia:
    - For example, smoking, primary ciliary dyskinesia

2.3 Lung compliance

- Compliance (Cl) describes the relationship between lung volume (V) and pressure (P).
- It is a change in volume (ΔV) per change in pressure (ΔP).
- Typically it is equated as: $Cl = \dfrac{\Delta V}{\Delta P}$
- As can be seen from Figure D.2.2, compliance will be measured from the *slope* of the curve. Many experiments use the expiration curve to measure this.

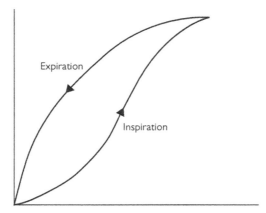

Figure D.2.2 Pressure–volume curve throughout respiratory cycle

2.3.1 Static lung compliance

- This describes the change in lung volume per unit change in pressure across the lung (i.e. from within the alveoli to the pleural surface of the lung); it is therefore a measure of distensibility:
  - This is affected by factors such as age, sex, size, and degree of 'stiffness' of the lung (e.g. pulmonary fibrosis increases lung stiffness)
  - Lower values of static compliance are found in women and children compared to men due to the smaller lung sizes
- Therefore a lung of high compliance expands more with the same degree of *transpulmonary pressure* (i.e. that generated across the lung pleura to alveoli).
- Compliance of the lung is affected by the size due to the differing effects a change in a specific volume will have on the different lung sizes. For example, entry of 1L of air into the lungs of a 2-year-old child will have different effects on pressure in the lungs compared to that of a 20-year-old male. Likewise the same can be said of healthy, compliant lungs vs stiff, elderly, fibrotic lungs. Some further examples of factors affecting static lung compliance are mentioned in Table D.2.2.

Table D.2.2 Factors affecting lung compliance

	High compliance	Low compliance
Lung of normal structure	Large size Active, healthy individuals	Small size Respiratory muscle weakness
Lung surfactant deficiency		Premature infant ARDS
Fibrous stroma	Age, COPD (esp. smokers and α1-antitrypsin deficiency)	Disorders of lung parenchyma (e.g. pulmonary fibrosis)
Visceral pleura		Thickened due to asbestosis, haemothorax, TB
Alveolar muscle tone	Bronchodilator drugs During exercise	Hypoxia, histamine (e.g. asthma)

2.3.2 Dynamic lung compliance

- The measurement of compliance can also be made during lung inspiration and expiration (i.e. when the lung isn't stationary).
- By measuring lung volume and pressures in the oesophagus at the end of inspiration or expiration, *apparent* lung stationary measurements can be taken. This gives *dynamic compliance*.
- Therefore, in patients with normal, healthy lungs the 2 recordings have similar values; however, in patients who suffer from changes to airway resistance the values are different:
  - For example, for patients with narrowing of the airways in asthma, the dynamic compliance is reduced. This difference is due to the airflow of gas within the lungs influencing the transpulmonary pressure
  - Dynamic compliance is therefore a measure of airway resistance

2.4 Surfactant

- As mentioned previously, it is important to have a volume of air within the lung to ensure that airways don't collapse (collapse is known as *atelectasis*). This principle is explained by **surface tension**:
  - As alveoli are spherical and moist they are affected by surface tension due to the gas–liquid interface that occurs on the inner surface of the alveoli. This tension acts to pull alveoli inwards
  - This tension is at its greatest when the alveoli volume is low, causing an unstable alveolus and collapse, whilst larger alveoli become more distended
  - Laplace's law calculates the pressure (P) created from surface tension (T, in dynes/cm) in relation to alveoli radius (r, in mm): $P = \dfrac{2T}{r}$
    - Thus if surface tension is constant then the pressure to collapse in a smaller alveolus is greater
- The mechanism by which the lung acts to counteract the collapse of the smaller alveolus is the production of **surfactant**:
  - Surfactant is made up of a lipid/protein material, the main component being phosphatidylcholine. This is secreted by specialized epithelial cells lining the alveoli, known as pneumocytes (type II)
  - Surfactant acts to drastically reduce surface tension. This means that alveoli are less prone to collapse and are kept more distensible (i.e. more compliant)
- In certain clinical situations there is a reduction in surfactant causing reduced compliance and collapse of airways leading to atelectasis:
  - One significant example of this, which highlights the importance of surfactant, is in premature neonates:
    - The lungs are one of the last organs to develop *in utero* given that a foetus relies on its oxygen supply via the placenta
    - Premature infants therefore have the correct anatomy; however, the lungs are not ready to be used owing to the fact that there is no production of surfactant yet
    - These infants consequently suffer from high surface tension within the lungs and have a poor ability to breathe spontaneously due to the high pressures needed to inflate poorly compliant (stiff) lungs. Therefore atelectasis and inadequate ventilation result
    - This is known as infant respiratory distress syndrome (IRDS)

- Another example is when the lungs suffer from an acute injury, for example, significant trauma (to lung or other parts of the body), sepsis, aspiration, or inhalation of a noxious substance:
  - In these situations, amongst others, the lung surfaces are injured leading to a decrease in surfactant
  - This causes the chain of events described earlier in this section, and can cause rapid death
  - The loss of surfactant is thought to be due to the aggregation of neutrophils causing capillary damage and releasing harmful toxic products
  - This is known as adult respiratory distress syndrome (ARDS)

2.5 Airway resistance

- Airway resistance (R_{aw}) is defined as the ratio of driving pressure of a gas against flow. The same formulae can be used as for electrical resistance (i.e. Ohm's law).
- Used in relation to airways, $R_{aw} = \Delta P/V$:
  - Where ΔP = pressure difference across an airway (in the lung this is mouth pressure − alveolar pressure) and V = airflow
- Airflow is also determined by the radius of the vessel by which it travels.
- Poiseuille's law dictates that flow = $\pi r^4/8\eta L$:
  - Where η = viscosity of fluid and L = length of tube
  - Therefore if the viscosity of fluid and length of tube are constant then the flow is inversely proportional to the radius to the power of 4. So if the airway is reduced in diameter by 50%, then flow is reduced 16-fold
  - For this reason the diameter of the airways in the lung are tightly regulated by the autonomic nervous system (ANS). The ANS innervates the smooth muscle found in the walls of airways from the trachea to the terminal bronchioles
  - **Parasympathetic** tone causes *constriction* of the vessels by smooth muscle contraction and increased mucus production. The neurotransmitter at the postganglionic fibres here is Ach
  - **Sympathetic** tone causes *dilatation* of the vessels by smooth muscle relaxation and reduced mucus production. The neurotransmitter at the postganglionic fibres here is epinephrine (adrenaline), acting on β_2 receptors
  - A combination of both parasympathetic and sympathetic innervation acts to maintain airway diameter. Sympathetic stimulation will occur during the 'fight or flight' response or during exercise, thus improving airflow as much as possible to help ventilate lower airways and improve gas exchange
- Patients with **asthma** suffer from an increase in bronchoconstriction, thus limiting the amount of airflow. Patients suffering an acute severe 'asthma attack' will have such drastic constriction of the airways that ventilation of the alveoli is severely compromised and this can be lethal if not treated.
- Patients with asthma can be treated by stimulation of the sympathetic system with the use of β_2 agonists, such as *salbutamol*, and by blocking parasympathetic stimulation with Ach antagonists, such as *ipratropium bromide*.
- In order to clinically measure a patient's airway resistance we can measure the patient's peak expiratory flow rate (PEFR).
- Normal values for PEFR are dependent on initial lung size:
  - The smaller the lung volume, the lower the PEFR. It is therefore difficult to know exactly what is normal for each individual

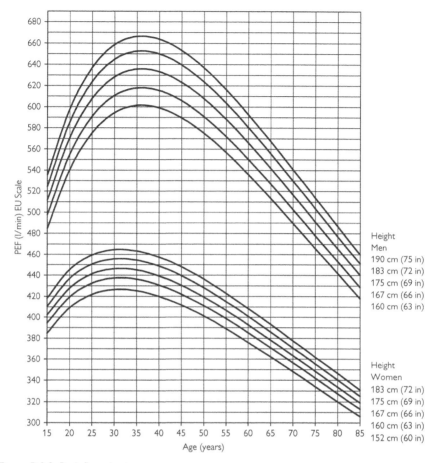

Figure D.2.3 Peak flow chart

Reproduced with permission from Clement Clarke. Adapted by permission from BMJ Publishing Group Limited by Clement Clarke for use with EN13826 / EU scale peak flow meters from *The BMJ*, 'New regression equations for predicting peak expiratory flow in Adults', A.J Nunn, I. Gregg. 298, pp. 1068–7, 1989.

- For this reason a chart (see Figure D.2.3) is used, using a patient's age, sex, and height as a guide to what the PEFR should be
- Another investigation is the calculation of forced expiratory volume over a 1sec period (FEV_1) compared to the total forced vital capacity (FVC):
  - This is completed with the use of spirometry and is useful clinically to differentiate those patients with obstructive lung defects (e.g. chronic obstructive pulmonary disease (COPD)), and those with restrictive disease (e.g. pulmonary fibrosis)
  - The normal ratio of FEV_1/FVC is around 0.8, i.e. in normal individuals 80% of their forced vital capacity can be exhaled in 1sec
  - Patients with an obstructive lung disorder have a reduced flow of air out of the lungs (e.g. COPD due to loss of elastic recoil or asthma due to poor airflow). In these patients the FVC remains normal or low but FEV_1 is markedly reduced, so the FEV_1/FVC ratio is also markedly reduced, i.e. <0.8 (see Figure D.2.4)

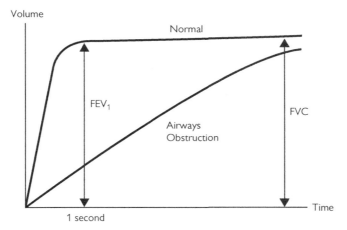

Figure D.2.4 Volume–time curve for a person with obstructive lung function

- Patients with restrictive lung disorders have difficulties with lung inflation; therefore both FEV$_1$ and FVC are reduced to similar levels, so that actually the ratio of FEV$_1$/FVC is 0.8 or above. However, the FVC is markedly reduced as can be detected on the spirograph (see Figure D.2.5)

2.6 Gas transfer

- When discussing lung physiology, different units are used to measure gas pressures.
  - These include mmHg (millimetres of mercury) and cmH$_2$O (centimetres of water):
    - 1mmHg = 1.36cmH$_2$O
    - 1cmH$_2$O = 0.74mmHg
- Barometric pressure (P$_B$) is also known as atmospheric pressure (atm): 1atm = 101.325kPa or 14.7lbf/sq in:
  - At 1atm, i.e. atmospheric pressure at sea level, P$_B$ = 760mmHg.

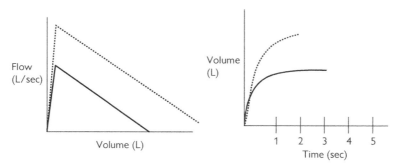

Figure D.2.5 Volume–time curve for a person with restrictive lung function (solid line) compared with normal (broken line)

- The total pressure of an 'atmosphere' is caused by the combination of all the pressures exerted by individual gases.
  - This is known as **Dalton's law**, so:
    - $P_B = PN_2 + PO_2 + PH_2O + PCO_2$
  - Therefore to calculate the PO_2, it is the fraction of O_2 in the atmosphere multiplied by the P_B. The fraction of O_2 in the atmosphere is 21%, so:
    - $PO_2 = P_B \times 0.21$
    - This is $760 \times 0.21 = 160mmHg$, i.e. the *partial pressure* of *oxygen* in the atmosphere.
  - If we take into account that the air in the lungs is humidified with water, this also exerts a partial pressure of 47mmHg.
  - So when taking this into account the *dry partial pressure* of oxygen is:
    - $PO_2 = 0.21 \times (760 - 47) = 150mmHg$
  - For **nitrogen** =
    - Humidified $PN_2 = 0.79 \times 760 = 600mmHg$
    - Dry $PN_2 = 0.79 \times (760 - 47) = 563mmHg$
  - For **carbon dioxide** =
    - Humidified $PCO_2 = 0.0003 \times 760 = 0.23mmHg$
    - Dry $PCO_2 = 0.0003 \times (760 - 47) = 0.21mmHg$

2.6.1 Alveolar gas transfer

- The alveoli are made of 2 different types of cells, known as pneumocytes. Type II cells produce surfactant as previously mentioned. Type I pneumocytes are involved in gas exchange. They:
  - Are large, thin cells
  - Have a large surface area
  - Are unable to replicate, so are affected by toxic gas inhalation
- Type I pneumocytes have the special ability to enable gas exchange within the lung due to their very thin structure. The distance between capillaries and alveoli is very small at only 1μm.
- The *permeability* to gases varies depending on the gas. CO_2 is non-polar and highly lipid-soluble so moves easily across plasma membranes:
  - The capillary–alveoli barrier is 20 times more permeable to CO_2 than to O_2
  - However, the diffusion *gradient* for CO_2 isn't as great as for O_2, i.e.:
    - Alveolar concentration: $CO_2 = 40$; $O_2 = 104$
    - Mixed venous blood: $CO_2 = 46$; $O_2 = 40$
  - The diffusion gradient of CO_2 **from the venous system into alveoli** = 6mmHg
  - The diffusion gradient of O_2 **from the alveoli into venous blood** = 64mmHg
- In order to calculate how well a gas moves across the alveolar membrane, i.e. the **transfer factor**, carbon monoxide is generally used:
  - This is because carbon monoxide is not normally found in the body at meaningful levels
  - As carbon monoxide can be measured both in inspired and exhaled air, and there is no 'back reaction' (no carbon monoxide travelling back across the membrane from capillary to alveolus), then calculations can be made to determine the diffusion of gas particles through the membranes and into fluid
- The transfer factor for carbon monoxide (TL_{CO}) is the quantity of the gas that is transferred from the alveolus into the capillaries per minute per unit gas tension difference between the 2 sites:
  - This then gives a measurement of how well gases, specifically carbon monoxide, can move across the lung into the blood

■ This has clinical implications as measurements can be used to compare those who are healthy and those who have pathological lung conditions, and to compare the severity of these conditions

2.6.2 Factors reducing gas exchange

- The factor that causes the largest reduction in TL_{CO} is the overall surface area of the lung available and not the thickness of the lung—this does have an effect but to a lesser degree. Therefore TL_{CO} is affected in patients with lung resections or patients with COPD, as normal alveoli are replaced by air spaces known as bulla.
- Another factor affecting TL_{CO} is the loss of 'effective' alveoli. Therefore in any condition where ventilation is reduced to alveoli, TL_{CO} is consequently diminished.
- Disease in pulmonary capillaries and a reduction in available Hb will also decrease TL_{CO}.
- The 'effective' volume of alveoli (i.e. the alveoli available for ventilation and gas exchange) can be calculated, therefore factoring loss of alveoli for various conditions. If this is combined with TL_{CO} this gives the *transfer coefficient* (K_{CO}):
    ■ So values for K_{CO} are actually normal for patients with asthma, as TL_{CO} is only reduced due to a decrease in ventilation to those areas of the lung affected by asthma
    ■ However, in COPD both K_{CO} and TL_{CO} are reduced due to not only the loss of effective alveoli from bulla but also the loss of gas exchange even in the relatively healthier parts of the lung
    ■ In some situations, TL_{CO} may increase due to greater blood flow to the lungs (therefore more red blood cell availability) and hence improved gas transfer:
        • This occurs in conditions such as polycythaemia or pulmonary haemorrhage
        • The K_{CO} will also increase in these conditions as there will be a greater proportion of pulmonary capillaries per volume of alveoli during this time
    ■ K_{CO} will also increase where there is a decrease in lung volume compared to alveolar perfusion, therefore increasing capillary density. This occurs in extrapulmonary conditions that restrict lung volume, such as pleural disease, ribcage deformity, and respiratory muscle weakness.

2.7 Gas transport within the circulation

2.7.1 Oxygen transport

- The uptake of oxygen from the air into circulation is limited by 2 stages:
    ■ Diffusion of oxygen through the blood–gas barrier
    ■ The transfer of oxygen to Hb
- The transport of oxygen in the blood mainly occurs via Hb. However, oxygen is also transported via the plasma of the blood in dissolved form.

2.7.2 Dissolved oxygen

- This only produces a very small fraction of oxygen transport.
- Oxygen dissolved in plasma follows Henry's law, which defines the amount of gas able to dissolve in a liquid given its partial pressure:
    ■ For O_2, $PO_2 = 100$, therefore dissolved $O_2 = 0.3mL/100mL$ of plasma (i.e. 0.003% vol.)
    ■ This would not provide tissues with an adequate amount of oxygen

2.7.3 Haemoglobin transport

- Oxygen forms an easily reversible combination with Hb to give oxyhaemoglobin.
- At the tissues, this oxyhaemoglobin once again dissociates to release O_2.

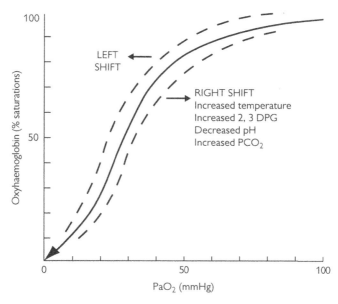

Figure D.2.6 Oxygen–haemoglobin dissociation curve

- Approximately 1g of Hb has the capacity to carry 1.34mL of O_2.
- Therefore for a normal haematocrit of 15g Hb/100mL of blood, the Hb carrying capacity of O_2 = 1.34mL × 15 = 20.1mL O_2/100mL
- For *whole blood* the total carrying capacity for O_2 = Hb transport + diffused = 0.3 + 20.1 = 20.4mL (i.e. around 20% vol.)
- In reality, the oxygen-carrying capacity is slightly less and saturation is calculated as:
  - %HbO_2 saturation = HbO_2 content/HbO_2 capacity × 100
  - When measured, a 'saturation curve' is created for the reaction of Hb with O_2 (see Figure D.2.6)
- As the curve shows in Figure D.2.6, Hb is nearly fully saturated under normal physiological conditions, where PO_2 = 104mmHg in the alveoli, Hb saturation is 97%, and the oxygen content is 20% vol.
- The O_2–Hb saturation is not a linear relationship; it is curvilinear:
  - This has physiological benefits—small drops in alveolar PO_2 will hardly affect the Hb saturation given its flattened upper portion
  - The steep lower part of the dissociation curve means that the peripheral tissues are able to obtain large amounts of O_2 for only a small drop in PO_2 in the capillaries
- There are 4 main factors that shift the O_2–Hb dissociation curve; these are:
  - Temperature
  - pH
  - PCO_2
  - Organic phosphate (i.e. 2,3-DPG)
- Most of these conditions are related to tissues requiring oxygen transport:
  - For example, a working muscle that is using O_2 to create energy will have an increasing temperature, increased output of CO_2, and hence decreased pH, thus will require more oxygen delivery
  - These conditions act to shift the dissociation curve to the *right*, thus increasing oxygen dissociation (see Figure D.2.6)

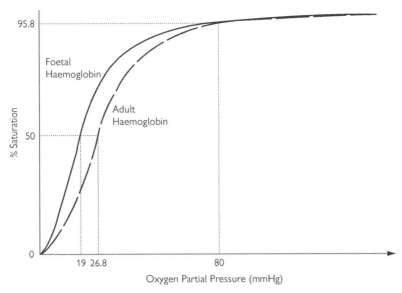

Figure D.2.7 Oxygen–haemoglobin dissociation curve of adult vs fetal haemoglobin

- A shift to the *left* has the opposite effect of decreasing oxygen dissociation (see Figure D.2.6)
- An increase in 2,3-DPG occurs in conditions of chronic hypoxia (e.g. at altitude) in chronic lung disease, and in anaemia, and therefore helps to acclimatize to the lower PO_2 or improve oxygen delivery in hypoxaemia.

2.7.4 Anaemia

- This is a condition where there is a reduction in Hb within the body.
- The oxygen-carrying capacity of the blood will therefore be reduced.
- This results in the O_2–Hb dissociation curve being shifted to the right.
- Another condition whereby a shift occurs in the dissociation curve is as a foetus:
  - From the age of 10 weeks' gestation to 12 weeks postnatally, the foetus has a different type of Hb (foetal Hb, HbF), which is then replaced by adult Hb at about 12 weeks after delivery
  - HbF has a higher affinity for O_2 giving the foetus better access to O_2 from the maternal bloodstream (see Figure D.2.7)

2.7.5 Carbon dioxide transport

- CO_2 is transported in blood in 3 ways:
  - As bicarbonate (HCO_3^-) (60%)
  - With Hb (30%)
  - Dissolved in plasma (10%)
- The majority of the transport of CO_2 is as bicarbonate. This is formed by the reaction of: $CO_2 + H_2O \leftrightarrow H_2CO_3 \leftrightarrow H^+ + HCO_3^-$
- Due to the presence of carbonic anhydrase (CA) in the red blood cells, the reaction is greatly enhanced, so that conversion of CO_2 to HCO_3^- is fast:
  - This occurs in the red blood cells (RBCs)

- HCO_3^- diffuses out of the RBCs leaving higher concentrations of H^+ within the cell. There is consequently a shift of Cl^- ions into the RBCs to maintain electroneutrality. This is known as the *chloride shift*
- There is some H^+ that requires buffering by the RBCs and this occurs by binding to Hb. Therefore Hb has a buffering effect: $H^+ + HbO_2 \leftrightarrow H\text{-}Hb + O_2$
  - The reduced (i.e. non-oxygen-carrying form) of Hb is a better H^+ binder
  - This means in tissues that are respiring, where there is a high concentration of CO_2 and low O_2, Hb is able to bind to H^+ more easily and improve CO_2 transport. This is known as the *Haldane effect*
- Another large proportion of CO_2 transport is via proteins such as Hb; more specifically it is the terminal amine group that the CO_2 binds to:
  $CO_2 + Hb\text{-}NH_2 \leftrightarrow Hb\text{-}NH\text{-}COOH \leftrightarrow Hb\text{-}NH\text{-}COO^- + H^+$
  - The reduced Hb can bind more CO_2 than HbO_2, again increasing the unloading in the lungs and pick-up at respiring tissues (Haldane effect)
  - The CO_2 doesn't bind directly to the iron molecule as O_2 does, but instead binds loosely to the amine group

2.8 Control of respiration

- Control of respiration is both an **automatic** *and* a **voluntary** process.
- Inspiration occurs with:
  - Contraction of the diaphragm (breathing at rest)
  - External intercostals (with extra demand required)
  - Cervical muscles (with extra demand required)
- Expiration occurs with:
  - Passive movement, i.e. elastic recoil of lung and chest wall (breathing at rest)
  - Abdominal wall movement (with extra demand required)
  - Internal intercostals muscles (with extra demand required)

2.8.1 Medullary respiratory centres

- 2 centres in the medulla oblongata have been associated with respiration:
  - **Dorsal respiratory group** (DRG)—thought to initiate *inspiration* via signals through the **phrenic nerve** to stimulate the diaphragm
  - **Ventral respiratory group** (VRG)—thought to be involved in inspiration and expiration
- The exact mechanisms of respiratory control are unclear and it is unlikely that it is produced from one discrete 'centre'.

2.8.2 Pontine respiratory centres

- The pontine respiratory group (PRG)—also known as the **pneumotaxic centre**—is made up of a group of nuclei that are thought to inhibit the actions of the inspiratory centres of the apneustic centre.
- Apneustic centre—this is responsible for generating a signal to the DRG to stimulate inspiration. It has inhibitory signals from **pulmonary stretch receptors**:
  - These are proprioceptors found in the smooth muscle of airways. They are activated when the lung is at the peak in inspiration, thus protecting against over-inflation and also regulating the respiratory cycle
- For voluntary control of breathing, cortical structures in the brain impose effects via the pyramidal tracts on respiratory muscle. It is thought that both the autonomic *and* voluntary control areas do have signals between each other.

2.8.3 Sensory inputs

- The respiratory centres need both an input and an output.
- The output is mainly stimulation of the phrenic nerve to stimulate diaphragm control for inspiration:
  - As expiration is a passive process the output for this is an 'off' signal (i.e. no stimulation of the phrenic nerve)
  - However, other muscles are initiated, and therefore other signals needed, when there is an increased demand required (e.g. during exercise)
- The inputs for the respiratory system involve:
  - Chemoreceptors:
    - These are receptors that respond to chemical changes in the bloodstream
    - Both peripheral and central
  - Stretch receptors
  - Irritant receptors
  - J-receptors

2.8.4 Central chemoreceptors

- These receptors are the major controller for ventilation and are found in the medulla near the exit of the cranial nerves IX and X.
- As explained earlier in this section, when there is an increase in CO_2 there is a formation of H_2CO_3, which dissociates into H^+ and HCO_3^-. The central chemoreceptors are sensitive to the H^+.
- Therefore with a rise in blood CO_2 there must be an increase in respiration to remove this waste product. This occurs by:
  - A rise in PCO_2 in the blood from tissues
  - CO_2 is converted via H_2CO_3 to $H_2CO_3^-$ and H^+ in the cerebrospinal fluid (CSF), as the blood–brain barrier is permeable to CO_2 but not to H^+ or HCO_3^-. CSF contains carbonic anhydrase to facilitate the conversion of CO_2 to H^+
  - H^+ consequently acts to stimulate the chemoreceptors in the medulla, which are surrounded by CSF
  - The chemoreceptors activate the respiratory centres and lead to enhanced respiration (i.e. hyperpnoea) which is an increase in alveolar ventilation with no change in arterial PCO_2 (Hyperventilation is an increase in alveolar ventilation with a fall in PCO_2.)
- The reverse process also occurs, where a fall in blood PCO_2 leads to a hypopnoea.
- The cerebral vasodilation that occurs with increased PCO_2 enhances the diffusion of CO_2 into the CSF.
- As the central chemoreceptors are sensitive to PCO_2 indirectly via H^+, they are therefore affected by the overall pH of the blood.
- This mechanism ensures that the pH of the blood is kept in strict regulation, as it has severe consequences on overall cellular function throughout the body.

2.8.5 Peripheral chemoreceptors

- These are located in the:
  - Arch of the aorta (**aortic bodies**)
  - Bifurcation of the common carotid artery (**carotid bodies**)
- These chemoreceptors are sensitive to changes in arterial PCO_2, H^+, and PO_2.
- Although not as significant as PCO_2, the levels of oxygen in the blood are monitored by the peripheral chemoreceptors.
- Therefore any hypoxaemia that occurs causes a stimulation of the peripheral chemoreceptors and consequently an increase in ventilation.

- When there is a decrease in levels of arterial oxygen, and to a lesser extent CO_2 and H^+, there is an increase in stimulation of the cranial nerves IX and X, which act on the medullary centres to increase ventilation.
- Direct measures of arterial H^+ can be made at the peripheral chemoreceptors.
- Therefore during acidaemic or alkalaemic situations (e.g. DKA) there is a subsequent change in respiration via the peripheral chemoreceptors.

2.8.6 Stretch receptors

- As already mentioned, the lung contains proprioceptors within the airways that, when stimulated, lead to an inhibition of the inspiratory centres.
- The stimulation from the stretch receptors is carried via the cranial nerve X (vagus nerve) to inhibit these centres in the apneustic centre. It is thought that this stimulation only occurs in humans with tidal volumes greater than 1L (i.e. during exercise).
- It is also thought that the signals carried via the vagus nerve also cause an inhibition of the cardiac vagal motor neurons, thus causing a tachycardia during inspiration, also known as *sinus arrhythmia*.

2.8.7 Irritant receptors

- These receptors act to protect the lung from noxious substances (e.g. smoke, particles, or cold air).
- When stimulated these receptors send signals via the vagus nerve to cause bronchoconstriction and hyperpnoea.
- It is thought that these receptors may have a role in patients with asthma.

2.8.8 J-receptors

- Juxta-capillary receptors are found in the alveolar walls next to capillaries and are innervated by the vagus nerve.
- It is thought that these receptors respond to pulmonary capillary engorgement and an increase in interstitial fluid volume in the alveolar walls.
- Therefore in clinical situations of pulmonary oedema, pulmonary emboli, pneumonia, and barotrauma, the receptors are activated.
- Once activated the J-receptors are thought to increase breathing rate, but also stimulate the sensation of dyspnoea (i.e. the feeling of shortness of breath).

2.9 Ventilation–perfusion relationship

- The ventilation–perfusion relationship describes a normal difference of ventilation and perfusion that occurs throughout the lung.
- The major cause of this is the effect of gravity, and therefore the position of the person is the most important factor.

2.9.1 Ventilation (V)

- A difference in ventilation occurs throughout the lung so that the base of the lung has better ventilation than the apex.
- This is due to the gravitational effect on the lung mass when a person is upright.
- Thus at the base of the lung there is an increased pleural pressure (making these areas less negative); this makes them more compliant, as they will be easier to inflate.
- The opposite is true for the apex, where the alveoli are under a higher negative pressure and therefore are more distended.
- The apex therefore will be less compliant, as the alveoli cannot distend any further.

2.9.2 Perfusion (Q)

- The perfusion pressure for the lungs is from the right side of the heart, and is said to be a 'low-pressure system', i.e. systolic/diastolic = 25/10mmHg.
- For the same reasons as with ventilation there is a difference that occurs throughout the lung according to whether a person is upright or lying down.
- Therefore the base of the lung receives the majority of blood flow and perfusion is high here.
- The converse is true for the apex.
- So for the apex of the lung the V/Q ratio is high, and for the base the V/Q is low.
- Taken into consideration as a whole, the V/Q of the lung is 0.8:
  - An area with no ventilation (V/Q = 0) is termed a 'shunt'
  - An area with no perfusion (V/Q = infinity) is termed 'dead space'

2.9.3 Hypoxic vasoconstriction

- When a mismatch occurs of V/Q, due to areas of poor ventilation, the lung is able to redirect blood to areas of better ventilation. This is known as a shunt.
- If an area of lung has poor ventilation (i.e. with pneumonia, pulmonary oedema, or even as a normal process), the arterioles feeding the under-ventilated alveoli are stimulated by the hypoxic conditions and therefore constrict.
- This hypoxic vasoconstriction acts to shunt blood away from poorly ventilated regions to better ventilated regions. In this way the V/Q relationship is maintained.
- When a V/Q mismatch occurs an arterial blood gas sample will show:
  - Hypoxaemia
  - An increased A–a gradient
- With a low V/Q there will be reduced alveoli ventilation but normal perfusion, thus lower oxygen in the blood (hypoxaemia) and an increased A–a gradient. This will occur in under-ventilated lung, for example:
  - Pneumonia
  - Pulmonary oedema
  - Acute asthma
- These are examples of shunt that occur within the lung and are pathological.
- Other examples include an arterial venous malformation within the lung.
- Intracardiac shunts also exist (e.g. right-to-left shunt such as a VSD).
- When oxygen is given to patients with intracardiac right–left shunts no difference is made to the hypoxaemia—the mixing of venous and arterial blood outside of the lung means there is no relationship to alveolar oxygen.
- In most other V/Q mismatches oxygen will improve the hypoxaemia.

Cardiovascular physiology

CONTENTS

3.1 Systemic overview

3.1.1 Appreciation of how cardiovascular components are suited to their primary functions

See Table D.3.1 and Figure D.3.1.

- Veins as thin-walled capacitance and return vessels:
  - The walls of veins are thinner in relation to their overall vessel diameter and therefore more distensible than arteries. This distension enables the venous system to act as a capacitor, holding most of the total blood volume (normally around 70%) and thereby regulating regional blood volume
  - The larger veins also possess valves at various intervals along their length, thereby preventing the backward flow of blood
- Arteries as elastic pulsation-dampening distribution vessels:
  - Arteries provide a dampening and resistance function
  - The arterial system normally holds around 12% of the total blood volume
  - The large elastic central arteries are able to distend in order to accommodate the pulsatile pressure of each stroke volume. Dampening is therefore a function of the aortic compliance
  - Although capable of constricting and dilating, the large arteries that branch directly off the aorta (e.g. the carotid, mesenteric, or renal arteries) serve virtually no role in the regulation of pressure and blood flow under normal physiological conditions. During diastole the elastic recoil maintains diastolic blood flow (*Windkessel effect*)
  - The smaller, more muscular arteries and arterioles fulfil the role of maintaining peripheral resistance and of effective blood flow distribution to various vascular beds. In this way, the smaller arteries and arterioles regulate arterial blood pressure through their innervation by the autonomic nervous system
- Capillaries and venules as sites of exchange and return:
  - The capillaries are the principal exchange vessels of the cardiovascular system and normally contain around 5% of the total blood volume

Table D.3.1 Relative sizes and functions of different blood vessels

Vessel type	Diameter (mm)	Function
Aorta	25	Pulse dampening and distribution
Large arteries	1.0–4.0	Distribution of arterial blood
Small arteries	0.2–1.0	Distribution and resistance
Arterioles	0.01–0.20	Resistance and flow regulation
Capillaries	0.006–0.010	Exchange
Venules	0.01–0.20	Exchange, collection, and capacitance
Veins	0.2–5.0	Capacitance
Vena cava	35	Collection of venous blood

- Capillaries have no smooth muscle, consisting of a single layer of endothelial cells and a basement membrane and thereby enabling the movement of solutes across their walls
- Capillaries coalesce to form postcapillary venules, which in turn merge to form the true venules and veins. Postcapillary venules also contribute to exchange, particularly of larger molecules and fluid, as well as to the regulation of capillary pressure

3.1.2 Normal adult values for total blood volume, cardiac output, and stroke volume

- Normal total blood volume is approximately 70mL/kg in adults—equivalent to around 5L in the 70kg male.

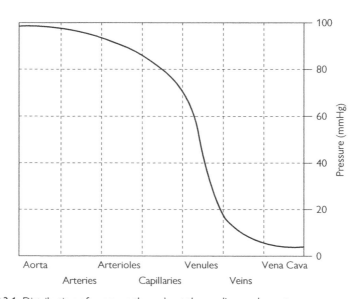

Figure D.3.1 Distribution of pressure throughout the cardiovascular system

- The stroke volume (SV) is the volume of blood ejected by the ventricles with each heartbeat, specifically that of the left ventricle for calculating cardiac output (CO):
  - The normal value of SV is 70–80mL for an average male at rest.
- CO is the volume of blood pumped from one side of the heart per minute, and is calculated by the product of stroke volume × heart rate:
  - The normal value for CO is around 5L/min in the average resting male
  - CO is affected by changes in heart rate, myocardial contractility, preload (venous pressure), and afterload (arterial pressure). This may be due to various physiological and pathological processes, such as a rise in metabolic rate (e.g. sepsis, exercise), and many different forms of therapeutic agents
  - Changes in CO vary with body surface area. The cardiac index is measured as the CO per square metre of body surface area.
  - Normal CO is distributed approximately in the following proportions:
    - Liver 25%
    - Kidneys 22%
    - Muscle 20%
    - Brain 14%
    - Heart 5%
    - Remainder 14%

3.1.3 Mean arterial pressure (MAP) as diastolic + one-third pulse pressure and the rationale for this

- The MAP represents the average arterial blood pressure throughout the cardiac cycle, and therefore the mean pressure available for tissue perfusion.
- As can be seen in Figure D.3.2, the area contained within the arterial waveform pressure trace above the MAP should be equal to the area below this line.
- This may be approximated to the diastolic pressure + one-third pulse pressure (pulse pressure = systolic pressure − diastolic pressure).

3.1.4 Values of mean blood pressure before and after capillary beds and of the central venous pressure

- Typical pressures within the capillary bed are around 30mmHg at the arteriolar end, falling to around 15mmHg at the venous end.
- These pressures are controlled by local autoregulatory mechanisms (see Chapter D3, Section 3.7.2).

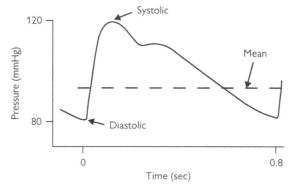

Figure D.3.2 Arterial waveform curve

- Normal central venous pressure (CVP) ranges from $-2cmH_2O$ to $+12cmH_2O$.
- CVP will vary with cardiac cycle, respiration, and the position of the patient.

3.2 Cardiac cycle I

3.2.1 Sinoatrial node as the originator of the cycle, modulated via autonomic nerves

- The sinoatrial (SA) node is located at the junction of the superior vena cava and right atrium.
- The SA node is innervated by both sympathetic (T1–4, spinal nerves) and parasympathetic (vagus) nerve fibres.
- Parasympathetic stimulation will result in a decreased SA nodal rate, while sympathetic stimulation will result in an increase in SA nodal rate.
- The SA node is formed by specialized myocytes that are responsible for initiation of the cardiac action potential.
- Although all cardiac myocytes possess the ability to generate action potentials and trigger cardiac contraction, the SA node generates impulses slightly faster than the other areas with pacemaker potential—thereby overriding these and controlling cardiac contraction.
- Activation of atrial myocytes via gap junctions and desmosomes:
  - Myocytes possess an array of T-tubules, which are finger-like invaginations of the sarcolemma with openings up to 200nm in diameter:
    - These are regularly spaced so that the tubules tend to lie alongside the Z lines of the myofibrils
    - The T-tubules allow the depolarization of the action potential to be transmitted into the interior of the cell
    - As with skeletal muscle, depolarization causes the opening of voltage-gated calcium channels and release of Ca^{2+} from the T-tubules. This influx of calcium causes calcium-induced calcium release from the sarcoplasmic reticulum, and free calcium causes muscle contraction. Compared to skeletal muscle, the T-tubules in cardiac muscle are larger and broader.
  - Gap junctions are specialized intercellular connections, which are responsible for electrochemical and metabolic coupling:
    - This enables the action potential to be passed efficiently and ensures that electrical impulses propagate freely between cells in every direction, so that the myocardium functions as a single contractile unit
    - Desmosomes are also found in cardiac muscle tissue where they provide cell-to-cell adhesion, ensuring organized force transmission during muscle contraction, as well as facilitating the rapid spread of action potentials and synchronized contraction of the myocardium
- Role of annulus fibrosus cordis in limitation of excitation:
  - The annulus fibrosus cordis are the fibrous rings of tissue that surround the atrioventricular (AV) and arterial orifices in both sides of the heart. These rings serve as the attachments of the muscular fibres of the atria and ventricles, and also provide a physical barrier to the propagation of the action potential between the atria and the ventricles
  - This 'insulating plane' thereby channels the action potential to the AV node
  - Defects in the annulus fibrosus may result in abnormalities of AV conduction, such as Wolff–Parkinson–White (WPW) syndrome

3.2.2 Atrioventricular node

- The AV node is a very compact mass (<5mm size) of specialized cardiac tissue that lies in the atrial septum, just above the coronary sinus opening.
- The AV node is normally the only means of conduction between the atria and ventricles.
- The AV node coordinates myocytic mechanical activity by delaying the received impulse from along the atrial internodal pathways by approximately 120ms. This delay provides 2 main functions:
  - Ensuring that atrial ejection is complete before the ventricular contraction
  - Protection from an excessively fast ventricular response to atrial arrhythmias
- The AV node also has the property of 'decremental conduction', meaning the more frequently the node is stimulated the slower it conducts. This property also prevents rapid conduction to the ventricle in cases of rapid atrial rhythms.
- The AV node is also innervated by parasympathetic and sympathetic nerve fibres:
  - Parasympathetic stimulation slows conduction, while sympathetic stimulation speeds it
  - The AV node's normal intrinsic rate without stimulation is 40–60 impulses/min

3.2.3 Propagatory fibres

- The distal portion of the AV node is known as the bundle of His.
- The bundle of His splits into 2 branches in the interventricular septum:
  - The left bundle branch and the right bundle branch, which pass on either side subendocardially
  - The left bundle branch further divides into anterior and posterior fascicles
- The Purkinje fibres spread from the end of the bundle branches and fascicles to the rest of the ventricles.
- This system conducts the cardiac impulse to the apex of the heart and thereby results in a depolarization wave outwards and upwards, encouraging upward expulsion of blood from the ventricles.

3.2.4 Basis of the electrocardiogram (ECG)

- The ECG may be thought of as a graphical representation of the electrical activity of the heart over time.
- Local electrical circuits produced by the spread of the action potential impulse may be measured at electrodes placed at specific points on the skin. The ECG then displays the voltage differences between pairs of these electrodes, which represent the muscle activity in different directions.
- These directions may also be referred to as vectors—see Figure D.3.3.
- A complete picture of the spread of excitation through the electrical conduction system of the heart and the myocardium may be gained by combining the graphical representations of a number of electrode placements (*leads*)—see Figure D.3.3.
- Lead arrangement:
  - Standard (bipolar) leads:
    - I = right arm ↔ left arm
    - II = left leg ↔ right arm
    - III = left leg ↔ left arm
  - Augmented unipolar leads:
    - aVR = right arm
    - aVL = left arm
    - aVF = left leg

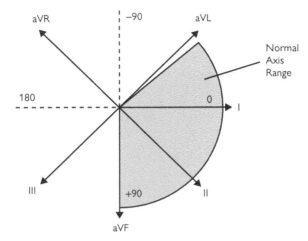

Figure D.3.3 Diagrammatic representation of ECG axis

- Unipolar chest leads (combined aV leads form reference electrode):
  - V_1 = 4th intercostal space, right sternal edge
  - V_2 = 4th intercostal space, left sternal edge
  - V_3 = midway between V_2 and V_4
  - V_4 = 5th intercostal space, left midclavicular line
  - V_5 = 5th intercostal space, left anterior axillary line
  - V_6 = 5th intercostal space, left midaxillary line
- Heart region representation by lead:
  - Inferior = aVF, II, and III
  - Anterolateral = aVL, I, and II
  - Right side = V_{1-2}
  - Septum = V_{3-4}
  - Left side = V_{5-6}

3.2.5 Normal ECG values and relevant calculations

- ECG should record patient's name, age, and the time/date of study.
- Usual speed of recording is 25mm/s.
- Standard calibration is 1mV/cm.
- Heart rate (HR): divide 300 by number of 5mm squares between QRS complexes.
- QTc: QT corrected for HR by dividing by square root of preceding R–R interval in seconds (*Bazett's formula*)—normal range = 350–430msec.
- Normal interval ranges:
  - PR 120–200msec
  - QRS 40–120msec
  - QTc 350–430msec

3.2.6 ECG interpretation

See Figure D.3.4.

- HR:
  - Normal range defined in adult as 60–100 beats/min

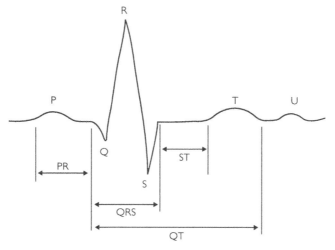

Figure D.3.4 ECG pattern

- ■ May be <50 beats/min in fit young subjects
- ■ Rate of 100 beats/min with loss of sympathetic and parasympathetic tone
- ● Rhythm features:
  - ■ Regular or irregular
  - ■ If irregular: may be irregularly irregular (e.g. atrial fibrillation, AF) or regularly irregular (e.g. 2 to 1 block)
  - ■ Presence or absence of P waves (i.e. AF):
    - ● In AF, ventricular rate depends upon conducting ability of AV node
    - ● P wave usually positive in I, II, and V_{4-6}
    - ● P wave usually negative in aVR
    - ● Normal P wave height < 2.5mm, width < 3mm
  - ■ Flutter waves with atrial flutter ('saw-tooth' appearance):
    - ● Caused by re-entrant circuit in atria
    - ● Rapid atrial discharge usually 300 beats/min
    - ● Commonly occurs with 4:1 or 2:1 AV block
    - ● Causes as for AF
  - ■ Atrial or ventricular ectopic beats
  - ■ Pacing spikes
- ● Axis:
  - ■ Represents the summation of electrical potentials from standard and aV leads, plotted as vectors (see Figure D.3.3)
  - ■ Normal axis lies between −30° and +90°
  - ■ Causes of left axis deviation (< −30°):
    - ● Normal in pregnancy, ascites
    - ● Left bundle branch block (LBBB)
    - ● Left anterior hemiblock
    - ● Left ventricular hypertrophy
  - ■ Causes of right axis deviation (> 90°):
    - ● May be normal finding
    - ● Right ventricular hypertrophy

- Right bundle branch block (RBBB)
- Left posterior hemiblock
- AV blocks:
  - 1st degree:
    - PR >0.2sec at normal HR
    - Usually clinically insignificant
    - May be caused by ageing, IHD, increased vagal tone, digoxin, cardiomyopathy, or myocarditis
  - 2nd degree (Mobitz type I—Wenckebach):
    - PR interval lengthens until complete AV block occurs
    - Usually due to AV conduction delay
    - Rarely progresses to complete heart block
  - 2nd degree (Mobitz type II):
    - Sudden block below AV node
    - May occur regularly (e.g. every 2nd complex)
    - Risk of developing complete heart block
  - 3rd degree (complete heart block):
    - At AV node or below—there is no continuity between atrial and ventricular contraction
    - ECG shows independent atrial and ventricular rhythms
    - Ventricular complexes usually wide and slow (rate <45 beats/min)
    - Caused by old age, ischaemic heart disease, myocarditis, cardiomyopathy, following cardiac surgery, increased vagal tone, digoxin, hyperkalaemia, or congenital abnormalities
- QRS complex:
  - Represents ventricular depolarization
  - Pathological Q waves: width >0.04sec and depth >4mm or >¼ of R-wave height in the same lead
  - QRS usually positive in I, II, and V_{4-6}
  - QRS usually negative in aVR and V_{1-2}
  - R-wave progression (smooth increase in amplitude from V_1 to V_6)
  - Left ventricular hypertrophy if R wave in V_6 + S wave in V_1 >35mm
  - Right ventricular hypertrophy if R:S ratio >1 in V_{1-2}
  - May be wide (>120msec) and is termed bundle branch block; due to problems with conduction of impulse down the His–Purkinje fibres
  - Extra waves:
    - J waves (positive deflection at end of QRS) seen in hypothermia
    - Delta waves seen in WPW syndrome (short PR interval and slurred upstroke of QRS)
    - U waves: positive deflection following T wave (slow repolarization of papillary muscle) made more prominent by hypokalaemia
- ST segment:
  - Usually level within 1mm of isoelectric line (between T and P wave)
  - Average duration 320msec
  - Pathological elevation:
    - Acute myocardial infarction (AMI)
    - Pericarditis
  - Pathological depression:
    - Myocardial ischaemia
    - Hypokalaemia
    - Digoxin therapy ('reverse tick')
    - Reciprocal leads following AMI
- T wave:
  - Represents ventricular repolarization

- Orientated as per QRS complexes
- Upper limit 5mm in standard leads, 10mm in chest leads
- Causes of T-wave inversion:
  - Myocardial ischaemia
  - Ventricular hypertrophy
  - Bundle branch block
  - Digoxin toxicity
- May be notched in pericarditis
- Tall peaked T waves suggest hyperkalaemia
- QT and QTc:
  - Measured from beginning of QRS to end of T wave
  - Represents duration of ventricular systole
  - Varies with heart rate, age, and gender
  - Corrected QT for heart rate (Bazett's formula—see Chapter D3, Section 3.2.5)
  - Shortened QTc:
    - Short QT syndrome (familial)
    - Hypercalcaemia
    - Hyperkalaemia
    - Digoxin therapy
  - Prolonged QTc:
    - Familial (e.g. Brugada syndrome, long QT syndromes)
    - Hypothyroidism
    - Hypokalaemia and hypocalcaemia
    - Hypothermia
    - Ischaemic heart disease
    - Tricyclic antidepressant toxicity
    - Other drugs including quinidine, amiodarone, phenothiazines, erythromycin, and non-sedating antihistamines

3.3 Cardiac cycle II

- The sequence of electrical and mechanical changes during the cardiac cycle is divided into 7 phases.
- Phase 1—atrial contraction:
  - 30% of ventricular filling occurs during this phase
  - Ventricular (end-diastolic) pressure at the end of atrial contraction sets the preload for the next ventricular contraction
  - ECG: PR interval and ends with the Q wave
- Phase 2—isometric ventricular contraction:
  - Starts with closing of tricuspid and mitral valves
  - Ventricular pressures exceed aortic and pulmonary artery pressures
  - Ventricular volume remains constant until ventricular ejection begins
  - Ends with opening of aortic and pulmonary valves
  - 1st heart sounds heard during phase 2 and 3
  - ECG: remaining ventricular depolarization (RS)
- Phase 3—rapid ventricular ejection:
  - Almost 70% of SV is ejected in the first one-third of systole
  - ECG: ST segment
- Phase 4—reduced ventricular ejection:
  - Ejection rate declines as ventricular and arterial pressures equalize

- Ends with closing of aortic and pulmonary valves
- ECG: T wave (repolarization)
- Phase 5—isometric ventricular relaxation:
  - Begins with closure of the aortic and pulmonary valves
  - Ventricular pressure falls below atrial pressure
  - Ends with opening of tricuspid and mitral valves
  - 2nd heart sound heard during phase 5
  - ECG: starts with end of T wave
- Phase 6—rapid ventricular filling:
  - Atrial pressure reaches its peak just as the AV valves reopen
  - Pressures in both the atrial and ventricular cavities fall as ventricles relax
  - Usually no ECG activity during phase 6, although U waves may be seen
- Phase 7—passive ventricular filling:
  - Atrial and ventricular pressures rise slowly as blood returns to the heart
  - ECG: marks the beginning of the next P wave

3.3.1 Normal intracardiac pressures

- Right atrium: 0–3mmHg
- Right ventricle (systolic): 15–30mmHg
- Right ventricle (diastolic): 2–8mmHg
- Pulmonary artery (systolic): 15–30mmHg
- Pulmonary artery (diastolic): 4–12mmHg
- Left atrium: 6–10mmHg
- Left ventricle (systolic): 100–140mmHg
- Left ventricle (diastolic): 3–12mmHg

3.3.2 Origin of heart sounds

- The 1st heart sound is due to closure of the AV valves (mitral and tricuspid):
  - It is louder in mitral stenosis, with a hyperdynamic circulation, and softer with mitral incompetence and severe heart failure
- The 2nd heart sound is due to closure of the semilunar valves (aortic and pulmonary):
  - It is louder in systemic or pulmonary hypertension and softer with aortic or pulmonary valve stenosis. Splitting of the 2nd heart sound may be caused by the following:
    - Physiological: effect of respiration
    - Fixed: increased volume load on right ventricle such as atrioseptal defect or pulmonary hypertension
    - Paradoxical: delayed or prolonged left ventricular systole (e.g. LBBB)
- 3rd heart sound heard early in diastole due to rapid filling of the left ventricle and may indicate constrictive pericarditis, or mitral or tricuspid incompetence.
- An abnormal 4th heart sound may be heard early in diastole due to forceful atrial contraction and ventricular distension, and may indicate hypertension, heart block, or myocardial infarction.

3.3.3 Venous pressure changes during cardiac cycle

- a wave: atrial systole. Increased with pulmonary hypertension, severe pulmonary stenosis, and tricuspid stenosis.
- c wave: bulging of tricuspid valve during ventricular contraction.
- v wave: rise in atrial pressure before tricuspid valve opens during diastole.
- x descent: drawing away of tricuspid valve during ventricular systole.
- y descent: fall in atrial pressure as blood enters ventricles. Deepened by high jugular venous pressures (e.g. constrictive pericarditis) and slowed by tricuspid stenosis.

3.4 Cardiac cycle III

3.4.1 Electrical basis of cardiac contractility

- Cell membrane potentials are determined primarily by 3 factors:
  - Concentration of ions on the inside and outside of the cell
  - Permeability of the cell membrane to those ions through specific ion channels
  - Activity of electrogenic pumps (e.g. Na^+/K^+-ATPase)
- The resting membrane potential of a ventricular myocyte is $-90mV$, which is near the equilibrium potential for K^+.
- The action potential of cardiac cells is divided into 5 phases (0–4)—see Figure D.3.5:
  - 0: rapid depolarization—rapid rise in sodium permeability (rise to $+20mV$)
  - 1: onset of repolarization—rapid fall in sodium permeability and small rise in potassium permeability
  - 2: plateau—due to increase in calcium permeability and the absence of any increase in potassium permeability
  - 3: repolarization—gradual increase in potassium permeability
  - 4: slow depolarization—restoration of resting potential by sodium/potassium exchange pumps
- The main determinant of the shape of the cardiac action potential, compared to that of neurons or skeletal myocytes, is changes in cell membrane permeability to both sodium and calcium ions.
- As the sodium concentration is higher outside the cell, sodium ions diffuse across the membrane down this chemical gradient.
  - During an action potential, the cell membrane becomes more permeable to sodium, which increases its entry into the cell through fast sodium channels
  - The sodium gradient is maintained by active transport out of the cell by energy-dependent Na^+/K^+-ATPase pumps
  - As these fast sodium channels become inactivated at peak depolarization there is a small efflux of potassium ions, producing the 'notch' at phase 1
- Like sodium, calcium also has a large chemical gradient across the cell membrane, and diffuses into the cells through calcium channels during the action potential:
  - The plateau of phase 2 is produced due to these slower calcium channels opening and holding the membrane voltage near the equilibrium potential even after the sodium channels have inactivated

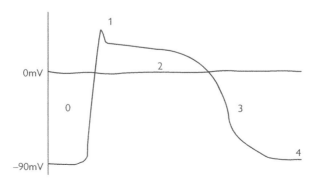

Figure D.3.5 Cardiac action potential

- This influx of calcium ions is balanced by the sustained slow movement of potassium out of the cell
- 2 voltage-dependent calcium channels are involved:
  - T-type (transient): initiates the action potential
  - L-type (long-lasting):
    - 'Voltage-gated'
    - Responding to higher membrane potentials
    - Slower opening and remain open longer than T-type channels
    - Sustains the action potential

3.4.2 SA node

- The action potentials of pacemaker cells (e.g. SA node) vary from other cardiac myocytes as follows:
  - Slow upstroke mediated by calcium channels
  - Smaller magnitude
  - Absence of fast sodium channels
  - Spontaneous depolarization during diastole (phase 4)
- Absence of fast sodium channels and implications of this:
  - Spontaneous depolarization of cardiac pacemaker cells is due to reduced cell membrane permeability to potassium while allowing the passive transfer of calcium ions
  - This allows a net charge to build via the relatively slow depolarizing calcium current rather than the fast sodium channels
  - This results in slower action potentials in terms of how rapidly they depolarize but produces automaticity by spontaneous depolarization
- Physiological basis of the pacemaker potential:
  - Pacemaker cells are characterized by having no true resting potential, but instead generate regular, spontaneous action potentials
  - SA nodal action potentials are divided into 3 phases—see Figure D.3.6
  - Phase 1—spontaneous depolarization (pacemaker potential):
    - Opening of slow sodium channels—'funny currents'
    - 'Transient' calcium channels open at around −50mV
    - Triggers the action potential at threshold (between −40 and −30mV)

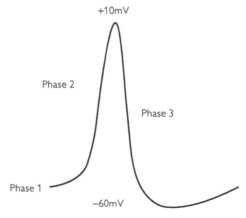

Figure D.3.6 Pacemaker action potential

- Phase 2—depolarization phase:
  - Increased calcium conductance through 'long-lasting' calcium channels
  - Sodium influx slows, 'transient' calcium channels close
- Phase 3—repolarization (−60mV):
  - Potassium channels open with increase in efflux
  - Calcium channels inactivated, slowing influx
  - Following this, the cycle is spontaneously repeated
- Effects of chronotropes upon potassium currents and hence rate of contraction:
  - The primary role of potassium channels in cardiac action potentials is cell repolarization
  - Potassium channels remain open until the next action potential is triggered
  - Therefore, agents that bind to and block the potassium channels will delay repolarization, leading to an increase in action potential duration and an increase in the effective refractory period (ERP)
  - Increasing the ERP causes suppression of tachyarrhythmias by preventing the re-emerging action potential from causing premature activation during the lengthened refractory phase
  - Potassium channel activation by parasympathetic muscarinic receptors also leads to a decrease in heart rate
  - Conversely, increasing activation of potassium channels will lead to a positive chronotropic effect by increasing the potassium current and speeding repolarization, thereby reducing the ERP.

3.4.3 Excitation–contraction (EC) coupling

- Fundamental role of calcium and its origin in sarcoplasmic reticulum:
  - Cardiac muscle contraction requires the presence of extracellular calcium ions
  - Influx of extracellular calcium ions through the L-type calcium channels leads to sustained depolarization of cardiac myocytes
  - Calcium-induced calcium release (CICR) from the sarcoplasmic reticulum must occur under normal EC coupling to cause contraction
  - As the intracellular concentration of calcium increases, calcium ions bind to the protein troponin, which initiates contraction by allowing the contractile proteins, myosin and actin, to associate through cross-bridge formation
- Sequestration of calcium via Ca-ATPase and sodium/calcium exchange pumps:
  - During relaxation, calcium ions are actively transported from the cytosol into the sarcoplasmic reticulum through the activity of a Ca^{2+}- and Mg^{2+}-dependent ATPase membrane and sodium/calcium exchange pumps
- Biochemical basis of the Treppe effect:
  - The Treppe effect (also known as the Bowditch effect) refers to the intrinsic regulatory mechanism whereby myocardial contractility increases with an increase in heart rate
  - The inability of the Na^+/K^+-ATPase pump system to maintain adequate influx of sodium at higher heart rates results in the accumulation of calcium in the myocytes (due to the sodium–calcium exchange system), thereby leading to an increased force of myocardial contraction

3.4.4 Effects of inotropes

- Effect of norepinephrine (noradrenaline) on calcium handling via β-receptors:
  - Norepinephrine enhances the activity of voltage-dependent calcium channels, this effect being mediated by β-adrenoceptors
  - β-adrenergic stimulation results in an increase in the intracellular concentration of cyclic AMP, which leads to phosphorylation of voltage-sensitive calcium channels in the myocardium

- During membrane depolarization this results in an increased influx of calcium across the sarcolemma, producing an increase in inotropy
- Effects of digoxin (via Na^+ pump) and of hypoxia (H^+/Ca^{2+} competition) on calcium handling:
  - The cardiac inotropic and bradycardic effects of digoxin are mediated by its inhibition of the Na^+/K^+-ATPase pump:
    - This induces a rise in sodium concentration inside myocytes, which in turn results in an increase in the intracellular calcium concentration via the sodium–calcium exchanger
    - This rise in intracellular calcium increases the force of contraction
  - Na^+/K^+-ATPase is the main route for Na^+ extrusion from cardiac myocytes and is a primary regulator under physiological conditions:
    - Early during ischaemia there is a rise in intracellular Na^+ concentration, mediated by Na^+/H^+ exchange and Na^+ channel entry
    - As with cardiac glycosides, this contributes to the increased sarcoplasmic reticulum Ca^{2+} content, larger Ca^{2+} transients, and thereby a positive inotropic effect
    - Intracellular protons strongly inhibit Na^+/Ca^{2+} exchange activity by competitive binding at regulatory sites, thereby causing a rise in intracellular calcium

3.5 Cardiac output

3.5.1 Relation of cardiac output, heart rate, and stroke volume

- Cardiac output (CO) is the volume of blood pumped from one side of the heart per minute, usually referring to the left ventricle, and is measured in L/min.
- **CO = stroke volume (SV) × heart rate (HR)**:
  - SV = end-diastolic volume (EDV) − end-systolic volume (ESV), representing the volume of blood ejected with each contraction
  - SV generally varies from 70 to 120mL
  - In comparison, HR can vary between 60 and 180 beats/min
  - Therefore, most of the increases in CO can be attributed to an increase in HR
- The main determinants of CO include myocardial contractility, preload, and afterload.
- Myocardial contractility:
  - Contractility is the force of myocardial contraction, determining stroke volume and cardiac output as well as myocardial oxygen demand
  - Extrinsic inotropic factors will affect contractility, i.e. positive inotropic factors increase contractility
  - Positive inotropic factors:
    - Increased sympathetic nervous system action
    - Circulating catecholamines
    - Inotropic drugs (such as digoxin, levothyroxine)
  - Negative inotropic factors:
    - Increased parasympathetic nervous system action (mild effect)
    - Hypoxia and hypercapnia
    - Acidosis and alkalosis
    - Hyperkalaemia, hypocalcaemia
    - Drugs (such as most anaesthetic agents, antiarrhythmic agents)
  - Intrinsic mechanisms also affect CO, for example, cardiac filling, or the presence of cardiac disease such as cardiomyopathy or ischaemic heart disease
- Preload:
  - Preload represents end-diastolic ventricular wall tension, itself inferred from ventricular end-diastolic pressure, which approximates to:

- Central venous pressure (CVP)—right side of the heart
- Pulmonary capillary wedge pressure (PCWP)—left side of the heart
■ Ventricular end-diastolic pressure is determined by:
  - Blood volume
  - Venous tone
  - Gravity
  - Respiratory and muscle pumps
■ It is related to myocardial contractility and CO by Starling's law (see Chapter D3, Section 3.5.2).
- Afterload:
  ■ Afterload is the ventricular wall tension required to eject the SV during systole.
  ■ It is represented by the arterial blood pressure and is determined by CO and total peripheral resistance.
  ■ SV is inversely proportional to afterload when the preload and contractility are constant.
  ■ Left ventricular afterload is increased by:
    - Anatomical obstructions (such as aortic valve stenosis)
    - Raised systemic vascular resistance
    - Decreased aortic and large vessel elasticity
    - Increased ventricular volume (Laplace's law)

3.5.2 Frank–Starling relation between stroke volume and end-diastolic volume

- Starling curve (*Frank–Starling mechanism*)—see Figure D.3.7:
  ■ Starling's law describes the intrinsic cardiac relationship between preload (thereby related to EDV) and SV
  ■ In general terms, the force developed in a muscle fibre depends upon the degree to which that fibre is stretched
  ■ As applied to cardiac function, the initial fibre length is represented by left ventricular EDV (several assumptions are made about the 3D shape of the ventricle)
  ■ The force of myocardial contraction is therefore proportional to initial fibre length
  ■ However, contractility falls when the EDV rises beyond a certain threshold
  ■ Preload influences contractile force by increasing the sarcomere length, which then increases troponin C calcium sensitivity and the rate of cross-bridge attachment and detachment
  ■ The amount of tension developed by the muscle fibre is therefore increased (EC coupling)

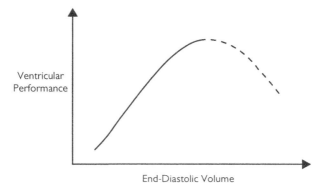

Figure D.3.7 Starling curve

- The effect of increased sarcomere length on the contractile proteins is termed length-dependent activation
- Changes in contractility will shift the curve's position; for instance, in cardiac failure the curve is moved downwards, while positive inotropy moves the curve upwards
- Shifts along a curve may be induced by a fluid bolus (to the right) or by vasodilators (to the left)
- In summary, changes in venous return cause the ventricle to move along a single Frank–Starling curve that is defined by the existing conditions of afterload and inotropy

3.5.3 Implications of imbalance in the Starling relationship—pulmonary oedema

- The normal ventricle is capable of increasing its stroke volume to match physiological increases in venous return:
  - However, this is not the case in heart failure
  - The loss of cardiac inotropy (i.e. decreased contractility) causes a downward shift in the Frank–Starling curve and a decrease in stroke volume
  - In an attempt to shift the curve to the right, there is a compensatory rise in preload (e.g. ventricular end-diastolic pressure or pulmonary capillary wedge pressure)
  - Stroke volume falls, leading to an increase in end-systolic volume
  - If the left ventricle is involved, then left atrial and pulmonary venous pressures will also rise, which may lead to pulmonary oedema
  - If the right ventricle is involved, the increase in end-diastolic pressure will be reflected back into the right atrium and systemic venous vasculature, leading to peripheral oedema and ascites

3.5.4 Baroreceptors as a determinant of CVP upon standing to correct the Starling relationship

- A change in posture from supine to standing results in a fall in cardiac output, as CVP drops from gravitational venous pooling and a subsequent decrease in stroke volume due to the Starling relationship.
- This fall in cardiac output is detected as a fall in blood pressure by cardiovascular baroreceptors.

3.5.5 Control of blood pressure

- Afferent control:
  - Baroreceptors (stretch receptors) in walls of aortic arch and carotid sinus respond to distension caused by increases in BP
  - Rate of receptor discharge increased by rise in BP, and increased rate of rise
  - Impulses via glossopharyngeal nerve (carotid sinus) and vagus (aortic arch)
  - Atrial stretch receptors discharge during diastolic distension (e.g. from increased venous return or during positive pressure ventilation) and this results in reduced sympathetic activity and inhibition of vasopressin release
- Central control:
  - Vasomotor centre:
    - Neurons in ventrolateral medulla
    - Control of arterial BP
    - Sympathetic preganglionic neurons in spinal cord
    - Normal continuous discharge provides resting vasomotor tone
  - Cardioinhibitory centre:
    - Mainly nucleus ambiguous and ventral medulla
    - Some input from dorsal motor nucleus and tractus solitarius

- Stimulated by increased baroreceptor discharge
- Receives afferents from higher centre
- Inhibits the vasomotor centre
- Produces resting vagal tone (via vagus nerve)
- Increased BP therefore inhibits vasomotor centre activity and will decrease BP, while stimulating the cardioinhibitory centre and reducing HR
- The reverse occurs with a fall in BP
- Pain and emotion leads to increased vasomotor centre activity, although the reverse occurs from prolonged pain and emotion
- Hypoxia will initially stimulate the vasomotor centre, but depression will rapidly follow if hypoxia is sustained
- Efferent control:
  - Efferent fibres of the sympathetic system emerge from spinal segments T1–L2 and pass via white ramus communicans into the sympathetic trunk at each level
  - Innervation of the heart is via the cardiac plexus
  - Stimulation of the sympathetic system results in tachycardia, increased myocardial contractility, and increased velocity of cardiac contraction
  - Relevant cervical ganglia include:
    - Superior (C2–3): superior cardiac nerve, internal carotid plexus
    - Middle (C6): middle cardiac nerve
    - Inferior (C7): inferior cardiac nerve, often fused as stellate ganglion
  - The vagus nerves carry the efferent parasympathetic fibres that innervate the heart, as well as many other organs
  - Stimulation of the parasympathetic system results in bradycardia and reduced velocity of cardiac contraction

3.5.6 Implications of the Starling relationship for increased afterload

- The pressure that the ventricle generates during systolic ejection is very close to aortic pressure (unless aortic stenosis is present).
- Afterload is increased when aortic pressure and systemic vascular resistance are increased.
- The ejection velocity after aortic valve opening is reduced because the velocity of cardiac fibre contraction is decreased and, as there is only a finite time period for electrical and mechanical systole, less blood is ejected.
- This results in an increase in end-systolic volume leading to a decrease in stroke volume.
- The Starling curve is therefore shifted downwards and to the right.
- Conversely, a decrease in afterload shifts the Frank–Starling curve upwards and to the left.

3.6 Peripheral vascular physiology I

3.6.1 Basis of vasoconstriction

- Appreciation of the role of G-protein mediated changes in intracellular calcium levels:
  - G-proteins (guanine nucleotide binding proteins) are cell membrane proteins that mediate the intracellular responses to activation of neighbouring surface receptors
  - Following receptor activation GDP is displaced by GTP causing splitting of the G-protein into its α and β subunits. The α subunit then initiates the relevant intracellular response
  - α_1-adrenoceptor activity involves a G-protein mediated signal transduction cascade, which increases the intracellular calcium ion concentration via the following steps:
    - Activation of phospholipase C (PLC)

- PLC cleaves phosphatidylinositol 4,5-bisphosphate (PIP2)
- Increase in inositol triphosphate (IP3) and diacylglycerol (DAG)
- IP3-mediated calcium release from the sarcoplasmic reticulum
- IP3-mediated calcium channel influx across the sarcolemma
  - As intracellular levels rise, calcium ions form complexes with calmodulin, which in turn activate myosin light chain kinase
  - This is responsible for phosphorylating the light chain of myosin to stimulate cross-bridge cycling and smooth muscle contraction via the sliding filament mechanism in order to produce vasoconstriction
- Effect of calcium-channel blocking drugs upon vasoconstriction:
  - Calcium channel blockers inhibit the movement of calcium ions into the cell by blocking voltage-gated calcium channels in both cardiac myocytes and blood vessels
  - As well as the direct negative chronotropic and inotropic effects on the heart, this also results in less contraction of arterial vascular smooth muscle
  - The subsequent vasodilation leads to a fall in total peripheral resistance, while a decrease in cardiac contractility decreases cardiac output

3.6.2 Endothelial function as a source of vasoactive mediators

- Endothelium releases various vasoactive mediators in order to modulate the vasomotor tone induced by the sympathetic system and other substances in order to maintain vascular homeostasis.
- Nitric oxide (NO) is the major endothelium-derived vasodilator.
- Prostacyclin (PGI2) and a theoretical substance named endothelium-derived hyperpolarizing factor (EDHF) also have a role.
- NO:
  - Synthesized in endothelial cells during oxidation of L-arginine to L-citrulline, catalysed by nitric oxide synthase (NOS)
  - 2 isoforms: cNOS and iNOS
  - Activates guanylate cyclase, which converts guanosine triphosphate (GTP) into cyclic guanosine monophosphate (cGMP) in vascular smooth muscle, causing relaxation
- Prostacyclin (PGI2):
  - Prostacyclin is produced in endothelial cells from prostaglandin H2 (PGH2) by the action of the enzyme prostacyclin synthase
  - Acts as a potent paracrine vasodilator
  - Acts within homeostatic mechanism in balance with thromboxane (TXA2) in relation to vascular damage
  - Binds to endothelial prostacyclin receptors and raises cAMP levels in the cytosol, leading to activation of protein kinase A (PKA)
  - PKA causes smooth muscle relaxation and vasodilation by phosphorylating and inhibiting myosin light-chain kinase
- Endothelium-derived hyperpolarizing factors (EDHF):
  - EDHF is proposed to be a substance and/or electrical signal generated by or synthesized in and released from the endothelium
  - Mechanism is to hyperpolarize vascular smooth muscle cells, causing vasodilation
  - Thought to involve the activation of endothelial K$^+$ channels
  - Effect appears to be greatest at level of small arteries

3.6.3 Endothelial function as stimulus to endothelial secretion

- Nitric oxide (NO):
  - NO is continually produced by cNOS under normal basal conditions—activity relies upon presence of calcium and calmodulin
  - Local shearing forces stimulate cNOS activity by release of calcium

- Calcium release also stimulated by Ach, bradykinin, substance-P, and adenosine
- iNOS activity is calcium independent, basal activity is very low
- Inflammatory processes stimulate iNOS activity (e.g. cytokines and interleukins)—may have 1000-fold activity compared to cNOS
- Prostacyclin (PGI2):
  - Production stimulated by local factors including endothelial trauma, thrombin, trypsin, and arachidonic acid
  - Effect may be augmented by additional substrate production by platelets
- Endothelium-derived hyperpolarizing factors (EDHF):
  - Release appears to be stimulated by local factors such as oxidative stress
  - Suggested as a 'backup mechanism' for endothelium-dependent relaxation in the presence of compromised NO contribution

3.7 Peripheral vascular physiology II

3.7.1 Overview of the structure of the microcirculation

- Terminal arterioles:
  - Small vessels (10–50µm) composed of an endothelium layer surrounded by one or more layers of smooth muscle cells
  - Highly responsive to sympathetic vasoconstriction via both α_1- and α_2-adrenoceptors
  - Vital component of the regulation of systemic vascular resistance
  - Spontaneous vasomotion may occur (rhythmical contraction and relaxation)
  - Primary function is flow regulation in organ tissue
  - Involved in regulation of capillary hydrostatic pressure and therefore influence capillary fluid exchange
- Capillaries:
  - Small vessels (6–10µm) composed of highly attenuated endothelial cells surrounded by basement membrane—no smooth muscle
  - Primary site of exchange for fluid, electrolytes, gases, and macromolecules due to large surface area and relatively high permeability (especially at intercellular clefts)
  - Precapillary sphincters (a circular band of smooth muscle at entrance to capillaries) can regulate the number of perfused capillaries in some organs
  - Classified into 3 types by structure:
    - Continuous: continuous basement membrane with intercellular clefts and tight junctions resulting in lowest permeability of capillaries (found in muscle, skin, lung, and CNS)
    - Fenestrated: fenestrated endothelium with relatively high permeability (found in exocrine glands, renal glomeruli, and intestinal mucosa)
    - Discontinuous: large intercellular and basement membrane gaps result in extremely high permeability (found in liver, spleen, and bone marrow)
- Lymphatic capillaries:
  - Composed of endothelium with intercellular gaps surrounded by highly permeable basement membrane
  - Similar in size to venules—terminal lymphatics end as blind sacs
  - Larger lymphatic vessels also have smooth muscle cells
  - Spontaneous and stretch-activated vasomotion is present, which serves to 'pump' the lymph proximally
  - Sympathetic activity modulates vasomotion and causes contraction
  - Valves ensure lymph is directed into the systemic circulation via the thoracic duct and subclavian veins

- Postcapillary venules:
  - Small exchange vessels (10–50µm) composed of endothelial cells surrounded by basement membrane
  - Larger venules also have smooth muscle
  - Fluid and macromolecular exchange occurs mostly at venular junctions
  - Sympathetic innervation of larger venules can alter vasomotor tone, which plays a role in regulating capillary hydrostatic pressure

3.7.2 Transcapillary exchange

- There are 2 primary fluid compartments in the body between which fluid, electrolytes, and small molecular weight solutes are readily exchanged:
  - The intravascular compartment consists of the blood within the cardiac chambers and vascular system of the body
  - The extravascular compartment consists of everything outside of the intravascular compartment. Subcompartments of the extravascular compartment include:
    - Intracellular
    - Interstitial
    - Lymphatic
    - CSF
- Transcapillary exchange relates to the movement of fluid, electrolytes, and other small molecular weight solutes between the tissue (interstitial) and the capillary (vascular) compartments.
- Movement of these is governed by several factors including oncotic pressure, hydrostatic pressure, membrane permeability, active transport mechanisms, presence of lipophilia/hydrophilia, and solute molecular size.
- The main determinants of fluid flow across capillary walls are oncotic pressure and hydrostatic pressure.
- Capillary hydrostatic pressure (P_C):
  - This pressure drives fluid out of the capillary and is highest at the arteriolar end of the capillary and lowest at the venular end
  - The usual pressure gradient (organ dependent) is 15–30mmHg
  - The average capillary hydrostatic pressure is determined by arterial and venous pressures (P_A and P_V), and by the ratio of post-to-precapillary resistances (R_V/R_A)
  - P_C is influenced more greatly by changes in P_V than by changes in P_A
- Tissue (interstitial) pressure (P_i):
  - This pressure is determined by the interstitial fluid volume and by the tissue compliance and is normally near to zero
  - Tissue compliance is generally low although small increases in tissue volume that may occur during states of enhanced filtration or lymphatic blockage can result in dramatic increases in P_i
- Capillary plasma oncotic pressure (π_C):
  - The osmotic pressure within the capillary is principally determined by plasma proteins that are relatively impermeable
  - Therefore, this pressure is referred to as the 'oncotic' pressure or 'colloid osmotic' pressure because it is generated by colloids
  - Albumin generates about 70% of the oncotic pressure, typically 25–30mmHg
  - The oncotic pressure increases along the length of the capillary, particularly in capillaries having high net filtration (e.g. in renal glomerular capillaries), because the filtering fluid leaves behind proteins leading to an increase in protein concentration

- The effects of capillary membrane permeability on the physiological oncotic pressure are determined by the reflection coefficient (σ) of the capillary wall:
  - If the capillary is impermeable to protein then $\sigma = 1$
  - If the capillary is freely permeable to protein then $\sigma = 0$
  - Continuous capillaries have a high σ (>0.9), whereas discontinuous capillaries have a very low σ
  - In the latter case, plasma and tissue oncotic pressures may have a negligible influence on the net driving force
- Tissue (interstitial) oncotic pressure (π_i):
  - The oncotic pressure of the interstitial fluid depends on the interstitial protein concentration and the reflection coefficient of the capillary wall
  - The more permeable the capillary barrier is to proteins, the higher the interstitial oncotic pressure
  - This pressure is also determined by the amount of fluid filtration into the interstitium
  - Tissue oncotic pressure is usually around 5mmHg
- The Starling equation describes the relationship between hydrostatic pressure, oncotic pressure, and fluid flow across a capillary membrane (see Chapter D3, Section 3.7.5).

3.7.3 Movement of lipophilic and hydrophilic substances

- Lipophilic:
  - Uncharged lipophilic molecules may cross a cell membrane simply by passing through its lipid core, for example, the gases oxygen and carbon dioxide
  - Polar lipophilic molecules, such as water, pass through intermolecular pores
- Hydrophilic:
  - Non-lipid-soluble, hydrophilic molecules must cross the membrane by interaction with specialized carrier or channel proteins
  - These include glucose, amino acids, and all ions (e.g. Na^+, K^+, Cl^-, HCO_3^-).

3.7.4 Role of tight junctions, glycocalyx, and pores in determining selective passage

- Tight junctions:
  - These intercellular structures prevent the passage of molecules and ions through the space between cells
  - This ensures that substances must enter the cells (either by diffusion or active transport) in order to pass through tissue
  - Epithelium may be classed as 'tight' or 'leaky' depending on the ability of the tight junctions to prevent water and solute movement
- Glycocalyx:
  - A glycocalyx (literally 'sugar coat') is made up of a network of polysaccharides that project from cellular surfaces
  - Its established roles include reducing friction to the flow of blood and serving as a barrier to loss of fluid through the vessel wall
  - The endothelial cell wall glycocalyx is sheared off in the presence of inflammatory response in order to permit attachment of leucocytes and movement of water from capillaries and other microvessels
- Pores:
  - The 'small pore' system ensures that substances greater than 10 000 daltons (such as plasma proteins) are prevented from diffusing across the capillary membrane
  - Another specialized form of pore protein structure is aquaporin, a cell membrane channel that regulates the flow of water, which is primarily found in renal tissue

3.7.5 Filtration

- The movement of fluid and accompanying solutes between compartments (mostly water, electrolytes, and smaller molecular weight solutes) is governed by hydrostatic and oncotic forces.
- These forces are normally balanced in such a manner that fluid volume remains relatively constant between the compartments (see Figure D.3.8).
- There are 2 important and opposing hydrostatic forces: capillary hydrostatic pressure (P_C) and tissue interstitial pressure (P_i).
- Because P_C is normally much greater than P_i the net hydrostatic pressure gradient across the capillary is positive, meaning that hydrostatic forces are driving fluid out of the capillary and into the interstitial compartment.
- There are also 2 opposing oncotic pressures influencing fluid exchange: capillary plasma oncotic pressure (π_C) and tissue (interstitial) oncotic pressure (π_i).
- As π_C is much greater than π_i the oncotic pressure gradient across the capillary, if unopposed by hydrostatic forces, will result in re-absorption of fluid from the interstitium into the capillary.
- The oncotic pressure difference ($\pi_C - \pi_i$) is dependent upon the reflection coefficient (σ) that represents the permeability of the capillary barrier to the proteins responsible for generating the oncotic pressure.
- Both hydrostatic and oncotic forces are normally expressed in units of mmHg.
- The net driving force (NDF) for fluid movement is the net pressure gradient determined by the sum of the individual hydrostatic and oncotic pressures.
- A positive NDF represents filtration and a negative NDF represents re-absorption.
- In most vascular beds, filtration occurs across the arteriolar end of the capillary and re-absorption occurs across the venular end.
- In general, there is a small net filtration across capillary beds (i.e. filtration > re-absorption).
- This excess is absorbed and removed by the lymphatic system.
- The kidneys are an exception in that renal glomerular capillaries filter large amounts of fluid along their entire length.
- Net fluid movement (J_V) is described by the Starling equation: $J_V = K_F\,[(P_C - P_i) - \sigma(\pi_C - \pi_i)]$
  - Where: NDF $= (P_C - P_i) - \sigma(\pi_C - \pi_i)$; and K_F = filtration constant

3.7.6 Role of interstitial oncotic pressure and capillary hydrostatic pressure

- Interstitial oncotic pressure is the force produced by interstitial proteins, which favours movement of fluid from the vascular compartment (capillary exchange vessel) into the interstitial compartment.
- Capillary hydrostatic pressure is the force by which fluid is driven along the pressure gradient from the vascular compartment into the interstitium.

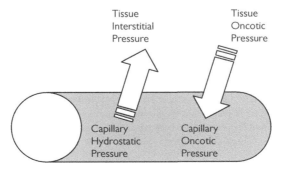

Figure D.3.8 Transcapillary flow of fluid

- Together these 2 forces may be referred to as 'outward pressures' influencing fluid movement out of the exchange vessel.
- These forces are usually predominant at the arterial end of the capillary, resulting in flow of fluid into the interstitial space.

3.7.7 Physiological basis of the net filtration of water within a capillary bed

- At the arterial end of the capillary, net intracapillary hydrostatic pressure exceeds the net interstitial oncotic pressure leading to the movement of fluid out of capillaries.
- At a variable point between the arterial end and venous end of the capillary these forces are in balance and there is no movement of fluid.
- As effective hydrostatic pressure falls towards the venous end, it is exceeded by the net plasma oncotic pressure resulting re-absorption.
- In most capillary systems of the body, there is a small net filtration (typically about 10%) of fluid from the intravascular to the extravascular compartment.

3.7.8 Clinical effects of poor endothelial quality, low oncotic pressure, and high venous pressure

- These are the typical factors that result in tissue oedema.
- A fall in endothelial quality (e.g. inflammation or ischaemia) will result in an increase in capillary permeability.
- A rise in venous pressure is readily transmitted back to the capillary, leading to a rise in capillary hydrostatic pressure.
- When combined with a low oncotic pressure this will lead to a rise in the NDF, causing more fluid to pass into the interstitial space.
- If the rise in interstitial fluid overwhelms the lymphatic capacity to transport this excess then tissue oedema will result.

3.7.9 Role of lymphatics

- There is around a 10% net filtration of fluid into the interstitial space from capillaries.
- The lymphatic system is responsible for removing this excess fluid and returning it to the intravascular compartment.
- If an imbalance occurs where net filtration exceeds the capacity of the lymphatics, then oedema will result.
- Lymph is formed when interstitial fluid enters the initial lymphatic vessels of the lymphatic system.
- This is moved along the lymphatic vessel network by either intrinsic contractions of the lymphatic vessels or by extrinsic compression of the lymphatic vessels via external tissue forces (e.g. the contractions of skeletal muscles).
- Other roles of the lymphatic system are to:
  - Absorb and transport fatty acids and fats as chyle to the circulatory system
  - Transport immune cells to and from the lymph nodes
  - Transport antigen-presenting cells to the lymph nodes
  - Carry lymphocytes from the efferent lymphatics exiting the lymph nodes
- Around 8L of fluid is filtered by the microcirculation and returned to the intravascular space by the lymphatic system per day.

3.8 Peripheral vascular physiology III

- Peripheral resistance is mainly determined by arteriolar vessel calibre—small changes lead to large changes in resistance.
- Arteriolar vasoconstriction leads to an increase in peripheral resistance while venous vasoconstriction leads to an increased stroke volume and cardiac output.

- Normal systemic vascular resistance is 700–1600 dyn/sec/cm^5.
- α-adrenergic receptors—vasoconstriction of most vessels
- β-adrenergic receptors—vasodilation of muscle and visceral arterioles
- Dopamine receptors—vasodilation of renal and splanchnic vessels
- Factors causing vasoconstriction:
  - Increased sympathetic tone
  - Increased circulating catecholamines
  - Angiotensin II
  - Vasopressin
  - Serotonin (inflammatory response, acts in some vascular beds)
  - Endothelin (response to mechanical/chemical stress, e.g. hypoxia)
  - Decreased local temperature
- Factors causing vasodilation:
  - Decreased sympathetic tone
  - Increased PCO$_2$
  - Decreased PO$_2$ (hypoxia causes vasoconstriction in lungs)
  - Acidosis
  - Increased local temperature
  - ANP
  - Endothelium-dependent vasodilation
  - NO

3.8.1 Local control of blood flow

- Autoregulation is a manifestation of local blood flow regulation and is defined as the intrinsic ability of an organ to maintain a constant blood flow despite changes in perfusion pressure.
- Autoregulation can occur in the absence of any neural and hormonal influences.
- When blood flow falls, arterial resistance will fall as the resistance vessels (small arteries and arterioles) dilate.
- Metabolic, myogenic, and endothelial mechanisms are responsible for this vasodilation.
- Range of pressures within which autoregulation occurs:
  - The lower limit of perfusion pressure for autoregulation of blood flow to occur is around 50–70mmHg, depending upon the organ, due to maximal vasodilation
  - Below this perfusion pressure, blood flow decreases passively in response to further reductions in perfusion pressure
  - Although there is a theoretical upper limit to the autoregulatory range, this is seldom reached physiologically. However, some texts state an upper limit of 160–170mmHg in normotensive subjects
  - Different organs have different autoregulatory limits and degrees of autoregulatory control:
    - Renal, cerebral, and coronary circulations all show excellent autoregulation, whereas skeletal muscle and splanchnic circulations show moderate autoregulation capacity
    - Skin shows little or no autoregulatory capacity
- Basis of the myogenic regulatory response and the effects of local vasodilatory factors:
  - The myogenic regulatory response theory postulates that vascular smooth muscle myocytes depolarize when stretched, leading to vasoconstriction as intraluminal pressure rises—as per Laplace's law
  - This effect is mediated by stretch-activated calcium channels
  - Conversely, a drop in pressure within the vessel will cause relaxation and vasodilation
  - Myogenic mechanisms are seen particularly in small arteries and arterioles. Although this effect has not been clearly identified in all vascular beds, it has been noted in the splanchnic and renal circulations and may be present to a small degree in skeletal muscle
  - Myogenic mechanisms may also contribute to the effect of reactive hyperaemia in some tissues

- Role of potassium, carbon dioxide, and adenosine in metabolic hyperaemia:
  - Active hyperaemia is a term used to describe dilatation of arteriolar smooth muscle to increase blood flow in response to an increase in metabolism and release of local vasoactive substances
  - Active hyperaemia is also influenced by competing vasoconstrictor mechanisms such as sympathetic stimulation which will reduce maximal hyperaemia
  - The most important of these include potassium, carbon dioxide, and adenosine
  - Potassium:
    - Released from active tissues and from ischaemia
    - Its effects of vasodilation are in part due to activity on Na^+ pumps and Ca^{2+} efflux, but also by hyperpolarization of myocytes
  - Carbon dioxide:
    - Induces vasodilation mediated by NO production and inhibition of Ca^{2+} cellular influx
  - Adenosine:
    - A potent vasodilator released from cardiac, skeletal, and brain tissue during periods of hypoxia and increased metabolism
    - It is produced from adenosine monophosphate and stimulates production of cAMP in smooth muscle
- Effects of inflammatory mediators in altering microcirculatory dynamics:
  - Autocoids (local hormones) cause vasodilation and increased vascular permeability in order to allow access of leucocytes and antibodies to tissues
  - These include histamine and bradykinin
  - Platelet activation induces vasoconstriction by the action of serotonin and thromboxane A_2, in order to reduce blood loss during clotting cascade

3.8.2 Pulmonary flow

- Mean pulmonary arterial pressure is 12–15mmHg while left atrial pressure is around 5mmHg, resulting in a pressure gradient across the pulmonary circulation of 7–10mmHg.
- Pulmonary vascular resistance (PVR) is around one-tenth that of the systemic circulation and is distributed more evenly with around 50% in the arteries and arterioles, 30% in capillaries, and 20% in veins.
- The pulmonary circulation lies in series with the systemic circulation, therefore receiving the whole cardiac output.
- The total gas exchange capillary surface area is around 70m^2.
- A separate bronchial circulation supplies the airways, local connective tissue, and visceral pleura, draining into the pulmonary veins via the azygos system, thereby representing an anatomical shunt.
- Extra-alveolar vessel diameter is mainly affected by lung volume.
- Alveolar vessel blood flow depends upon arterial, venous, and alveolar pressures, as well as gravity.
- Pulmonary blood flow is influenced by the following factors:
  - Sympathetic and parasympathetic activity
  - PVR is increased by both low and high extremes of lung volumes
  - PVR is lowest when lung volume is at functional residual capacity (FRC)
  - Increased cardiac output with reduced PVR
  - Gravity and posture
  - Vasomotor tone is minimal due to maximal dilatation in the resting state
  - Blood viscosity
  - Local changes:
    - Hypoxic pulmonary vasoconstriction
    - Hypercapnia and acidosis increase PVR

- Therapeutic agents (e.g. vasoconstrictor agents)
- Pulmonary embolus, trauma/surgery, atelectasis, or pleural effusion
- The pulmonary circulation acts in the manner of a vascular capacitor during postural changes; falls in pulmonary blood volume of around 25–40% are observed when moving from a supine to a standing position.
- Hypoxic pulmonary vasoconstriction:
  - This mechanism, whereby small arteries constrict in response to hypoxia, is unique to lung tissue as hypoxia usually causes vasodilation in systemic arteries.
  - This results in the diversion of blood away from poorly ventilated areas of the lung and optimizing of ventilation–perfusion matching.

3.8.3 Cutaneous flow

- Role of arteriovenous anastomoses in thermoregulation:
  - Thermoregulation is the main function of the cutaneous circulation. Arterioles and venules are linked by arteriovenous anastomoses (AVAs), which provides a high blood flow into the venous plexus and thereby the radiation of heat
  - These are found mainly in the skin of the hands, feet, and face
  - A fall in core temperature will be detected by the hypothalamus and causes sympathetic stimulation, which results in cutaneous vasoconstriction and a reduction of cutaneous blood flow
- Contributory factors to enhanced local blood flow:
  - The net increase in cutaneous blood flow may be up to 30 times normal
  - A rise in core temperature causes vasodilation due to decreased vasomotor tone, thereby increasing cutaneous blood flow
  - Local release of endothelium-dependent vasodilators will also cause cutaneous vasodilation
  - For example, the release of bradykinin is promoted by the sympathetic cholinergic pathway as part of the sweating mechanism

3.8.4 Coronary flow

- Cardiac tissue has a high metabolic demand.
- Normal myocardial O_2 consumption is around 30mL/min and normal coronary blood flow is around 200mL/min at rest, representing about 5% of the CO.
- This may increase up to 5 times during exercise.
- As O_2 extraction from blood is unusually high at around 70%, increased O_2 demands must be met by increased blood flow.
- Metabolic hyperaemia (see Chapter D3, Section 3.8.1) is the main mechanism responsible for intrinsic coronary blood flow regulation to maximize oxygen uptake, aided by a dense capillary network.
- This process overrides vasomotor tone mediated by the sympathetic system.
- Circulating epinephrine also causes vasodilation via β_2-adrenoceptors.
- Cardiac muscle is well adapted to be resistant to fatigue although it relies heavily upon aerobic metabolism.
- At basal metabolic rates, about 1% of energy is derived from anaerobic metabolism.
- This can increase to 10% under moderately hypoxic conditions.
- Under basal aerobic conditions, 60% of energy comes from free fatty acids and triglycerides, 35% from carbohydrates, and 5% from amino acids and ketone bodies.
- Left ventricular coronary flow only occurs during diastole, as ventricular pressure is greater than aortic pressure during systole.
- Coronary flow to the right ventricle and atrium occurs during both systole and diastole.

- Left ventricular coronary blood flow is influenced by the following factors:
  - The difference between aortic end-diastolic pressure and left ventricular end-diastolic pressure
  - Duration of diastole (inversely proportional to HR)
  - Patency of the coronary arteries (e.g. thrombosis)
  - Diameter of the coronary arteries (e.g. spasm, stenosis)
  - Autoregulation usually maintains flow above a MAP of 60mmHg
  - Therapeutic agents such as GTN
  - Blood viscosity
- Autonomic neural activity has little direct effect on coronary arteries.

3.8.5 Brain circulation

- Normal cerebral blood flow (CBF) is 700 mL/min, representing about 15% of the CO.
- CBF is influenced by the following factors (see Figure D.3.9):
  - Arterial PCO_2:
    - Hypercapnia increases CBF by vasodilation
    - A reduction of PCO_2 from 5.3 to 4.0kPa decreases CBF by 30%
  - Arterial PO_2: hypoxia reduces CBF (minimal effect until <6.7kPa)
  - Cerebral metabolic rate for oxygen ($CMRO_2$)
  - Cerebral perfusion pressure (CPP): autoregulation at MAP of 60–160mmHg
  - Intracranial pressure (ICP): relationship CPP = MAP − ICP
  - Autoregulation is impaired with cerebral disease or trauma
  - Sympathetic and parasympathetic activity appear to have little effect
  - Hypothermia reduces CBF by 5% per 1°C drop from normal
  - Various drugs—especially anaesthetic agents:
    - Ketamine will increase CBF
    - Benzodiazepines, thiopentone, and propofol will reduce CBF
- The Cushing reflex occurs in response to an increase in ICP and involves systemic vasoconstriction to increase arterial pressure in order to maintain blood flow to the brain. Compensatory bradycardia is also noted.
- Main components of blood–brain barrier:
  - Endothelial cells of the brain's highly dense capillary network have very tight junctions and membrane transporters that closely regulate the composition of CSF

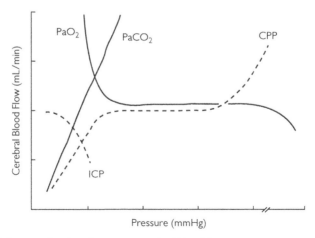

Figure D.3.9 Influence of various factors on cerebral blood flow

- This 'blood–brain barrier' is continuous except in locations where substances must be absorbed from, or released into, the circulation
- Key roles of CO_2 and potassium in determination of cerebral autoregulation:
  - CO_2 and K^+ are important intrinsic metabolic regulators of cerebral circulation
  - Increases in either of these will result in vasodilation and a 'functional hyperaemia'
  - In general terms, functional hyperaemia is the term given to an increase in blood flow due to the presence of metabolites and/or a change in local conditions
  - Increased tissue activity results in a rise in these metabolites, resulting in vasodilation. A rise in temperature also produces the same effect
  - The mechanism for the vasodilation is unclear, but is thought to be due to the opening of precapillary sphincters

3.8.6 Skeletal muscle flow

- Skeletal muscle blood flow represents around 15–20% of the CO at rest, and at exercise may rise to more than 80%.
- Capillary recruitment via metabolic hyperaemia:
  - At rest, most skeletal muscle capillaries are not perfused as arterioles are constricted
  - Capillaries are recruited during exercise by metabolic hyperaemia caused by the release of tissue metabolism products, CO_2 and K^+
  - This process overrides sympathetic vasoconstriction
- Role of skeletal muscle beds in generating total peripheral resistance:
  - As a widespread vascular bed, skeletal muscle provides a significant contribution to total peripheral resistance

CHAPTER D4

Gastrointestinal physiology

CONTENTS

4.1 Functional anatomy of the gastrointestinal tract: outline of structure

- The GI tract has a fairly consistent general structure that is arranged into 4 concentric layers (see Figure D.4.1)—described from innermost to outermost as follows.

4.1.1 Mucosa

- The innermost layer, which lines the lumen.
- Functions include:
  - Secretion of mucus and enzymes into the tract's lumen
  - Secretion of hormones into the plasma
  - Protection against infectious disease
  - Absorption of digestive end products into plasma
- The mucosa consists of 3 layers:
  - Epithelium:
    - Lines the lumen
    - Typically simple columnar, often with goblet cells
  - Lamina propria:
    - Loose connective tissue underneath the epithelium
    - Contains capillaries for nutrient absorption, and lymphoid tissue
  - Muscularis mucosa:
    - Underlies the lamina propria
    - Consists of a thin layer of smooth muscle that produces local movements of the mucosa

4.1.2 Submucosa

- Lies deep to the mucosa.
- Is made up of connective tissue containing blood and lymphatic vessels, lymphoid nodules, and nerve fibres.
- Provides vascular supply to most structures of the GI tract wall.

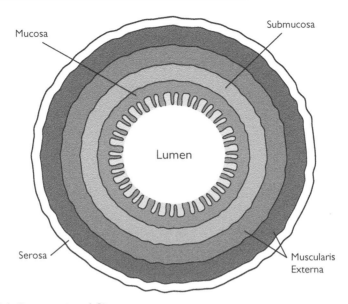

Figure D.4.1 Cross-section of GI tract

4.1.3 Muscularis externa

- Lies deep to the submucosa.
- Consists of smooth muscle responsible for peristalsis and segmentation.
- Is divided into 2 layers:
  - An inner circular layer
  - And an outer longitudinal layer
- In several sites the circular layer thickens to form a sphincter, which regulates passage of contents and prevents backflow.

4.1.4 Serosa

- The outermost layer of the GI tract.
- Also known as the visceral peritoneum.
- Histologically consists of a simple squamous epithelium overlying thin areolar connective tissue.
- The oesophagus has an adventitia rather than a serosa.
- Associated fibrous connective tissue firmly holds the relevant section of the tract in place.
- Retroperitoneal structures have both a serosa and an adventitia.

4.2 Saliva

4.2.1 Sites of production, composition, and functions in health
Production

- Saliva is produced by the 3 main exocrine salivary glands (see Figure D.4.2):
  - The parotid glands are a pair of glands located in the subcutaneous tissues of the face overlying the mandibular ramus and anterior and inferior to the external ear:
    - Around 20–25% of saliva in the oral cavity is produced by the parotid glands

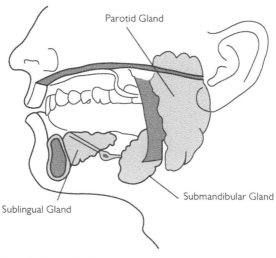

Figure D.4.2 Location of salivary glands

- The submandibular glands are a pair of glands located beneath the lower jaws, superior to the digastric muscles:
  - The submandibular glands contribute around 70–75% of the saliva in the oral cavity
- The sublingual glands are a pair of glands located beneath the tongue near to the submandibular glands:
  - The sublingual glands are classified as a mixed gland—both serous and mucous
  - Approximately 5% of saliva entering the oral cavity comes from the sublingual glands
- A healthy person will produce an estimated 0.75–1.5L of saliva per day
- During sleep this production of saliva falls to almost zero

Composition

- 98% of human saliva is composed of water.
- The remaining 2% consists of:
  - Electrolytes:
    - Sodium: 2–21mmol/L (lower than plasma)
    - Potassium: 10–36mmol/L (higher than plasma)
    - Calcium: 1.2–2.8mmol/L (similar to plasma)
    - Chloride: 5–40mmol/L (lower than plasma)
    - Bicarbonate: 25mmol/L (higher than plasma)
    - Phosphate: 1.4–39mmol/L
    - Magnesium: 0.08–0.5mmol/L
  - Mucus: consisting of mucopolysaccharides and glycoprotein
  - Antibacterial compounds (thiocyanate, hydrogen peroxide, and secretory immunoglobulin A)
  - Enzymes:
    - Amylase: starts the digestion of starch with an optimal pH of 7.4
    - Lingual lipase: has an optimal pH of around 4.0 so not activated until entering the acidic environment of the stomach

- Others:
  - Including lysozymes, salivary lactoperoxidase, lactoferrin, immunoglobulin A, and proline-rich proteins (involved in enamel development)

Function

- Saliva has 3 main functions: aiding swallowing, initiating digestion, and maintaining oral hygiene.
- Swallowing:
  - When added to food in the mouth, saliva helps to soften and bind the food bolus in order to aid swallowing
  - Saliva also solubilizes dry food, assisting swallowing and enabling taste
- Digestion:
  - The main 2 enzymes, amylase and salivary lipase, when added to food in the oral cavity begin the process of digestion—breaking down starch and fat molecules
- Hygiene:
  - Salivary lysozymes help to prevent overgrowth of oral microbial populations, while constant flow of saliva 'flushes' the mouth and teeth of food debris

4.2.2 Control of salivary secretion via taste (and additionally smell) receptors

- Secretion of saliva is under the control of the autonomic nervous system, which controls both the volume and type of saliva secreted.
- Potent stimuli for increased salivation include the presence of food or irritating substances in the mouth, and thoughts of or the smell of food.
- Secretory stimuli generate afferent nervous impulses to the higher salivary centres.
- Salivary glands are innervated by both the parasympathetic and sympathetic autonomic systems.
- Stimulation results in an increased amylase output and volume flow.
- Parasympathetic innervation:
  - Carried via cranial nerves
  - The parotid gland is innervated by the glossopharyngeal nerve (CN IX) via the otic ganglion, while the submandibular and sublingual glands receive their parasympathetic input from the facial nerve (CN VII) via the submandibular ganglion
  - Ach and substance P are released, which activates the IP3 and DAG pathways respectively
- Sympathetic innervation:
  - Via preganglionic nerves in the thoracic segments T1–T3
  - These synapse in the superior cervical ganglion with postganglionic neurons that release norepinephrine, which is then received by ß-adrenergic receptors on the acinar and ductal cells of the salivary glands. This leads to an increase in cAMP levels and a corresponding increase in saliva secretion
  - The sympathetic nervous system also affects salivary gland secretions indirectly by innervating the blood vessels that supply the glands

4.3 Swallowing (deglutition)

4.3.1 Phases (voluntary and reflex), control, and functional anatomy of the swallowing process

- The oesophagus may be divided into 3 functional sections:
  - Upper third—containing skeletal muscle

- Middle third—containing both skeletal and smooth muscle
- Lower third—containing smooth muscle
- Swallowing occurs in 2 phases—voluntary and reflex:
  - In the voluntary phase, the tongue presses against the palate, thereby pushing the food bolus into the oropharynx
  - Swallowing is then continued by reflex activity via afferent fibres of CNs IX and X with impulses passing to the tractus solitarius and nucleus ambiguous of the medulla
  - Efferent fibres transmit a contractile response to pharyngeal and tongue muscles via CNs IX, X, and XII
  - Food is propelled along the oesophagus by peristalsis
- During swallowing, the nasopharynx is sealed by elevation of the soft palate and superior constrictor muscle contraction.
- The larynx is covered by elevation and closure of the glottis, with posterior movement of the epiglottis and cessation of respiration.

4.3.2 Function of the upper and lower oesophageal sphincters and of peristalsis

- Upper oesophageal sphincter:
  - The upper oesophageal sphincter refers to the upper part of the oesophagus and consists of striated muscle under conscious control
  - The primary muscle of the upper sphincter is the cricopharyngeus portion of the inferior pharyngeal constrictor
  - During swallowing the upper sphincter opens so the food bolus can pass into the oesophagus
  - A secondary role of the sphincter is to reduce backflow from the oesophagus into the pharynx
- Lower oesophageal sphincter:
  - The lower oesophageal sphincter may also be referred to as the cardia, Z-line, or gastro-oesophageal junction and is an anatomical junction at the orifice of the stomach and the oesophagus
  - In this region, the mucosa of the oesophagus (non-keratinized stratified squamous epithelium) transitions into gastric mucosa (simple columnar epithelium) in the stomach
  - During peristalsis, the lower sphincter relaxes to allow the food bolus to pass into the stomach
  - It prevents chyme, a mixture of bolus, stomach acid, and digestive enzymes, from returning up the oesophagus
- At the beginning of the reflex swallowing activity, the food bolus is propelled into the upper oesophagus by inferior constrictor muscle, thereby initiating oesophageal peristalsis. 2 types of peristaltic waves occur:
  - Primary peristaltic wave:
    - Occurs once the bolus enters the oesophagus during swallowing
    - This forces the bolus down the oesophagus and into the stomach in a wave lasting about 8–9sec
    - The wave travels down to the stomach even if the bolus of food descends at a greater rate than the wave itself, and will continue even in the case of obstruction
  - Secondary peristaltic wave:
    - In the event that the bolus moves slower than the primary peristaltic wave, or stops, stretch receptors in the oesophageal walls are stimulated and a local reflex response causes a secondary peristaltic wave around the bolus, forcing it further down the oesophagus
    - These secondary waves will continue indefinitely until the bolus enters the stomach

4.4 Stomach

- The stomach is a 'J'-shaped organ continuous with the lower oesophagus above and the duodenum below, lying against the diaphragm at its uppermost end and in front of the pancreas.
- It is surrounded by an autonomic nerve plexus, which regulates secretory activity and integral muscular function.
- In the stomach, food is mixed with water and gastric secretions in order to produce a creamy semi-liquid material called chyme.
- Very little absorption occurs in the stomach.
- However, ethyl alcohol and certain unionized organic substances, such as aspirin, are absorbed.

4.4.1 Overview of functions

- Storage:
  - The wall of the stomach has many folds (called 'rugae') that enable it to expand in capacity from just 50mL when empty up to 4L when fully distended
  - Due to the relaxation of smooth muscle in these areas, the fundus and body of the stomach can accommodate large increases in volume without a significant change in intragastric pressure
  - This temporary storage allows time for mixing with gastric secretions, and for the gradual release of resultant chyme into the small intestine at a rate compatible with digestion and absorption
- Digestion:
  - There are 2 main processes of digestion in the stomach—physical and chemical
  - The stomach has 3 layers of smooth muscle in the muscularis externa, instead of the usual 2 seen in the rest of the GI tract
  - This extra layer is the inner oblique layer, responsible for producing the vigorous contractions of the antral and pyloric regions that churn and physically break down food into smaller particles
  - Intrinsic nervous innervation is formed by the submucosal plexus ('Meissner's plexus') and myenteric plexus ('Auerbach's plexus')
  - Chemical processes include the protease enzyme pepsin, secreted in the form of pepsinogen by the chief cells, which breaks proteins down into polypeptides
  - The addition of hydrochloric acid (HCl) leads to denaturing of proteins and the dissolving of intercellular bonds
  - The low pH also kills most bacteria that may accompany the food
- Chyme regulation:
  - A layer of thick circular smooth muscle at the exit of the stomach, the pyloric sphincter, controls the movement of chyme into the duodenum
  - Release of chyme from the stomach is controlled by the interaction of the enteric nervous system, autonomic nervous system, and local hormones
- Intrinsic factor:
  - Parietal cells are scattered along the neck and lower walls of the ducts
  - They secrete HCl and the glycoprotein intrinsic factor:
    - Intrinsic factor is essential for the absorption of vitamin B12 in the small intestine
    - Intrinsic factor binds B12 in the food in the small intestine and protects it from enzymatic action
    - This complex is later absorbed by mucosal epithelial cells of the lower ileum

4.4.2 Role of the chief and parietal cells

- The surface epithelium of the gastric mucosa contains gastric glands, which empty into depressions in the surface called gastric pits.
- There are around 100 pits per square millimetre of mucosa, occupying around 50% of the total gastric mucosa surface.
- The gastric glands contain chief cells, which secrete pepsinogen, and parietal cells, which produce gastric acid and intrinsic factor.
- Chief cells, as well as other stomach cells, are protected from self-digestion because chief cells produce and secrete the inactive precursor of pepsin—pepsinogen.
- Pepsinogen is converted to pepsin by the HCl produced and released by the parietal cells.
- Proteolytic enzymes, or pepsins, are secreted in the form of membrane-bound zymogen granules by exocytosis by stimulated gastric glands.
- Pepsins show their greatest proteolytic enzyme activity at pH values <3.
- Fat digestion by the stomach is negligible, although gastric glands do secrete a lipase active in the range of pH 4–7.

4.4.3 The crucial role of the proton (H^+/K^+-ATPase) pump in hydrogen ion management

- The pH of gastric juice is very low, maintained at between 1 and 3.
- This highly acidic environment is required for several reasons:
  - Assists the breakdown of connective tissue and muscle fibres of ingested meat
  - Activates pepsinogen and produces optimal conditions for the activity of pepsins
  - Aids absorption of calcium and iron
  - Bactericidal effects
- Gastric acid is secreted by the parietal cells, predominantly in the fundus and body of the stomach.
- Deep invaginations of the parietal cell membrane, called secretory canaliculi, enable a large surface area, bringing a large number of proton pump sites into contact with the luminal fluid.
- The process of acid production by the parietal cells is highly energy dependent, relying upon the H^+/K^+-ATPase pump to drive hydrogen ions against a high concentration gradient.
- As a result, parietal cells contain numerous mitochondria.
- Chloride leaves the cell by chloride channels in the secretory canaliculi and a potassium–chloride co-transport system.

4.4.4 Protective mucosal barrier mechanisms within the gastric lumen

- 3 factors contribute to the gastric mucosal barrier:
  - Tight junctions between epithelial cells preventing leaking of gastric secretions to underlying tissue
  - Alkaline mucus secreted by the epithelial cells and mucous neck cells of gastric glands forms a protective layer between 5 and 200μm thick
  - Prostaglandin ('E' series) release increases the thickness of the mucus layer and production of bicarbonate and optimizes conditions for tissue repair in damaged areas of mucosa
- The constant growth and desquamation of gastric epithelium also ensures mucosal protection against the highly acid environment.

4.4.5 Secretion patterns and their stimulant pathways

- Cephalic:
  - The cephalic phase takes place before ingestion—due to anticipation of food (sight, smell, and taste)

- The contribution of this phase is dependent upon mood and appetite, and may be up to 30% of total gastric secretion
- The stimulant pathway originates in the cerebral cortex or appetite centres of the amygdala/hypothalamus
- Efferent fibres of the vagus nerve reach the myenteric plexus where postganglionic parasympathetic activity of Ach stimulates secretion by the gastric glands
- Vagal stimulation also causes the release of gastrin from G-cells, which in turn stimulates release of gastric acid and pepsinogen
- Vagal activity and gastrin also cause the release of histamine, which stimulates parietal cells to secrete acid
- Gastric:
  - The gastric phase accounts for around 60% of total gastric secretion
  - The 2 main triggers are stomach wall distension and the chemical content of food
  - Stimulation of mechanoreceptors of the stomach wall smooth muscle by stretching initiates local myenteric and vaso-vagal reflexes
  - Both reflexes lead to Ach release that stimulates the gastric glands
  - Vagal mediated reflexes account for around 80% of this activity
  - Sympathetic stimulation (e.g. fear, pain, anxiety) will lead to inhibition of gastric secretion
  - Vagal stimulation also leads to release of gastrin, which increases acid, enzyme, and mucus secretion
  - As the pH of the stomach contents falls to 2–3, gastrin secretion is inhibited
  - Gastrin secretion is therefore maximal at the time of food entry to the stomach and then declines as digestion continues and pH falls
  - This inhibitory pathway is mediated by somatostatin release from the D cells of the gastric mucosa
  - As a result, gastric acid secretion is self-limiting—usually the gastric phase lasts around 3–4 hours
- Intestinal:
  - The intestinal phase accounts for the smallest proportion of gastric secretion (around 5%) and takes place due to the entrance of partially digested food into the duodenum
  - Gastrin is released from G-cells of the small intestine mucosa
  - However, this effect is short-lived as the enterogastric reflex is initiated, thereby inhibiting gastric secretory activity
  - This reflex is mediated by several hormones:
  - Secretin:
    - Secreted by duodenal mucosa in response to acid
    - Local effect reaching stomach via bloodstream
    - Inhibits the release of gastrin
    - Inhibits effect of gastrin on parietal cells
  - Cholecystokinin (CCK):
    - Released in presence of the products of fat digestion in duodenum and proximal jejunum
    - Inhibits the release of gastrin and gastric acid
  - Gastric inhibitory peptide (GIP):
    - Released in presence of the products of fat digestion in duodenum and proximal jejunum
    - Like CCK, inhibits the release of gastrin and gastric acid

4.4.6 Chyme production and its effects upon the pyloric sphincter

- Chyme is a semi-liquid mixture of food, water, and gastric secretions produced by both the chemical and mechanical action of the stomach.
- Forceful contractions of the antrum cause retrograde movement of food through the antral ring—a process called retropulsion.

- This helps to break down food and enhance mixing with gastric secretions.
- The pylorus itself usually holds around 30mL of chyme, and with each peristaltic contraction of the stomach, around 3mL is squirted through the pyloric sphincter into the duodenum.

4.4.7 Factors affecting gastric emptying

- The enterogastric reflex is the collective term for the hormonal and neural mechanisms that affect gastric emptying.
- Duodenal luminal pH:
  - A very acidic gastric chyme will delay gastric emptying
  - This is thought to be mediated by a combination of vagal activity and secretin release
  - Secretin delays gastric emptying by the inhibition of antral contraction and constriction of the pyloric sphincter
  - Secretin also stimulates production of a bicarbonate-rich pancreatic secretion in order to neutralize duodenal acid
- Fats (and protein):
  - Presence of fatty acids or monoglycerides in the duodenum will delay gastric emptying due to an increase in pyloric contractility
  - This ensures that the delivery of fats to the small intestine does not occur more quickly than the bile salts can deal with
  - This is mediated by the action of CCK and GIP. A similar inhibitory effect is also seen with the products of protein digestion
- Distension:
  - Distension of the stomach wall activates stretch receptors and gastrin-secreting cells, which both enhance the force of peristaltic contractions
  - The rate of gastric emptying is proportional to gastric volume

4.5 Small intestine

- Once processed and digested by the stomach, chyme passes through the pyloric valve into the duodenum.
- Once past the stomach peristaltic action continues to mix the chyme in the intestine.
- Through this process of mixing and continued digestion and absorption of nutrients, chyme gradually works its way through the small intestine to the large intestine.

4.5.1 Duodenally mediated inhibition of gastric juice release and its hormonal components

- The presence of fatty acids, protein, and acid in the duodenum results in the inhibition of gastric secretion and gastric emptying.
- The hormones involved include secretin, CCK, and GIP.

4.5.2 Effects of addition of water, bicarbonate, and bile upon duodenal chyme

- Water:
  - Around 2L of fluid are ingested per day
  - Secretion of gastric juices adds a further 2L to the chyme
  - Most of the water absorption by the small intestine takes place in the jejunum and ileum
  - Iso-osmotic gastric contents empty from the stomach faster than hypo- or hyperosmotic contents due to feedback inhibition from duodenal osmoreceptors
  - Isotonicity of chyme in the small intestine is maintained by osmosis, which either favours the gradient created by active ion transportation or the constituents of chyme
  - Water is either taken up by, or diffuses across, the enterocyte membrane

- Bicarbonate:
  - The addition of bicarbonate, from either the brush border or pancreatic secretions, to the chyme will raise the pH to maintain the optimal conditions for enzymic action and absorption of nutrients
- Bile:
  - Addition of bile to the chyme results in emulsification of fats, similar to a detergent effect, to enable digestion and absorption of fatty acids, monoglycerides, and cholesterol

4.5.3 Functional anatomy of the intestinal villus

- The small intestine presents a huge surface area (estimated 200m²) due to its length and structural modifications resulting in deep folds of mucosa and submucosa ('valvular conniventes'), particularly in the jejunum.
- The folded mucosal surface of the small intestine is also covered in villi.
- These are finger-like projections of columnar epithelial cells (enterocytes) that perform the absorptive function of the GI tract.
- Each projection is around 1mm high and its mucosal surface consists of many tiny processes called microvilli (1.0μm long and 0.1μm diameter), which constitute the 'brush border', thus increasing the available surface area even further.
- The villi differ in appearance throughout the small intestine: broad in the duodenum, narrow and flat in the jejunum, and short and finger-like in the ileum.
- Each villus contains a lacteal (modified lymphatic vessel), artery, vein, and a small amount of smooth muscle. See Figure D.4.3.
- Regular isolated clusters of lymph nodules are also found in the walls of the ileum. Called 'Peyer's patches', they form the collective of lymphoid tissues referred to as mucosa-associated lymphatic tissue (MALT).

4.5.4 Importance of the sodium pump in creating the osmotic gradient of the small intestine

- The movement of water occurs by passive osmosis secondary to the active reabsorption of electrolytes.
- Sodium absorption in the small intestine is chiefly due to coupled Na^+/Cl^- co-transport at the luminal membrane, as well as Na^+ channels and Na^+/glucose or amino acid-coupled co-transporters.
- A sodium gradient is created by a low enterocyte intracellular sodium concentration—maintained by the basolateral Na^+-ATPase pump.

4.5.5 Carbohydrate handling

- All monosaccharides are normally fully absorbed from the chyme in the small intestine before the end of the terminal ileum.
- Brush border enzymes:
  - Although some starch digestion occurs by α-amylase in the stomach, most occurs in the small intestine
  - Pancreatic α-amylase hydrolyses dietary carbohydrates to maltose, maltriose, and α-dextrans, which are then further broken down by the brush border enzymes
  - These include disaccharidases (maltase, sucrase), peptidases, and phosphates
  - One of these, the peptidase 'enteropeptidase', breaks down pancreatic trypsinogen in order to activate it
  - The brush border enzymes produce fructose, glucose, and galactose for absorption

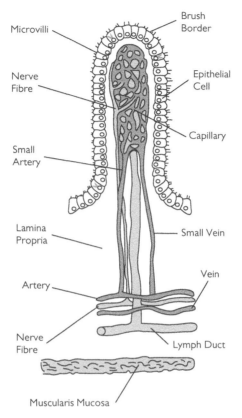

Figure D.4.3 Schematic view of intestinal villus

- Co-transporters:
  - Once carbohydrates are broken down into monosaccharides they are absorbed either by passive diffusion (80% of glucose) or carrier-mediated transport (around 20% of glucose, all galactose, and fructose)
  - The active transport system involves a Na^+ carried mediated co-transporter mechanism
  - The sodium gradient that drives this system is maintained by Na^+/K^+-ATPase cellular membrane pump
  - Fructose is absorbed by a sodium-independent facilitated diffusion process
- Diffusion:
  - Around 80% of the glucose is absorbed by passive diffusion
  - Once the luminal glucose level falls below 5mmol/L the active glucose co-transport mechanism becomes dominant
  - The process of transportation of monosaccharides across the basolateral membrane occurs via facilitated diffusion

4.5.6 Functional effects of proteases and carboxypeptidase

- Proteases, secreted by the pancreas, cleave internal peptide linkages in order to produce small peptide chains such as dipeptides and tripeptides.

- Carboxypeptidases are produced by the pancreas and intestinal epithelial cells.
- These cleave the ends of protein chains, thereby producing free amino acids, which are readily absorbed by the intestine.

4.5.7 Calcium absorption via Ca^{2+}-ATPase and Na^+/Ca^{2+} antiporter (exchanger) mechanisms

- Calcium is absorbed by enterocytes via 2 main mechanisms:
  - Passive—'paracellular' and more efficient with a high intraluminal Ca^{2+}
  - Active—rate limited but better with a relatively low intraluminal Ca^{2+}
- This action is subject to the presence of parathyroid hormone acting with vitamin D to enhance absorption in the gut.
- Vitamin D also has a direct effect on enterocytes by increasing the synthesis of basolateral Ca^{2+}-ATPase pumps and brush border Ca^{2+} cytosol binding proteins.
- The diffusion of luminal Ca^{2+} is facilitated by passage along a gradient created by the maintenance of a low intracellular Ca^{2+} by 2 basolateral transport pump systems—the Ca^{2+}-ATPase and Na^+/Ca^{2+} exchanger.

4.5.8 Iron absorption via ascorbate complexes and carrier proteins

- The haem from dietary meat is more easily absorbed as it is already in a soluble form.
- This is taken up by facilitated diffusion and the action of intracellular xanthine oxidase then releases Fe^{2+} ions.
- Soluble iron in the ferrous state is absorbed across the brush border of the mucosal cells, mainly of the duodenum and upper jejunum.
- Around 10% of dietary iron is absorbed in the normal person (although this may be increased to 20–30% in pregnancy or iron-deficiency states).
- Complexes with ascorbate prevent the precipitation of the normally insoluble Fe^{3+}.
- Iron is then readily transferred from these compounds into enterocytes.
- A ferric reductase enzyme on the enterocyte's brush border reduces ferric Fe^{3+} to Fe^{2+}.
- The protein divalent metal transporter 1 (DMT1) then transports the iron across the enterocyte's cell membrane and into the cell.
- Factors that favour the absorption of iron include gastric acid and reducing agents—both of which maintain the availability of soluble iron in the ferrous state.
- Iron is transported in plasma bound to transferrin, which is synthesized in the liver.

4.5.9 Fat handling (emulsification agents, micelles) and the handling of fat-soluble vitamins

- The first step of fat digestion is emulsification.
- Fat globules are broken down into smaller particles by the detergent actions of bile salts and lecithin.
- Fatty acids and monoglycerides produced by the action of pancreatic lipases and esterases then form micelles with the bile salts.
- Micelles consist of a central fat globule containing monoglycerides and free fatty acids, along with fat-soluble vitamins and cholesterol, surrounded by bile salts that project outwards and cover the surface of the micelle.
- Small intestine contractions allow micelles to come into contact with, and adhere to, the enterocyte surface.
- Lipids, cholesterol, and fat-soluble vitamins then diffuse freely from the core of the micelle into the apical membrane of the enterocyte.
- Monoglycerides and fatty acids enter the ER to be recombined to form triglycerides.
- Phospholipids are formed from phosphatides and fatty acids.

- Cholesterol is re-esterified and combined with triglycerides and phospholipids into globules called 'chylomicrons' within the Golgi apparatus.
- These are miscible with water due to the arrangement of the phospholipids around the globule.
- They pass by exocytosis into the basolateral space and then into lymph via the central lacteal of the villus.
- By this method, fat is transported by the lymph into the central circulation via the thoracic duct.

4.6 Pancreas

4.6.1 Principal constituents of the exocrine pancreatic juice

- Exocrine secretions of the pancreas are produced by the acinar and ductal cells.
- Around 1.5L of pancreatic secretions are produced per day. The principal constituents are:
  - Aqueous—containing water, sodium, potassium, and bicarbonate
  - Digestive enzymes
- The aqueous components of pancreatic secretions are formed by the columnar epithelial cells that line the intercalated and interlobular ducts.
- The constituents of this fluid are similar to that of plasma, although slightly hypertonic with a pH of around 8.
- Bicarbonate is produced in increasing amounts with greater demand following ingestion of food—at rest the pancreas secretes a mainly plasma-like solution.
- At low flow rates, bicarbonate is exchanged for chloride ions from the ductal fluid.
- At higher flow rates, this fluid is barely altered resulting in a greater bicarbonate concentration.
- The aqueous components of pancreatic secretions appear to be regulated by cAMP, via stimulation of proton pump activity in the basolateral membrane.
- Bicarbonate diffuses down a concentration gradient, as well as being produced from hydration of plasma CO_2 and the products of cellular metabolism.
- Water diffuses freely to maintain osmotic balance.
- The bicarbonate-rich secretions of the pancreas help to neutralize the acidic chyme as it enters the duodenum, together with the intestinal secretions.
- The other main function is to promote the optimal pH for pancreatic enzyme activity in the small intestine.
- Pancreatic enzymes are synthesized as proenzymes in the ribosomes that line the ER of acinar cells.
- Zymogen granules are created in the Golgi complex—proenzymes are secreted by exocytosis.
- Distinct receptors binding Ach, gastrin, and CCK result in the release of pancreatic enzymes via the phosphatidylinositol system.
- Secretin receptors promote the release of pancreatic enzymes via the cAMP pathway.
- The 3 main types of pancreatic enzymes are proteolytics, α-amylase, and lipases.
  - Proteolytics:
    - Trypsinogen and chymotrypsinogen are secreted as inactive proenzymes
    - These are activated either by the action of enteropeptidase (conversion to trypsin) or by trypsin itself (autocatalysis) at the brush border
    - Activation may also occur spontaneously in the more alkaline environment of the small intestine
    - Their main function is the cleavage of peptide linkages in order to break down proteins into free amino acids and smaller polypeptides
    - Carboxypeptidases, elastase, and aminopeptidases then break these down further

- α-amylase:
  - Pancreatic amylase is secreted in its active form
  - It is stable between pH 4 and 11, with an optimal pH of 6.9
  - Its main function is the hydrolysis of complex carbohydrates into disaccharides
- Lipases:
  - Pancreatic lipases hydrolyse triglycerides into glycerol and fatty acids, which (along with bile salts rendering them water soluble) allows them to be absorbed
- Other enzymes include:
  - Carboxypeptidase: cleaves peptides at C-terminal end
  - Elastase: cleaves internal peptide bonds
  - Colipase: binds to micelles to anchor lipase to lipid
  - Phospholipase A2: cleaves fatty acids from phospholipids
  - Cholesterol esterase: releases esterified cholesterol
  - RNAse and DNAse: cleave RNA or DNA into short fragments
- Most of the zymogen precursor forms of enzymes are activated by trypsin, with the exception of trypsin itself, which is activated by enteropeptidase (also referred to as 'enterokinase').
- In order to prevent damage to the pancreas tissue from autodigestion by activated trypsinogen, an acid environment is maintained within the zymogen granules by way of a proton pump system and the presence of a trypsin inhibitor that binds trypsin to form an inactive complex.
- Similar to gastric secretion, pancreatic secretion is regulated by both vagal activity and local hormones.
- However, the endocrine control of pancreatic secretion is more significant.
- The main 2 chemical regulators of exocrine pancreatic function are CCK and secretin.
- Parasympathetic vagal efferent fibres innervate the pancreatic acinar and ductal smooth muscle cells, stimulation of which causes the release of zymogen granules and an increase in local blood flow.
- The stimulus originates from the sight, smell, or taste of food—the cephalic phase, accounting for around 20% of the total exocrine pancreatic secretion.
- This effect is also mediated by the release of gastrin from stomach antral cells—accounting for around 5–10% of the total exocrine pancreatic secretion.
- Around 70% of the total exocrine pancreatic secretion function is in response to CCK and secretin release.

4.6.2 Function and origin of CCK

- CCK increases the secretion of pancreatic enzymes and chloride-rich fluid by acinar cells.
- It is secreted by the upper intestinal mucosa in response to the presence of monoglycerides, fatty acids, peptides, amino acids, and acid.
- CCK also potentiates the effect of secretin.
- CCK is released from the duodenum in response to the breakdown products of fat and protein digestion.
- It is synthesized by I-cells in the mucosal epithelium of the small intestine.
- The effects of CCK are also stimulated by Ach, gastrin, and substance P.

4.6.3 Function and origin of secretin

- Secretin increases the secretion of bicarbonate-rich fluid from duct cells.
- As with CCK, it is secreted in response to the presence of monoglycerides, fatty acids, peptides, amino acids, and acid in the upper intestinal mucosa.

- Secretin is synthesized and released by specialized amine precursor uptake and decarboxylation cells in the duodenum.
- The effects of secretin are also stimulated by vasoactive intestinal polypeptide (VIP) and peptide histadine-isoleucine (PHI).

4.7 Liver

- The main functions of the liver include:
  - Metabolic:
    - Carbohydrates
    - Protein and lipoproteins
    - Fatty acids
    - Drug biotransformation—exogenous and endogenous compounds
  - Storage:
    - Vitamins A, D, E, and K
    - Iron and copper
    - Glycogen
  - Excretion of bilirubin and production of urea
  - Immunological:
    - Immunoglobulin synthesis
    - Kupffer cell phagocytosis
  - Filtration of bacteria and degradation of endotoxins
  - Haematological:
    - Foetal haemopoiesis
    - Blood volume reservoir

4.7.1 Constituents of a portal triad

- The hepatic lobule is the basic anatomical unit of the liver, consisting of a central hepatic efferent venule onto which cords of hepatocytes and sinusoids converge.
- Each functional unit, the acinus, is made up of a parenchymal mass between 2 centrilobular veins.
- The centre of the acinus is formed by the portal triads.
- The portal triads are made up of the portal vein, hepatic artery, and bile duct, and are supplied by terminal branches of the hepatic artery and portal veins (see Figure D.4.4).
- Portal veins drain into the sinusoids, and thence into the hepatic venules.
- Sinusoids represent a low pressure microvascular system that can act as a significant reservoir for blood—dependent on the vascular tone of the arteriolar and venous vessels.
- The liver is made up of 2 distinct types of cells—hepatocytes and Kupffer cells:
- Hepatocytes:
  - Form around 60% of the liver cell mass
  - Arranged in laminae through which sinusoids connect
  - Cells are polygonal in shape, having 3 surface types:
    - Facing space of Disse (sinusoid)
    - Facing bile canaliculi
    - Facing adjacent hepatocytes
  - Have projecting microvilli to increase surface area
  - Contain numerous organelles and mitochondria
- Kupffer cells:
  - Macrophages that are part of reticuloendothelial system lining sinusoids

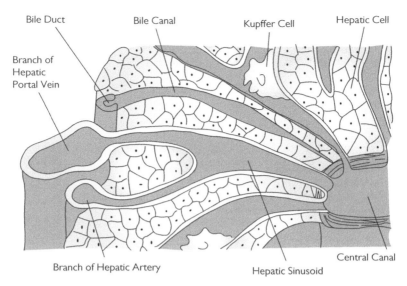

Bile Duct   Bile Canal   Kupffer Cell   Hepatic Cell

Branch of
Hepatic
Portal Vein

Branch of Hepatic Artery   Hepatic Sinusoid   Central Canal

Figure D.4.4 Liver lobule and portal triad

■ Functions include:
  ● Phagocytosis of bacteria, viruses, immune complexes, thrombin, fibrin complexes, and tumour cells
  ● Destruction of endotoxins
  ● Protein denaturation
  ● Accumulation of ferritin and haemosiderin
  ● Haemopoiesis in the foetus

4.7.2 Origin and constituents of hepatic bile

● The liver produces around 1L of bile per day.
● Bile is an isotonic fluid resembling plasma in its constituents with a pH of 7–8.
● During storage in the gallbladder, bile is concentrated to around one-fifth of its volume.
● Bile constituents include:
  ■ Electrolytes
  ■ Protein
  ■ Bilirubin
  ■ Bile salts
  ■ Lecithin
  ■ Lipids
● Bile acids:
  ■ The primary bile acids, cholic acid and chenodeoxycholic acid, are produced from cholesterol by the addition of hydroxyl and carboxyl groups
  ■ Secondary bile acids, including deoxycholic acid and lithocolic acid, are produced by the action of intestinal bacteria
● Bile salts:
  ■ Bile acids conjugate with glycine or taurine to form bile salts, which limits the passive absorption of bile in the gut due to their greater water solubility and reduced lipid solubility
  ■ The main function of bile salts is to emulsify dietary fat to aid its absorption and that of the fat-soluble vitamins

- ■ Bile acids also stimulate pancreatic secretion via release of CCK
- ■ Bile salts are re-absorbed at the terminal ileum by a sodium-dependent transporter
- ■ These are returned to the liver via the portal circulation, bound to plasma proteins
- ■ This recirculation is referred to as enterohepatic circulation
- ● Water and electrolytes:
  - ■ These are secreted by the hepatocytes and ductal epithelial cells
  - ■ Sodium is actively transported into the ductal lumen, followed by the passive movement of chloride and water
  - ■ Bicarbonate ions are actively secreted into bile by ductal cells
- ● Bilirubin:
  - ■ The steps of bilirubin production are as follows:
    - ● 'Old' red blood cells are phagocytosed by the reticuloendothelial cells of the spleen, releasing free Hb
    - ● Haem is broken down in the reticuloendothelial system by haem oxygenase and NADPH-cytochrome P450 to form biliverdin
    - ● Biliverdin is converted to bilirubin by a reductase enzyme
  - ■ Bilirubin is bound to serum albumin and transported to the liver, where unbound bilirubin enters the hepatocyte before conjugation with glucuronides by glucuronyl transferase, rendering it water soluble—as bilirubin diglucuronide
  - ■ Around 80% of bilirubin is conjugated in this way
  - ■ The conjugated form is secreted in the bile, where it is broken down by bacteria to form urobilinogen, which undergoes enterohepatic circulation and is excreted in urine
  - ■ Bilirubin is also converted to stercobilin and urobilin, which give faeces its typical brown colour

4.7.3 Pathway of enterohepatic circulation

- ● Around 94% of the bile salts are re-absorbed into the portal circulation by active transport mechanisms from the distal ileum.
- ● Most of bile salts are returned to the liver unaltered and recycled, while a small proportion are deconjugated in the gut before being returned to the liver for reconjugation and recycling.
- ● The remainder is deconjugated and undergoes modification by intestinal bacteria to secondary bile acids.
- ● Relatively insoluble secondary bile acids (lithotomic acid) are excreted in the faeces. Recirculation occurs around 6 times a day.
- ● Bile acids may be recycled up to 20 times before finally being excreted in the faeces.

4.8 Gallbladder

4.8.1 Appreciation of both its storage and metabolic roles (bile concentration region)

- ● The gallbladder protrudes from the inferior margin of the liver and stores bile that is not required immediately for digestion, as well as concentrating it by the absorption of water, sodium, chloride, and bicarbonate.
- ● This process occurs mainly via active transport of sodium from the lumen by the gallbladder mucosa.
- ● Chloride and bicarbonate are absorbed in order to maintain electroneutrality.
- ● Water follows via passive diffusion along a 'standing osmotic gradient' created by high salt content within intercellular channels between the epithelial columnar cells.

- The relatively high tone of the sphincter of Oddi between meals leads to diversion of hepatic bile into the gallbladder.
- The gallbladder can usually accommodate up to 60mL of bile.

4.8.2 Stimulants to bile formation

- Bile salts:
  - The rate at which bile salts are actively secreted is dependent upon the rate of return to the liver via the enterohepatic circulation
  - This may be referred to as the bile acid-dependent fraction
- Secretin, glucagon, and gastrin:
  - The production of bicarbonate-rich watery fluid by ductal epithelial cells is enhanced mainly by secretin, and to a lesser extent by glucagon and gastrin
  - This may be referred to as the bile acid-independent fraction

4.8.3 Role of CCK and vagal stimulation in bile release

- Within a few minutes of ingestion, particularly of food rich in fats, the muscular wall of the gallbladder contracts causing bile to flow towards the duodenum due to the increased pressure against a relaxed sphincter of Oddi.
- The initial response is stimulated by the vagal nerves (cephalic phase) although the major stimulus for gallbladder contraction and emptying is CCK.
- CCK is released in response to the presence of fatty acids and acid in duodenal chyme.
- CCK also relaxes the sphincter of Oddi, in order to allow the entry of bile and pancreatic secretions into the duodenum.
- The gallbladder is usually emptied completely by around 1 hour following a fat-rich meal.
- Hepatic bile production is also stimulated by the increases in liver blood flow that follow ingestion of a meal, as well as the increase in rate of re-absorption of bile salts via enterohepatic circulation.
- Emptying of the gallbladder is inhibited by sympathetic activity.

4.9 Large intestine

- In adults the large intestine is around 1.2m long, with a greater diameter than the small intestine.
- The main functions of the large intestine are:
  - Storage of unabsorbed/unusable food residue prior to excretion
  - Secretion of mucus to lubricate faeces
  - Secretion of bicarbonate to neutralize acid produced by bacteria
  - Absorption of remaining water (400–1000mL/day) and electrolytes
  - Synthesis of vitamin K and some B vitamins by colonic bacteria
- Around 100–150mL of water is normally left in the faeces by the time it reaches the sigmoid colon.
- Food residues are usually stored in the colon for no more than 72 hours, although up to 30% may remain for up to a week or more.
- Structurally, the large intestine is similar to the small, although the longitudinal smooth muscle layer of the muscularis externa is thickened into 3 bands called the 'taeniae coli'.
- Contraction of these leads to the 'haustra'—pocket-like sacs along the caecum and colon.
- Haustra are absent from the rectum.
- Also, as opposed to the small intestine, the mucosal surface is smooth and lacking in any villi.
- Instead, there are a large number of crypts—which contain columnar absorptive cells and mucus-secreting goblet cells.

- As opposed to the more continuous peristalsis of the small intestine, faecal contents are propelled into the large intestine by periodic mass movements.
- These mass movements occur 1–3 times per day in the large intestine and colon, and help propel the contents from the large intestine through the colon to the rectum.

4.9.1 Factors affecting opening of the ileo-caecal sphincter

- The function of the ileo-caecal sphincter is to prevent reflux of colonic contents into the ileum.
- It represents a thickening of the muscularis mucosa at the junction of the small and large intestine.
- Peristalsis propels chyme towards the ileo-caecal valve.
- Both gastrin and CCK result in relaxation of the ileo-caecal sphincter, which facilitates ileal emptying.
- Distension or irritation of the caecum results in increased tone of the sphincter.

4.9.2 Functional role of the taeniae coli via autonomic innervation

- The large intestine receives both parasympathetic and sympathetic innervation.
- The vagus supplies the caecum and colon up to the distal third of the transverse colon.
- Parasympathetic fibres beyond this point are supplied by pelvic nerves from the sacral nerve roots.
- Sympathetic input is derived from coeliac and superior mesenteric ganglia (caecum/colon), and the superior hypogastric plexus (rectum/anal canal).
- The smooth muscle tone of the taeniae coli results in 'puckering' of the wall of the large intestine—forming haustra.
- These are necessary for motility.
- Bundles of muscle from the taeniae coli penetrate the circular layer at irregular intervals.
- The coordinated contraction of circular and longitudinal smooth muscle results in various non-propulsive and propulsive movements.
- The smooth muscle is under both intrinsic and autonomic control.

4.9.3 Handling of chyme as being a combination of mixing and propulsion

- Around 1500mL of chyme pass from the ileum to the caecum each day.
- Both non-propulsive and propulsive movements occur in the colon.
- Motility is coordinated by fast (6–12 cycles/min) or slow (2–4 cycles/min) rhythms of slow-wave electrical activity in the colon.
- The intraluminal pressure waves correspond to this slow-wave activity.
- Colonic contents typically travel along the colon at around 5–10 cm/hour.
- Non-propulsive:
  - Non-propulsive movements commonly occur during fasting and consist of haustral segmentation due to alternating regional muscular contractions
  - These 'haustrations' result in a squeezing movement of chyme backwards and forwards along the colon
  - This improves mixing and enhances absorption by 'rolling' the material around the absorptive surfaces of the colonic mucosa
  - Haustrations mainly occur in the caecum and proximal colon
- Propulsive:
  - Involve coordinated contractions that slowly push colonic contents along the large intestine.

4.9.4 Role of Na⁺/K⁺-ATPase in water absorption against a concentration gradient

- Aldosterone-sensitive active transportation of sodium ions from the intestinal lumen creates an osmotic gradient along which water can diffuse.
- Chloride ions are also absorbed, linked to the secretion of bicarbonate, which also maintains this osmotic gradient.
- Potassium absorption is passive, due to an electrochemical gradient maintained by the energy-dependent Na^+/K^+-ATPase pump.

4.9.5 Overview of the role of colonic bacteria

- The colon contains up to 10^3 times the number of bacteria in the small intestine.
- Over 400 species are usually present including *Bacteroides* and coliforms (e.g. *E. coli*).
- This is partly due to longer transit times due to reduced peristalsis.
- Bacterial residues constitute around one-third of the total dried weight of faeces.
- For comparison, the bacterial flora of the small intestine includes:
  - Duodenum:
    - Relatively few microflora
    - Mainly Gram-positive cocci and rods
  - Jejunum:
    - Greater than duodenum
    - Usually *Enterococcus faecalis, Lactobacilli*, and diphtheroids
  - Ileum:
    - Larger number than proximal GI tract
    - Mainly *Bacteroides, Clostridia*, and *Bifidobacterium*
- The main roles of colonic bacteria include:
  - Vitamin synthesis:
    - Many bacteria, such as *E. coli* found in the large intestine, can synthesize vitamin K2 (menaquinone)
    - Biotin (one of the B vitamins) is also produced by the action of bacteria in the large intestine
    - Although this source of vitamins generally provides only a small part of the daily requirement, it makes a significant contribution when dietary vitamin intake is low
  - Bilirubin handling:
    - Bilirubin is converted to non-pigmented metabolites, urobilinogens, as part of the enterohepatic circulation
  - Fermentation of indigestible carbohydrates:
    - Indigestible carbohydrates, such as cellulose, entering the large bowel are fermented by action of the bacteria to produce short-chain fatty acids as well as a number of waste gases (mainly nitrogen, methane, and carbon dioxide)
    - These gases account for the composition of flatus—approximately 100mL is present in the colon
    - The short-chain fatty acids are readily absorbed by colonic enterocytes, which utilize them for energy
    - Water and sodium also follow the absorption of these molecules

4.9.6 Functional basis of colonic mass movement (based upon mid-zone GI distension)

- There are several types of propulsive colonic movements:
  - Haustral: slowly move colonic contents
  - Multihaustral: seen as fresh ileal effluent passes over more solid contents
  - Intrahaustral: annular constrictions in distal colon that loosen solid faeces

- 'Mass movements' are more vigorous propulsive movements than the more frequent short-range peristaltic waves of the transverse and descending colon.
- They are due to a modified peristaltic wave that slowly carries chyme along the colon, and usually occur 3–4 times per day.
- These contractions last longer than normal peristaltic waves and result in the emptying of a large portion of the proximal colon.
- Mass movements are initiated by intrinsic reflex pathways from distension of the stomach and duodenum following meals—termed the gastro-colic and duodeno-colic reflexes.
- These intrinsic mechanisms may be modulated by the autonomic nervous system and hormone release.
- Vagal stimulation, gastrin, and CCK all enhance colonic motility.

4.9.7 Basis of the defecation reflex

- The rectum is normally empty but if a mass movement results in faecal material being pushed into the rectum, this causes a desire for defecation by the stimulation of sensory nerve fibres from rectal wall distension.
- The internal and external anal sphincters border the anal canal, into which the rectum opens to allow defecation.
- The external anal sphincter is composed of skeletal muscle, is supplied by the pudendal nerve, and is under voluntary control (learned voluntary control from around age 18 months).
- The internal anal sphincter is supplied by both sympathetic and parasympathetic neurons.
- Sympathetic stimulation of the internal sphincter causes contraction and parasympathetic stimulation results in relaxation.
- Defecation is a complex process involving both reflex and voluntary actions.
- The defecation reflex may be consciously inhibited, under which circumstances the urge to defecate will slowly subside until the next mass movement causes further rectal distension.
- In order to defecate, an increase in parasympathetic tone results in contraction of the smooth muscle of the sigmoid colon and rectal walls in order to push the faeces towards the anus.
- Both anal sphincters relax and expulsion is assisted by voluntary diaphragmatic and abdominal wall contraction.
- Glottic closure enables a Valsalva manoeuvre that raises intra-abdominal pressure to aid faecal material in passing through the relaxed sphincters.
- Muscles of the pelvic floor relax in order to straighten the rectum and anus and help prevent prolapse.

CHAPTER D5

Renal physiology

CONTENTS

5.1 Kidneys

For the full anatomy of the kidneys see Chapter A4, Section A.4.11.

5.1.1 Functional anatomy of the renal tract

- Within the dense, connective tissue of the renal capsule, the kidney substance is divided into:
  - Outer cortex:
    - Contains glomeruli, Bowman's capsules, and proximal and distal convoluted tubules
    - It forms renal columns, which extend between medullary pyramids
  - Inner medulla:
    - Consists of 10–18 striated pyramids and contains collecting ducts and loops of Henle
    - The apex of each pyramid ends as a papilla where collecting ducts open
  - Calyces:
    - The minor calyces receive one or more papillae and unite to form major calyces, of which there are 2–3 per kidney
  - Renal pelvis:
    - The dilated upper portion of the ureter that receives the major calyces

5.1.2 Composition of the nephron

- 1.0–1.5 million nephrons per kidney
- 85% glomeruli are cortical (short loops of Henle)
- 15% glomeruli are juxtamedullary (close to the medulla with long loops of Henle)

5.1.3 Glomerular or Bowman's capsule

- Function is to filter crystalloids from plasma into tubule
- Filter 125mL/min
- Consists of 3 layers:
  - Capillary endothelium: similar to normal capillaries but with fenestrae
  - Basement membrane: no cells but collagen and proteoglycans
  - Epithelial cell layer of the Bowman's capsule: contains foot processes or podocytes

5.1.4 Tubule

- Made up of proximal tubule, loop of Henle, and distal nephron. Several distal nephrons make up a collecting duct.
- Function is to reduce the volume and modify the contents of the filtrate.
- Reabsorbs and excretes.
- Reabsorbs over 99% of the filtered water and solutes.

5.1.5 Proximal tubule

- Reabsorbs:
  - 66% of water and Na^+
  - 100% of glucose and amino acids
- Secretes:
  - Organic acids and bases such as drugs and drug metabolites
- Improvement in the function of re-absorption and secretion due to epithelial cells here having:
  - A brush border in the luminal surface
  - Basal processes in the basal surface area
  - Abundant mitochondria

5.1.6 Loop of Henle

- Thin descending limb:
  - Flat epithelial cell layer with short microvilli and few mitochondria
  - Very permeable to passive water transport into peritubular fluid
- Thin ascending limb (not in long loops):
  - Similar to thin descending limb
- Thick ascending limb:
  - At the junction of inner and outer medulla
  - Epithelial cells are cuboidal and extensively digitated
  - Contain multiple mitochondria
  - Actively transports Na^+ and Cl^- into peritubular fluid
  - Impermeable to water

5.1.7 Distal nephron

- Remarkably the distal nephron returns to its own original glomerulus.
- Made up of:
  - Distal convoluted tubule (DCT): cuboidal cells; have basal and lateral interdigitations and contain multiple mitochondria
  - Connecting tubule: epithelial cells; taller and more granular than those of the DCT
  - Collecting ducts (CD): now cells become columnar and have multiple mitochondria for active transport. The collecting ducts then pass from the cortex into medulla and then papillary collecting ducts. Several papillary collecting ducts form into a common collecting duct, which they drain into a minor calyx
- The distal nephron is responsible for the final transformation of tubular fluid into urine.
- Its functions include the re-absorption of Na^+ and Cl^-, the secretion of H^+ and K^+, and an important role in the concentration and dilution of urine.

5.1.8 Juxtaglomerular (JG) apparatus

- Found where the distal tubule meets the glomerulus.
- Involved in producing renin due to *tubuloglomerular feedback* as the relation of the JG apparatus allows for regulation from filtered substrate to blood flow to the glomerulus.

5.1.9 Renal blood supply and drainage

- Kidneys receive 20–25% of the total cardiac output.
- Therefore in an average adult with a cardiac output of 6L/min the renal blood flow exceeds 1.2L/min or 1700L/day.
- Of this renal blood flow approximately 125mL of plasma are filtered each minute at the glomerulus.
- This means that 180L of plasma are filtered each day.
- Therefore the kidneys have a rich blood supply
- Arterial supply:
  - The paired renal arteries are branches of the abdominal aorta
  - Interlobar arteries travel in renal columns in the cortical areas between pyramids
  - Arcuate arteries run parallel to bases of pyramids
  - Interlobular arteries are branches of arcuate arteries
  - Afferent arterioles lead to capillary tufts of glomeruli
- Venous drainage:
  - The venous drainage picks up from the peritubular capillaries and the vasa recta and then follows the same pattern as the arteries
- The blood flow to the kidney has a unique pattern:
  - The *afferent arterioles* that enter into the glomeruli capillary beds don't form a vein afterwards but form another arteriole named the *efferent arteriole*
  - This then follows the peritubular capillary bed, from the proximal tubule to the distal tubule, and eventually forms the vasa recta
  - Therefore the kidney has 2 arterioles and 2 capillary networks
  - This unique formation allows for tubular secretion of products from blood and re-absorption of water and solutes from the tubules, and thus has an important role in the concentration of urine
  - Another major role of this structure is for regulation of renal blood flow

5.1.10 Autoregulation

- This is the maintenance of renal plasma flow (RPF) despite changes in systemic arterial pressure. The maintenance of RPF therefore ensures GFR is maintained.
- Renal blood flow (RBF) = arteriovenous pressure difference/vascular resistance.
- An increase in arterial pressure must therefore be accompanied by an increase in vascular resistance to maintain RPF at a constant level without changing the pressures for filtration; this is achieved mainly at the afferent arteriole.
- This can be from *intrinsic* or *extrinsic* factors.
- Intrinsic:
  - Myogenic mechanism:
    - As the arteriole is stretched the smooth muscles of the arteriole are contracted via Ca^{2+} channel stimulation
    - This causes afferent arteriolar constriction
  - Tubuloglomerular feedback (TGF):
    - This occurs via the distal tubule and the juxtaglomerular apparatus
    - As the flow of tubular fluid is reduced through this area, there is a signal (possibly Na^+ or Cl^-) to the macula densa causing release of another signal (adenosine or thromboxane), leading to local constriction of the afferent arteriole as well as renin release
    - This leads to the release of angiotensin II, which also causes afferent constriction and efferent dilatation

- Extrinsic:
  - Nervous:
    - As the BP falls there is an increase in sympathetic tone via baroreceptors, which in the kidneys causes constriction of both the afferent and efferent arterioles to maintain both RPF and GFR as the SAP falls
  - Hormonal:
    - With increased sympathetic tone there is increased circulating *norepinephrine*, which causes afferent arteriolar constriction. At high levels this causes RPF to be reduced more than GFR and so blood flow to the kidney is reduced. This helps preserve essential SAP to vital organs during crises (e.g. massive hypovolaemia)
    - *Angiotensin II* via the renin–angiotensin–aldosterone system is released when the BP is low. Angiotensin II acts to cause efferent arteriolar constriction to maintain GFR
    - *Prostaglandins*—help to reduce vasoconstrictor effects of sympathetic nerves and angiotensin II, and that way help to maintain RBF and prevent renal ischaemia
    - *Nitric oxide*—produced by shear forces in endothelial cells and by other hormones (Ach, histamine, bradykinin, and ATP). Causes vasodilation of afferent and efferent arterioles as well as decreasing total peripheral resistance

5.2 Mechanism of filtration

5.2.1 Glomerular filtration

- In normal adults, GFR is around 90–140mL/min for males and 80–125mL/min for females.
- After the age of 30 the GFR decreases, but this does not affect the kidneys' function.
- Therefore in 24 hours as much as 180L/day of plasma is filtered at the glomerulus.
- The portion of the plasma in the blood that is filtered is known as the *filtration fraction* and is determined as: filtration fraction = GFR/RPF
- In normal conditions this is 0.15–0.2, i.e. only 15–20% of plasma is filtered. This is known as the *ultrafiltrate*.
- Ultrafiltration occurs due to the unique structure of the Bowman's capsule. The filtration barrier is made of only 3 layers:
  - Capillary endothelium
  - Basement membrane
  - Filtration slits of the podocytes
- This stops any molecules moving across into the nephron on the basis of size and electrical charge:
  - Molecules <20Å and neutral are filtered
  - Molecules 20–42Å are filtered to different degrees
  - Molecules >42Å are not filtered
- Cationic (positive charges) are filtered more readily than anionic. This is due to the negatively charged glycoproteins on all the surfaces of the filtration barrier. Most of the proteins in the plasma are therefore stopped by the barrier, as these are mainly negative.
- In patients with immunological and inflammatory diseases of the glomerulus, the negative charge on the filtration barrier is reduced and so protein leaks into the urine.
- For this reason the ultrafiltrate doesn't contain any cellular elements and is protein free. It is isotonic with normal plasma but driven out of the bloodstream by Starling's forces.
- This involves the balance of *hydrostatic pressure* (force from vascular resistance giving water movement out of the capillary lumen) and *oncotic pressure* (force from protein molecules pulling water molecules into the capillary lumen).
- In the kidneys, the main driving force for ultrafiltration is the hydrostatic forces in the glomerular capillary (PGC) due to the relative difference in protein content from the capillary lumen (100%) to the Bowman's space (0%).

- The forces against the movement of fluid out of the lumen are the hydrostatic pressure in the Bowman's space (PBS) and the oncotic pressure in the glomerular capillary (πGC).
- Due to the unique structure of the glomerulus the filtration is much greater than in any other systemic capillary network:
  - The permeability of the capillary (Kf) is large due to the thin filtration barrier and large surface area
  - The large hydrostatic pressure is because of the structure of the capillaries in the capsule
  - GFR = Kf [(PGC − PBS) − (πGC − πBS)]
  - Where = the reflection coefficient
- In normal individuals the GFR is altered by changes in PGC. These changes are brought about by arteriolar resistance. PGC is affected in 3 ways:
  - Changes in afferent arteriolar resistance: ↓ = ↑ PGC and GFR
  - Changes in efferent arteriolar resistance: ↓ = ↓ PGC and GFR
  - Changes in renal arteriolar pressure: ↑ = ↑ PGC and GFR
- The mechanisms regarding afferent and efferent resistance were discussed earlier (see Chapter D5, Section 5.1.10).

5.2.2 Creatinine clearance

- Assessment of renal function represents the 3 functions that occur in each nephron as one coordinated action. These are:
  - Glomerular filtration
  - Re-absorption of the substance from the tubules into the blood
  - Secretion of some substances from the blood into the tubules
- *Renal clearance* is the theoretical basis of GFR and RBF measurements. GFR can be seen as a direct measure of kidney function.
- In order to measure GFR, a substance that will act as an appropriate marker is needed that meets the following criteria:
  - Must be freely filtered across the glomerulus into Bowman's space
  - Must not be reabsorbed or secreted by the nephron
  - Must not be metabolized or produced by the kidney
  - Must not alter GFR
- *Creatinine* is an organic base that is produced from muscle metabolism. It is filtered by the glomerulus and only 10–15% is secreted into the tubule.
- For that reason it is the best clinical marker used to measure GFR, so: mass of creatinine excreted/time = mass of creatinine filtered/time
- Or: GFR × Pcr = Ucr × V
- Therefore: GFR = Ucr × V/Pcr
  - Pcr = plasma concentration of creatinine
  - Ucr = urine concentration of creatinine
  - V = rate of urine flow
- 10–15% of creatinine is *secreted* into the tubule, meaning that values given will be incorrect as the value for Ucr will be greater by 10%. However, the method used by laboratories to quantitate the Pcr overestimates the true value by 10%, so therefore they cancel each other out, providing a reasonable source for GFR.

5.2.3 Tubular transport

- In the nephron a substance can be re-absorbed or secreted:
  - *Through* cells from the basolateral membrane to the apical membrane (known as the **transcellular pathway**)

- *Between* the cells via the tight junctions that hold the cells together (known as the **paracellular pathway**)
- There are different mechanisms by which solutes can be transported:
  - Passive transport:
    - All movement of water is by this method (osmosis) and can create a 'solvent drag' pulling substances with it
    - Uncharged solutes move from high to low concentrations (chemical gradient)
    - Charged ions can move due to electrical potential differences (electrical gradient)
  - Facilitated diffusion:
    - Still a passive process but solutes are moved by specific membrane transporters for that substance, for example, aquaporins for water transport, **uniports** for urea or glucose, or Na^+, K^+, and Cl^- in coupled transport
    - Coupled transport of 2 or more solutes in opposite directions is by an **antiport** mechanism
    - Here one of the solutes is usually transported *against* its chemical gradient, the energy for which is provided by the other solute travelling *with* its concentration gradient
    - This is termed **secondary active transport** as ATP is not involved
  - Active transport:
    - This is transport that is directly coupled to energy derived from a metabolic process
    - Usually involves solutes moving against their concentration gradients
    - Most common is the Na^+/K^+-ATPase at the basolateral membrane
    - Also H^+-ATPase, H^+/K^+-ATPase, and Ca^{2+}-ATPase
    - This is **primary active transport**
- For many substances that are actively reabsorbed or use a transporter there is a maximum rate that is achieved. This is termed *transport maximum* (Tm):
  - Glucose, amino acids, phosphate, and sulphate are examples that exhibit such Tm-limited re-absorption
  - Usually the entire filtered load of these substances is reabsorbed as long as the transporters aren't saturated
  - However, when the transport system is saturated the excess load will be excreted
- Theoretical data collected show an abrupt change once the saturation of glucose transport has been reached. Actual glucose titration curves show more of a gradual change. This is known as **splay**. It means that due to this splay the renal threshold for glucose is approximately 11mmol/L instead of the saturation 16mmol/L measured.
- This is usually much greater than the plasma glucose level of around 5mmol/L and so glucose should normally be absent from the urine, as saturation should not occur and therefore *all* glucose will be reabsorbed.
- There are 2 reasons why splay may occur:
  - Although the affinity of the transporter for glucose is very high, some will still 'slip' through
  - Due to the heterogeneity of each nephron there is considerable variation in filtration and re-absorption. So while some nephrons are poorer at re-absorbing glucose, and so excrete glucose at lower plasma concentrations, others do the opposite
- For these reasons glucose will be found in the urine before saturation occurs, i.e. splay.

5.2.4 Proximal tubule (PT)

- Involved in the re-absorption of:
  - Approximately 60% of water and Na^+
  - 100% of glucose and amino acids
  - Also involved in secretion of organic acids and bases

- Sodium transport:
  - Sodium (Na^+) must be accompanied by an anion to maintain electrical neutrality. Approximately 75% is with Cl^-, and 25% with HCO_3^-
  - With the re-absorption of Na^+ in the PT comes the re-absorption of the majority of water also, due to the generation of the osmotic gradient. Na^+ is transported via the following mechanisms:
    - 1: Na^+-solute symport
    - 2: Na^+/H^+ exchange (antiport)
    - 3: Cl^--driven Na^+ transport
  - Both 1 and 2 are examples of active transport. The entry of Na^+ into the apical (luminal) membrane of the cell surface is carrier mediated via its electrochemical gradient. It is then removed at the basement membrane via the Na^+/K^+-ATPase channel against its gradient. This mainly occurs in the first half of the PT, due to an abundance of the transporters
  - In the second half of the PT Na^+ is transported with Cl^- via transcellular and paracellular routes:
    - Transcellular Na^+Cl^- re-absorption occurs via parallel H^+ transport
    - Paracellular NaCl re-absorption occurs because the rise in Cl^- in the tubular fluid in the first half of the PT creates a concentration gradient. This favours the movement of Cl^- from the lumen across tight junctions into intercellular space
    - This means that the tubular fluid becomes positively charged, forcing Na^+ movement also into intercellular space. This process is by passive diffusion
- Glucose transport:
  - As mentioned previously, solutes are linked to the transport of Na^+ (e.g. glucose). The energy for the transport of glucose is therefore provided by the Na^+/K^+-ATPase, which establishes the electrochemical gradient for the entry of Na^+.

5.2.5 Loop of Henle (LoH)

- Involved in:
  - Reabsorbing approximately 20% filtered Na^+ and 20% filtered water
  - Adds urea to tubular fluid
  - Involved in urinary concentration and dilution
- LoHs have different lengths—short or long.
- In general it is considered that the osmolality of the surrounding peritubular fluid is greater for long loops than short loops:
  - The peritubular fluid in the cortex is deemed isotonic as its osmolality is similar to that of plasma, i.e. 300mOsmol/kg H_2O.
  - At the tip of short LoH the osmolality of peritubular fluid is 600mOsmol/kg H_2O
  - At the tip of long LoH the osmolality of peritubular fluid is 1200mOsmol/kg H_2O
- This difference across the LoH is known as the *medullary gradient* (see Figure D.5.1).
- Thin descending limb:
  - This has a relatively low permeability to solutes and lacks mechanisms for active transport, but is highly permeable to water. Therefore, as the tubular fluid travels down the thin descending limb, it travels through regions of increasingly hypertonic peritubular fluid
  - As the descending limb is so permeable the tubular fluid becomes the same tonicity as the peritubular fluid
  - Therefore the fluid osmolality in the tubular fluid also increases. In long LoHs the osmolality at the tip of the nephron is around 1200, and in short LoHs it is around 600
  - This effect from the re-absorption of water causes a concentration of the solutes in the tubule so that in both short and long LoHs the predominant solutes in *tubular* fluid are Na^+ and Cl^-, but the main solute in *peritubular* fluid is urea

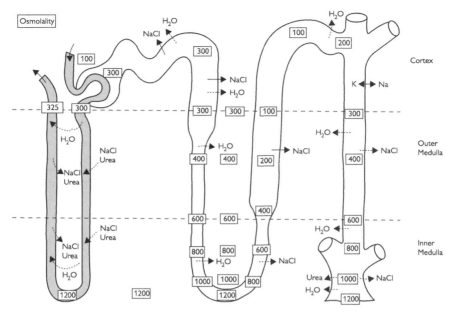

Figure D.5.1 Counter-current multiplier in the loop of Henle

- Thin ascending limb:
  - In the long LoH, a thin ascending limb is present. This is virtually impermeable to water but highly permeable to Na⁺, Cl⁻, and urea. Therefore Na⁺ and Cl⁻ diffuse passively from the highly concentrated tubular fluid into the surrounding peritubular fluid. Urea passes in the opposite direction
  - There is a greater permeability to Na⁺ and Cl⁻ than to urea, so the number of moles leaving the tubule is greater than the number of moles entering. Despite this net solute exit the *volume* of the tubular fluid stays the same, as water is unable to move out. Therefore the osmolality of the tubular fluid of the thin ascending limb falls slightly lower than that of the surrounding peritubular fluid.
- Thick ascending limb:
  - Here the water and urea permeability is low
  - Also, Na⁺ and Cl⁻ are **actively** transported from the lumen into the peritubular space
  - This means that the thick ascending limb *lowers* both the osmolality of the tubular fluid and the concentration of Na⁺ and Cl⁻ in the tubular fluid to levels below those in the surrounding peritubular fluid
  - In both nephron types (long and short) the tubular fluid that leaves the LoH is hypotonic and has a urea concentration greater than that of plasma and peritubular fluid
  - The active mechanism by which Na⁺ and Cl⁻ are actively reabsorbed is by the symporter of Na⁺, K⁺, and 2 Cl⁻ ions. This is termed the Na⁺/K⁺/2Cl⁻ symport (see Figure D.5.2)
  - The K⁺ is then leaked back across the apical membrane, therefore creating a potential difference by making the lumen positive
  - The transport of Na⁺ at this channel is *load dependent* so that if more Na⁺ arrives at the thick ascending limb, more Na⁺ is transported
  - Loop diuretics such as furosemide and bumetanide act at the Na⁺/K⁺/2Cl⁻ symport by inhibiting its action. This increases Na⁺ and to some extent K⁺ excretion, and therefore also water, due to its passive movement with Na⁺ ions

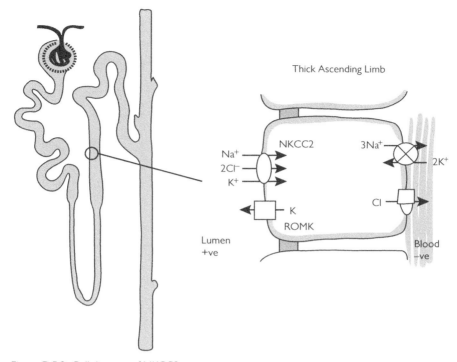

Figure D.5.2 Cell diagram of NKCC2

5.2.6 Distal collecting system

- Involved in finite modification of final urine production.
- Re-absorption of 5–10% of filtered Na^+.
- Re-absorption of urea.
- Secretion of H^+ and K^+.
- Re-absorption of 15% of filtered water.

5.2.7 Distal convoluted tubule (DCT) and connecting tubule

- Here the entry of Na^+ is coupled with Cl^- and it is removed at the basement membrane actively by the Na^+/K^+-ATPase channel (see Figure D.5.3).
- This is therefore by active transport and again the channel is load dependent.
- This is where thiazide diuretics act, by inhibiting the Na^+/Cl^- symporter.
- In a similar way to the thick ascending limb, the DCT and collecting tubule have low permeability to water and urea.
- This, combined with the active transport of Na^+, *lowers* the osmolality and electrolyte concentration in the fluid, increasing the hypotonicity further.

5.2.8 Collecting duct (CD)

- The Na^+ entry into cells in the various parts of the CD is not linked with other solutes and it is via an epithelial Na^+ channel (ENaC).
- This movement of Na^+ across the tubular membrane causes a potential difference.

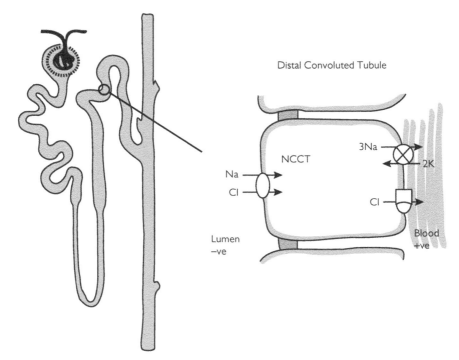

Figure D.5.3 Cell diagram of NCCT

- ENaC is stimulated by aldosterone, thus this acts to increase Na⁺ re-absorption (and therefore that of water) and increase the potential difference across the apical membrane.
- ENaC is inhibited by atrial natriuretic factor and diuretics including amiloride.
- Also, ENaC is produced via aldosterone acting on the nucleus of the cell to upregulate ENaC production.
- Spironolactone acts to inhibit this upregulation process.
- Water and urea permeability in the CD are regulated by a hormone known as antidiuretic hormone (ADH).
- This is a nonapeptide produced by the hypothalamus and stored in the posterior pituitary.
- When ADH levels are low, a large volume of urine is excreted (diuresis) and the urine is dilute.
- When ADH levels are high, a small volume of urine is produced and the urine is concentrated.

5.2.9 ADH action

- Increases the CD permeability to water and medullary portion to urea.
- ADH binds to a receptor on the basolateral membrane of the CD cells known as V2 receptor (V1 receptor being responsible for vasocontraction).
- This leads to the production of water channels known as aquaporins that insert into the apical membrane and increase the re-absorption of water.

5.2.10 K⁺ excretion and tubular flow

- A rise in the tubular flow of fluid acts to stimulate K⁺ excretion, by secretion of K⁺ into the tubular fluid in the DT and CD.

- This is thought to occur by 2 mechanisms:
  - As the flow of tubular fluid increases, then the difference in K^+ concentration across the apical membrane is increased, making it easier to secrete K^+ into the lumen due to the improved electrochemical gradient
  - A rise in tubular flow increases the Na^+ available at the DCT and CD so more Na^+ is reabsorbed. This causes an increase in Na^+/K^+-ATPase activity and so more K^+ is secreted apically
- As diuretics increase the tubular flow of tubular fluid they therefore act to enhance K^+ excretion.

5.2.11 Calcium regulation

- Calcium homeostasis (see Chapter D6, Section 6.5) occurs in the kidney and is directly affected by PTH, calcitriol (vitamin D analogue), and calcitonin:
  - PTH acts to dramatically stimulate the re-absorption of Ca^{2+} in the thick ascending limb and DCT, therefore urinary excretion declines
  - Calcitonin *and* calcitriol also act to enhance the re-absorption of calcium in the thick ascending limb and DCT
  - PTH acts at the proximal tubule to produce calcitriol from 25-hydroxy vitamin D3

5.2.12 Regulation of plasma osmolality

- Dilute urine—with low or absent ADH:
  - Fluid entering the LoH from the PT is essentially isotonic to the plasma
  - The descending LoH is permeable to water but not to solutes so water moves out as the loop descends into the medulla. Therefore at the bend of the LoH the osmolality is the same in the tubule compared to the peritubule but the concentrations of solutes differ:
    - That is, tubular NaCl concentration > peritubular
    - Tubular urea concentration < peritubular
  - The ascending limb is impermeable to water, but not to NaCl and urea
  - Therefore NaCl moves out of the tubule and urea moves in. But NaCl movement out is greater than urea in, so diluting the tubular fluid
  - The thick ascending limb is impermeable to water and urea and actively reabsorbs NaCl, therefore diluting the tubular fluid
  - Fluid leaving the thick ascending limb is hypo-osmotic (150mOsmol/kg H_2O) compared to plasma
  - The DCT and cortical CD actively reabsorb NaCl, but are impermeable to urea *and* are **impermeable to water in the absence of ADH**:
    - So the osmolality of the tubular fluid is reduced further. Fluid entering the cortical CD is now 100mOsmol/kg H_2O
  - The medullary CD actively reabsorbs NaCl. Even in the absence of ADH there is permeability to water and urea, so some urea moves into the tubule and some water is reabsorbed
  - The final urine composition without ADH secretion is therefore:
    - Osmolality = 150mOsmol/kg H_2O
    - Non-urea solutes = 20mmol/L
    - Urea = 50mmol/L
- Concentrated urine—with high ADH:
  - Due to the effect of the **counter-current multiplier** and the **medullary gradient** that occurs due to the re-absorption of NaCl from the ascending thin and thick LoH (which accumulates in the interstitium), a difference in osmolality is created. This creates the driving force for water re-absorption. See Figure D.5.1

- At the CD fluid in the tubule is therefore hypo-osmolar with respect to the interstitium
- In the presence of ADH and therefore water permeability (due to aquaporins) here, water moves *out* of the tubular lumen, and the tubule fluid becomes concentrated
- This concentration continues to occur across the medulla as the permeability to water continues
- Urea permeability is also increased with ADH, and therefore the urine becomes urea-rich
- The final urine concentration in the presence of ADH is therefore:
  - Osmolality = 1200mOsmol/kg H_2O
  - Non-urea solutes = 600mmol/L
  - Urea = 600mmol/L

5.2.13 Regulatory mechanisms for plasma osmolality

- Hypothalamus:
  - Cells involved in sensing changes in blood osmolality are found in the supraoptic hypothalamic nucleus and are known as **osmoreceptors**
  - When the osmolality of body fluids increases, osmoreceptors send signals to ADH-synthesizing cells and ADH production is stimulated
  - When the osmolality of body fluids is reduced the signal is then inhibited
  - The plasma half-life of ADH is about 15–30min. This means that when secretion stops, ADH is *quickly* metabolized and inactivated. It is inactivated by plasma and in the kidney and liver
  - This fast mechanism of secretion and fast breakdown means that the ADH system can respond quickly to changes in body osmolality
- Blood pressure:
  - A decrease in blood pressure, either by hypovolaemia or a drop in arterial pressure, also stimulates ADH release
  - **Baroreceptors** for this mechanism are found in the left atrium and pulmonary vessels, i.e. the *low pressure system*, and in the aortic arch and carotid sinus, i.e. *high pressure system*
  - The low pressure system responds to volume loss
  - The high pressure system responds to arterial pressure
  - Signals from these baroreceptors travel via the cranial nerves IX and X and enter the brainstem in the medulla oblongata at the solitary tract nucleus. (This area also affects regulation of blood pressure via direct cardiac mechanisms.)
  - These signals then cause the secretion of ADH from the hypothalamus
- Thirst:
  - The earlier-mentioned stimuli that alter ADH secretion also alter the perception of *thirst*
  - Of these stimuli, an increase in plasma osmolality is the most powerful
  - The 'thirst centre' is found in the anterolateral region of the hypothalamus
  - Similar to the ADH-secreting cells, the thirst centre responds to the osmolality of body fluid; it is also affected by changes in blood volume and arterial pressure and by angiotensin II levels
  - Therefore if the body is depleted of fluids these stimuli act on the thirst centre, which stimulates the person's desire to drink

5.2.14 Renin–angiotensin–aldosterone system (RAAS)

- **Renin** is a catalytic *enzyme* secreted from the juxtaglomerular apparatus, which is stimulated by:
  - Decreased renal perfusion pressure as sensed by the stretch receptors of smooth muscle in the afferent arterioles

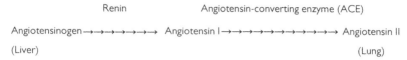

Figure D.5.4 The renin–angiotensin–aldosterone system (RAAS)

- Changes in the volume composition of the tubular fluid reaching the macular densa, i.e. *tubuloglomerular feedback*
- Stimulation of renal sympathetic nerves
- When renin is *secreted* due to these mechanisms, caused by *volume depletion*, it converts the reaction seen in Figure D.5.4
- **Angiotensin II** is an active peptide that causes:
  - Peripheral arteriolar vasoconstriction, increasing total peripheral resistance
  - Stimulation of ADH secretion and thirst in the hypothalamus
  - Enhancement of NaCl re-absorption by the proximal tubule
  - Stimulation of aldosterone secretion at the zona glomerulosa of the adrenal cortex
- Angiotensin II thus creates negative and positive feedback effects:
  - Negative feedback so that it increases blood pressure from the earlier-mentioned effects, thus reducing its own stimulation via renin
  - Positive feedback as it causes the stimulation of aldosterone and other actions in the kidney
- **Aldosterone** is a steroid hormone also produced by these mechanisms:
  - Increased angiotensin II
  - Decreased plasma atrial natriuretic peptide (ANP)
  - Increased plasma K^+ concentrations
  - Increased adrenocorticotrophic hormone (ACTH)
  - Decreased plasma Na^+ concentrations
- Aldosterone acts to stimulate the re-absorption of NaCl at the DCT and CD. The steroid hormone enters cells easily and binds to a cytoplasmic receptor, which enters the nucleus and causes the transcription of mRNA, which codes for membrane proteins.
- This causes the increased production of ENaC and Na^+/K^+-ATPase, so that entry of Na^+ into the cell and exit out of it is enhanced, due to more channels being produced.
- **Atrial natriuretic peptide (ANP)** is produced in states of increased body fluid volumes:
  - As the larger volumes of blood return to the heart, the atria are stretched, which causes a release of ANP from the myocytes of the heart
  - ANP causes the following effects, which act to antagonize that of the RAAS:
    - Vasodilation of the afferent arterioles and vasoconstriction of the efferent arterioles, thus increasing GFR and filtered load of Na^+
    - Inhibition of aldosterone via direct inhibition of the secretory cells in the adrenal cortex and via inhibition of renin secretion
    - Inhibition of NaCl re-absorption at the CD
    - Inhibition of ADH secretion and action in the CD
  - ANP therefore causes the excretion of water and Na^+ from the kidneys, thus reducing the blood volume circulation and reducing stretch at the atrium.

5.3 Acid–base balance

- The homeostasis of acid–base balance is essential in humans.
- In conditions outside of the normal pH of 7.35–7.45 in arterial blood, proteins are rapidly denatured meaning that cell structure and metabolic function are significantly affected. This would not be compatible with life if pH were not maintained within the normal range.

5.3.1 Henderson–Hasselbalch equation

- This equation describes the derivation of pH; in human physiology it is used to calculate the pH of a buffer solution (plasma) and find the equilibrium pH in acid–base reactions.
- $pH = pK_a + log\left(\dfrac{[conjugate\ base]}{[acid]}\right)$.
  - Where K_a = acid dissociation constant
- Applying this equation to plasma, where acid (H^+) is buffered by bicarbonate (HCO_3^-), the 2 following reactions occur:
  - $CO_2 + H_2O \xrightarrow{\text{Carbonic anhydrase}} HCO_3^- + H^+$
    - This occurs in tissues where high levels of CO_2 are produced
    - The reverse reaction then occurs in the lungs and kidneys where CO_2 levels are low, so H^+ is buffered
  - $HCO_3^- + H^+ \rightarrow H_2CO_3 \rightarrow CO_2 + H_2O$
- The 2 main components in acid–base balance are:
  - Acid = **CO_2**
  - Base = HCO_3^-
- Applying to the equation: $pH = pK_a + log\ ([HCO_3^-]/CO_2])$
- In plasma at 37°C the CO_2 concentration = $0.03 \times PCO_2$.
- To calculate the pH of plasma with a HCO_3^- level of 24 and CO_2 of 40mmHg:
  - $pH = 6.1 + log\ 24/(0.03 \times 40) = \textbf{7.40}$.

5.3.2 The anion gap

- The anion gap is a calculation used to find a differential diagnosis for a metabolic acidosis.
- It is calculated by subtracting the main cations from the main anions:
  - $([Na^+] + [K^+]) - ([Cl^-] + [HCO_3^-])$
- The normal gap is 3–11mEq/L.
- A *high anion gap* (>11) metabolic acidosis means that there is a loss in HCO_3^- without a loss in Cl^-, due to the presence of acid.
- The HCO_3^- is replaced by anions not measured, therefore causing the high anion gap.
- This is usually caused by the following substances/conditions:
  - Methanol
  - Uraemia
  - DKA
  - Propylene glycol
  - Lactic acidosis
  - Ethylene glycol
  - Salicylates
- A *normal anion gap* metabolic acidosis means there is a loss of HCO_3^- that is replaced by an increase in Cl^-. This is also known as hyperchloraemic acidosis.
- This is usually caused by the following substances/conditions:
  - Fistula (pancreatic)
  - Uretogastric conduits
  - Saline administration
  - Endocrine (hyperparathyroidism)
  - Diarrhoea
  - Carbonic anhydrase inhibitors (acetazolamide)
  - Ammonium chloride
  - Renal tubular acidosis
  - Spironolactone

5.3.3 Disturbances to acid–base balance

- Arterial blood samples are taken in order to measure the levels of different components and work out the causes of changes in acid–base balance. These are called arterial blood gases (ABGs).
- There are 2 causes for each condition (acidosis or alkalosis): respiratory and metabolic.
- Respiratory acidosis:
  - Caused by a reduction in adequate ventilation causing an increase in CO_2 and therefore creating an acidosis
  - Typical ABG:
    - pH <7.35 (acidosis)
    - PCO_2 >6.0kPa (45mmHg) (high)
    - PO_2 = 9.3–13.3kPa (80–100mmHg) = normal (or can be <9.3 = low)
    - HCO_3^- = 22–26mmol/L = normal (or can be >26 = high if chronic)
    - Base excess = −3 to +3 = normal (or can be >+3 if chronic)
- Respiratory alkalosis:
  - Caused by an increase in ventilation leading to a reduction in CO_2 and therefore creating an alkalosis
  - Typical ABG:
    - pH >7.45 (alkalosis)
    - PCO_2 <4.7kPa (35mmHg) (low)
    - PO_2 = 9.3–13.3kPa (80–100mmHg) = normal (or can be >13.3 = high)
    - HCO_3^- = 22–26mmol/L = normal (or can be >22 = low if chronic)
    - Base excess = −3 to + 3 = normal (or can be <−3 if chronic)
- Metabolic acidosis:
  - Caused either by an increase in acid within the body *or* by the inability to produce any alkali to buffer acids
  - Typical ABG:
    - pH <7.35 (acidosis)
    - PCO_2 = normal or low
    - PO_2 = normal or high
    - HCO_3^- <22mmol/L (low)
    - Base excess <−3 (low)
- Metabolic alkalosis:
  - Caused either by a decrease in acid within the body *or* by the increased production of HCO_3^-
  - Typical ABG:
    - pH >7.45 (alkalosis)
    - PCO_2 = normal or high
    - PO_2 = normal or low
    - HCO_3^- >26mmol/L (high)
    - Base excess >+ 3 (high)
- When an acidosis or an alkalosis does occur in the body, due to various different causes, the body has different mechanisms to attempt to return the pH to within the normal range.
- This helps to minimize the disturbance to pH, but ultimately the cause will need to be dealt with.
- Usually, in broad terms, if it is a metabolic condition then the *lungs* will provide some compensation. If it is a respiratory condition then the *kidneys* will provide some compensation *plus* also are affected in metabolic conditions.
- This proves that one of the major organs involved in acid–base balance are the kidneys.

5.3.4 Lung primary compensation

- In basic terms, therefore, if there is a metabolic acidosis, then the lungs will *increase* the removal of CO_2 from the bloodstream via an *increase* in ventilation.
- This increase in ventilation due to metabolic acidosis is known as **Kussmaul breathing**.
- This works to 'blow off' the excess CO_2 produced from the metabolic acidosis.
- The reverse is true for a metabolic alkalosis—i.e. ventilation is reduced so that CO_2 is retained and not as much is 'blown off' in an attempt to buffer the alkalosis.
- In some cases the change in ventilation also affects pO_2 levels.
- These effects can take place rapidly as ventilation changes are made during each respiratory cycle.

5.3.5 Kidney primary compensation

- The kidneys' role in the primary compensation for maintaining pH involves HCO_3^- production and H^+ excretion.
- In acidosis, secretion of H^+ by the nephron is stimulated, and the entire filtered load of HCO_3^- is reabsorbed. The production and excretion of NH_4^+ is also stimulated.
- These processes ensure that more acid is secreted and more alkali is retained in the body to help maintain the normal pH. This will cause a rise in HCO_3^- during an acidosis.
- The opposite effects occur when there is an alkalosis.
- These mechanisms usually take hours to days to take effect and sometimes conditions are referred to as **acute** (i.e. no renal compensation) or **chronic** (i.e. with renal compensation). For example:
  - pH = 7.30 (acidosis)
  - PCO_2 = 8.0kPa (high)
  - PO_2 = 10.1kPa (normal)
  - HCO_3^- = 24mmol/L (normal)
  - Base excess = 0 (normal)
  - This would be **acute respiratory acidosis**
  - pH = 7.33 (acidosis)
  - PCO_2 = 8.0kPa (high)
  - PO_2 = 10.1kPa (normal)
  - HCO_3^- = 30kPa(high)
  - Base excess = +4 (high)
  - This would be **chronic respiratory acidosis**

5.3.6 Urinary acidification

- The kidney can regulate pH with the promotion of urine acidification using the following processes:
  - Bicarbonate re-absorption:
    - This process occurs mainly at the PCT with the use of carbonic anhydrase (CA)
    - CA is found at the brush border of the PCT, thus leading to the production of carbonic acid. At the basolateral membrane of the PCT bicarbonate is co-transported *out* of the cell back into the blood
    - When there is an acidosis then this reaction is enhanced. H^+ is excreted at the lumen via a H^+/Na^+ exchanger
  - Excretion of acid:
    - The production of acid in the urine uses the same process as just listed for bicarbonate re-absorption. H^+ in the tubular fluid then combines with filtered buffers, the main one being phosphate

- This process acts to remove H^+ from the body, but also helps to reabsorb more HCO_3^- back into the blood due to the promotion of the Henderson–Hasselbalch equation (see Chapter D5, Section 5.3.1) towards the acidic side
- Excretion of ammonia:
  - Ammonia (NH_3) is synthesized mainly in the PCT; when combined with H^+ it forms ammonium (NH_4^+)
  - As the pK_a of NH_4^+ is so high, the direction of the reaction is in favour of NH_4^+ production
  - In the PCT the metabolism of amino acids leads to the production of NH_4^+ and NH_3
  - NH_3 diffuses readily through cell membranes into the tubular fluid, whereas NH_4^+ relies on a $Na^+/NH4^+$ exchanger at the luminal surface
  - This means that once in the acidic urine most ammonia is in the form of NH_4^+ and cannot diffuse back out of the tubular fluid due to its polarity
  - Once again this process is enhanced by acid conditions in the blood due to the shift in the equilibrium towards CO_2 production, as more H^+ is available

5.4 Potassium balance

5.4.1 Normal values

- Potassium is regulated so that there is a difference between intracellular and extracellular concentrations:
  - Intracellular = 150mmol/L
  - Extracellular = 4.5mmol/L (range 3.5–5.O)

5.4.2 Hypokalaemia

- This describes the condition whereby K^+ levels are low, i.e. <3.5mmol/L. Clinically this can produce the following effects:
  - Muscle weakness
  - Muscle cramps
  - Muscle paralysis
  - Cardiac conduction abnormalities (i.e. arrhythmias) which can progress to VF
- The following changes can occur on an ECG with hypokalaemia:
  - Prolonged QT intervals
  - Prominent U waves
  - Narrow QRS complex
  - T-wave flattening
  - Can evolve to sinusoidal shape

5.4.3 Hyperkalaemia

- This occurs when K^+ levels are high, i.e. >5.0mmol/L. This can produce the following effects:
  - Nausea
  - Fatigue
  - Muscle weakness or paralysis
  - Paraesthesia
  - Cardiac conduction abnormalities
- The following changes occur on an ECG for patients with hyperkalaemia:
  - Reduced P-wave size
  - Peaked T waves
  - Widened QRS complex
  - Can evolve to sinusoidal shape

5.5 Calcium balance

Please also see Chapter D6, Section 6.5.

- The normal values for total serum calcium are 2.25–2.5mmol/L.
- This equates to around 10mg/100mL of calcium in human plasma.
- In the normal state the serum calcium can be divided into 2 types:
  - Calcium that is *filtered* by glomeruli (50% of total serum calcium)
  - Calcium that is *not filtered* by glomeruli (50% of total serum calcium)
- Calcium that is filtered at the glomeruli is found in 2 forms:
  - **Ionized calcium** (50% of total serum calcium): this is the physiologically active form of calcium. It is regulated tightly as it is involved in many cellular functions
  - **Anion-bound calcium** (10% of total serum calcium): usually bound to bicarbonate/phosphate/citrate and others
- The unfiltered calcium is protein-bound (40% of total serum calcium).
- As this calcium is bound to the large proteins found in the plasma it is unable to travel out via cell membranes or glomeruli.
- Majority bound to albumin (40kDa) but also to globulins.
- Therefore in order to calculate a patient's serum calcium levels, adjustments need to be made for their protein content in the plasma also.
- This is done by:
  - +0.1mmol/L to calcium concentration for every 4g/L that albumin is below 40g/L
  - −0.1mmol/L to calcium concentration for every 4g/L that albumin is above 40g/L
  - Note: when the measured albumin concentration is less than 20g/L measurement becomes inaccurate
  - These levels will *not* be measuring ionized calcium

5.5.1 Calcium handling

- The average intake of calcium is 1g per day. This is primarily from dietary sources, most of which will be dairy produce.
- Foods rich in calcium include:
  - Cheese
  - Milk
  - Yogurt
  - Bony fish
  - Some vegetables and nuts

5.5.2 Calcium and the kidney

- The kidneys excrete approximately 150mg of calcium into the urine per day.
- This is around 1% of the total filtered load via the glomerulus, meaning that around 99% is reabsorbed back into the bloodstream.
- The 3 main areas where this occurs are:
  - PCT (60%)
  - LoH (30%)
  - DCT (10%)
- The re-absorption of calcium in these areas is mainly by an active process.
- The 'fine tuning' or tight regulation of calcium levels occurs at the DCT and this is therefore where hormones affect.

5.5.3 PTH and the kidney

- PTH is stimulated when serum levels of ionized calcium are low.
- In the kidneys PTH acts to:
  - Increase activity of 1α-hydroxylase, which catalyses the formation of 1,25-OH-vitamin D3 (another active hormone for calcium metabolism)
  - *Increase* active re-absorption of *calcium* at DCT
  - *Decrease phosphate* re-absorption at the PCT
- The kidney is the only organ of the body where calcium can be reabsorbed whilst phosphate is excreted.
- This enables an *increased availability* of serum *ionized calcium*, as it will not precipitate to the crystal form of hydroxyapatite (see Chapter D6, Section 6.5) as less phosphate is available.
- In the kidneys 1,25-OH-vitamin D_3 acts to:
  - *Increase* tubular re-absorption of both calcium *and* phosphate
  - Although its main effects occur at *bone*

5.5.4 Calcitonin

- This is stimulated when levels of calcium are low. However, it only has a very small role to play in calcium and phosphate homeostasis, and it is thought that it is only really for 'fine tuning' of calcium levels.
- In the kidneys calcitonin acts to:
  - *Decrease* re-absorption of both calcium and phosphate
  - Although its major action is again at *bone*

Endocrine physiology

CONTENTS

6.1 Pituitary function

6.1.1 Functional anatomy of the pituitary

- The pituitary sits in the sella turcica (pituitary fossa, part of the sphenoid bone) (see Figure D.6.1):
  - Separated from the brain by the diaphragma sellae (a reflection of dura mater)
  - Controlled by the hypothalamus and connected to the hypothalamus through the neural stalk
  - Because the pituitary fossa is small and sits just below the optic chiasm, the most common symptoms of a pituitary tumour are headache and visual loss
- Anterior pituitary (the adenohypophyses):
  - Composed of glandular cells
  - Releases a number of hormones:
    - Luteinizing hormone (LH)
    - Follicle-stimulating hormone (FSH)
    - Growth hormone (GH)
    - Prolactin
    - Adrenocorticotrophic hormone (ACTH)
    - Thyroid-stimulating hormone (TSH)
    - Melanocyte-stimulating hormone
- Posterior pituitary (neurohypophyses):
  - Essentially an extension of the hypothalamus composed of neural cells
  - Secretes oxytocin and ADH (vasopressin)
- Hypothalamus:
  - Situated directly above the pituitary
  - Receives signals from the brain including:
    - The reticular activating system
    - The thalamus
    - The limbic system
    - The optical system
- This means pituitary function is altered by wakefulness, senses, and emotion among other stimuli.

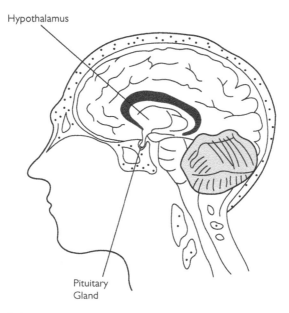

Hypothalamus

Pituitary
Gland

Figure D.6.1 The pituitary

6.1.2 Hypothalamic-releasing hormones and their effect on anterior pituitary

- Corticotrophin-releasing hormone (CRH):
  - Released from the paraventricular nucleus of the hypothalamus in response to stress
  - Stimulates the release of ACTH from the anterior pituitary
  - ACTH in turn stimulates the adrenal glands to produce cortisol
  - Cortisol prepares the body for stress by mobilizing energy stores and increasing blood pressure
  - CRH has an important role in the CNS, including central arousal and increased sympathetic response
- Thyroid-releasing hormone (TRH):
  - Released from the paraventricular nucleus of the hypothalamus
  - In response to thermal and energy requirements
  - Stimulates the anterior pituitary to release TSH
  - TSH stimulates thyroid gland to produce triiodothyronine (T3) and thyroxine (T4)
  - Leads to an increase in metabolic rate
  - T3 and T4 negatively feed back on both the pituitary and hypothalamus
- Dopamine:
  - Has many functions and is released from multiple sites throughout the brain
  - Released from the arcuate nucleus of the hypothalamus
  - Main role in pituitary function is to inhibit the release of prolactin from the anterior pituitary:
    - Prolactin plays a key role in lactation and sexual gratification
    - Counteracts the effects of dopamine, which is responsible for sexual arousal

6.1.3 Posterior pituitary hormones

- Antidiuretic hormone (ADH):
  - Produced in the supraoptic nucleus of the hypothalamus
  - Transported down the axons of these cells and stored in their terminals in the posterior pituitary
  - When the neurons are activated, ADH is released into the circulation via the inferior hypophyseal artery
  - ADH regulates body water volume by acting on the distal collecting ducts of the kidney to retain water
  - The stimulus for ADH release comes from osmoreceptors in the hypothalamus in response to a change in plasma osmolality (neuroendocrine reflex) and ADH acts over a shorter time period (minutes to hours) than most other hormones
  - Reduction in plasma osmolality is detected by osmoreceptors in the hypothalamus of the brain, which then switch off the release of ADH

6.1.4 Effect of disordered function

Anterior pituitary

- Hypopituitarism:
  - Commonest causes:
    - Pituitary and hypothalamic tumours
    - Surgery or radiotherapy
  - Dependent on which hormones are affected.
    - Mild deficiencies may go unnoticed
    - Hypoprolactinaemia rare and clinically unimportant
    - Reduced ACTH causes hypoadrenalism (aldosterone not deficient and patient does not become pigmented)
    - Reduced TRH and TSH cause hypothyroidism, but without the weight gain as usually accompanied by hypoadrenalism
  - A patient with panhypopituitarism is:
    - Pale and hairless
    - Hypotensive, lethargic, and weak
- Pituitary over-activity:
  - Hyperprolactinaemia:
    - Primary, for example, pituitary tumour
    - Secondary, for example, non-pituitary tumours preventing inhibition of prolactin, drug induced, and endocrine causes (e.g. polycystic ovarian syndrome)
    - Presents differently in women and men: women get galactorrhoea and infertility and condition is caused by a microadenoma. Men present later in life with larger tumours and present with impotence and infertility
  - Acromegaly:
    - Excess GH usually from pituitary adenoma
    - Presents with mass effect and effects of excess GH such as: headache; prominent and enlarged features—hands, feet, and face

Posterior pituitary

- Diabetes insipidus (DI):
  - Caused by either:
    - A lack of ADH production (neurogenic DI)
    - The kidneys' failure to respond to ADH (nephrogenic)
  - Patients are unable to retain water:
    - Polyuria

- Polydipsia
- Dehydration
  - Commonest causes are benign tumours to the hypothalamus and pituitary, head trauma, and iatrogenic (surgery and radiotherapy)
- Syndrome of inappropriate antidiuretic hormone hypersecretion (SIADH):
  - The release of ADH is not inhibited by a drop in plasma osmolality
  - Excess ADH secretion
  - Ongoing drop in plasma osmolality and hyponatraemia as excess water is retained
  - Caused by:
    - CNS disease (such as meningitis, head trauma, cancer)
    - Side effect of certain drugs
  - Features:
    - Headache and vomiting
    - At extremes, seizures and coma

6.2 Adrenal function

6.2.1 Functional anatomy
- The adrenal glands are found at the upper poles of each kidney and consist of:
  - The medulla:
    - Developed from neuronal tissue
    - Secretes epinephrine and norepinephrine
  - The cortex:
    - Developed from mesodermal tissue
    - Secretes steroid hormones

6.2.2 Adrenal cortex
- The cortex is made up of 3 layers (from outer to inner):
  - Zona glomerulosa—produces aldosterone:
    - A mineralocorticoid
    - Increases the reabsorption of sodium and water and secretion of potassium from the kidney
    - Acts on the distal tubules and collecting ducts
    - Part of the renin–angiotensin system
    - Increases blood volume and blood pressure
  - Zona fasciculate—produces cortisol:
    - Most important glucocorticoid
    - Released in pulses during normal physiological activity
    - Controlled by ACTH–CRH
    - Usually a peak in cortisol levels an hour after waking
  - Zona reticularis:
    - Secretes dehydroepiandrosterone (DHEA)

6.2.3 Effects of glucocorticoids
- Reduce immune response:
  - Inhibit pro-inflammatory mediators
  - Stimulate anti-inflammatory mediators
- Maintain blood glucose:
  - Stimulate gluconeogenesis in the liver

- Inhibit uptake of glucose into muscle (mediated by insulin)
- Increase appetite and truncal fat distribution
- Inhibit collagen synthesis (leads to thin skin and osteoporosis in long-term steroid use)

6.2.4 Clinical effects of disordered glucocorticoid secretion

Cushing's syndrome

- Cushing's syndrome is caused by an excess of glucocorticoids. (Cushing's disease is specific to a pituitary adenoma that produces ectopic ACTH.)
- The patient typically presents with non-specific features of:
  - Depression
  - Weight gain
  - Weakness
  - Malaise
- Classical signs include:
  - Moon face
  - Plethora
  - Thin skin
  - Truncal obesity
  - Muscle wasting
- Commonest causes are:
  - Pituitary adenoma
  - Adrenal tumours
  - Ectopic ACTH production (from carcinoid tumour)
  - Prolonged steroid use
- Diagnosis is from increased plasma or urinary cortisol levels. Investigation is via dexamethasone suppression test and through MRI scanning.

Adrenal insufficiency

- Adrenal insufficiency can be either primary (Addison's disease) or secondary either to pituitary disease or to prolonged steroid use.
- Addison's disease:
  - Causes:
    - Autoimmune >80%
    - Infection (TB, AIDS)
    - Tumour (uncommon)
  - Main features:
    - Hyperpigmentation (increased ACTH through feedback)
    - Weight loss
    - Weakness
    - Postural hypotension
    - Hyponatraemia and hyperkalaemia (lack of aldosterone)
    - Hypoglycaemia
  - Investigation is through Synacthen testing, CT, and MRI

6.2.5 Medullary function

- The adrenal medulla mainly consists of chromaffin cells:
  - Secrete epinephrine and norepinephrine
  - Directly connected to the sympathetic nervous system through the preganglionic neurons of the spinal cord

- Epinephrine and norepinephrine act on alpha and beta adrenoceptors:
  - Mobilize the body for activity by:
    - Vasoconstriction (alpha 1)
    - Inhibiting insulin, stimulating glucagon (alpha 2)
    - Increasing cardiac output (beta 1)
    - Increasing lipolysis (beta 2 and 3)
    - Airway dilatation (beta 2)
- Degradation of catecholamines:
  - Various metabolites
  - Mainly by monoamine oxidase (MAO) and catechol-O-methyltransferase (COMT) in:
    - Chromaffin cells when storage is saturated
    - Plasma catecholamines metabolized in liver and kidney
- Phaeochromocytoma:
  - Tumour of chromaffin cells; usually benign (90%)
  - Most release epinephrine and norepinephrine
  - Symptoms are paroxysmal and of excess catecholamines:
    - Palpitations
    - Headache
    - Sweating
    - Tremor
    - Weight loss
    - Anxiety
  - Signs:
    - Hypertension
    - Tachycardia
    - Flushing

6.3 Endocrine pancreas

- Normal value of blood glucose is 4–7mmol/L; <10mmol/L 90min after meals.

6.3.1 Functional anatomy of the endocrine pancreas

- Depending on whether we have recently eaten or are fasting, our metabolism is in 2 states:
  - Anabolic state:
    - The fuel that we consume is converted into storage molecules such as glycogen, triglycerides, and small amounts of protein
    - Controlled by insulin
  - Catabolic state:
    - When fasting
    - Convert above-mentioned energy stores to glucose, through gluconeogenesis
    - Controlled by glucagon
- Insulin and glucagon are hormones produced in the islets of Langerhans within the pancreas. Glucagon is produced by alpha cells and insulin by beta cells.

6.3.2 Insulin physiology

- Stimulants to production:
  - Insulin production is stimulated when eating by:
    - The parasympathetic nervous system
    - Gut hormones such as secretin (released in response to an increase in acid)

- Biggest release of insulin:
  - In response to an increase in plasma glucose
  - In a matter of seconds of exposure to glucose, a large amount of insulin is released
  - 10min later there is a second, slower phase of secretion
- Proinsulin:
  - Produced in ER of the beta cells of the pancreas in the islets of Langerhans
  - Guided to the Golgi apparatus:
    - Packed into granules
    - Slowly cleaved into insulin and C-peptide
    - Measurements of C-peptide levels tell us whether the body is producing insulin or not. It is also thought that C-peptide has important physiological effects in preventing nephropathy and autonomic neuropathy
    - The insulin receptor:
  - Tyrosine kinase receptor:
    - 2 alpha subunits (which are extracellular)
    - 2 beta subunits penetrate across the plasma membrane
  - When insulin binds to the alpha subunits:
    - Beta subunits autophosphorylate and there is activation of tyrosine kinase
    - This phosphorylates a number of intracellular substrates including insulin receptor substrate
    - Activates membrane signals and glucose transporter
    - Increased uptake of glucose and amino acids through the plasma membrane
    - In the cytoplasm glucose is then converted to glycogen and fatty acids, and amino acids into protein

6.3.3 Glucagon physiology

- Glucagon release is stimulated:
  - Directly by low blood sugar
  - Through catecholamine release:
    - Activates beta adrenoreceptors on the alpha cells to further increase glucagon release
- Glucagon synthesis is inhibited by insulin and glucose.
  - The main effect of glucagon is on the liver where it stimulates:
    - Glycogenolysis
    - Gluconeogenesis
    - Metabolism of free fatty acids to ketones
  - Glucagon binds to a hepatic plasma membrane glycoprotein receptor:
    - Signal is transmitted through G-protein
    - Stimulates a release of cAMP
    - Activates protein kinase A
  - Glucagon also acts on the kidneys, inhibiting sodium resorption causing a natriuresis
  - An increase in urea inhibits glucagon release

6.3.4 Diabetes mellitus

- Type 1 DM:
  - Caused by an autoimmune process that destroys the beta cells in the islets of Langerhans
  - Seen in younger patients, with a rapid onset
  - Untreated high glucose levels lead to a DKA
  - Insulin deficiency is necessary for DKA as only small levels of insulin inhibit hepatic ketogenesis

- High levels of blood glucose lead to:
  - An osmotic diuresis
  - Increased lipolysis by the hepatocytes, which leads to increased ketones in the blood
- Therefore the patient with DKA will present with:
  - Polyuria and polydipsia
  - Vomiting (attempt to reduce pH)
  - Dehydration
  - Metabolic acidosis (tachypnoea to compensate, Kussmaul breathing)
- All patients with type 1 DM will require insulin therapy.
- Type 2 DM:
  - Caused by an increased resistance to insulin, mostly associated with obesity
  - Usually presents in later life and has a more insidious onset than type 1 DM
  - Often presents with the complications of diabetes
  - Hyperosmolar hyperglycaemic non-ketotic coma (HHNK) can occur in type 2 DM, which can lead to severe dehydration and coma
- Complications of diabetes:
  - Caused by glycation:
    - A glucose molecule attaches to a protein molecule
    - Glycalated molecules are poorly excreted
    - Causes damage to collagen, stiffening arterial walls, and to the eyes, nerves, and kidneys leading to diabetic retinopathy, neuropathy, arterial disease, and nephropathy
  - Glycation is dependent on the level of glucose in blood and we can measure diabetic control over a time period (e.g. HbA1c)

6.4 Thyroid physiology

6.4.1 Functional anatomy

- The thyroid gland is found in the anterior part of the neck below the thyroid cartilage sitting around the larynx and trachea.
- Made up of 2 lobes, which are connected by an isthmus.
- The thyroid synthesizes T4 (90%) and T3 (10%), which is controlled through TRH and TSH by negative feedback (see Figure D.6.2).
- T3 is mostly responsible for the tissue actions of thyroid hormone, but up to 80% of T4 is converted to T3 in peripheral tissues (mostly liver and kidneys).

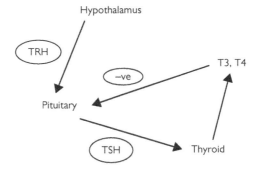

Figure D.6.2 Thyroid feedback loops

- Nearly all T3 and T4 in plasma are bound to the binding proteins thyroxine-binding globulin (TBG), albumin, and transthyretin.
- Only a very small percentage is unbound and therefore active.
- TBG allows a large circulating reservoir of T4:
  - Acts as a buffer if there is any change in thyroid function
  - Prevents excretion of T4 and T3 through the kidneys
- Free T3 and T4 in the blood easily cross the cell membrane:
  - They bind to thyroid hormone receptors, attached to DNA
  - Leads to transcription of thyroid-responsive genes
  - Synthesis of Na^+/K^+-ATPase:
    - Requires large amount of metabolic energy
    - Increased heat production
- T3 and T4 also:
  - Cause upregulation of beta adrenoreceptors:
    - Increase response to catecholamines, increasing cardiac output
  - Increase lipolysis by enhancing response to cortisol, glucagon, growth hormone, and epinephrine

6.4.2 Hypothyroidism

- Caused by disease of the thyroid or from hypothalamic–pituitary disease.
- Commonest cause is autoimmune:
  - Leads to lymphocytic infiltration into the gland, atrophy, and fibrosis
- Symptoms and signs are numerous, but indicate a reduced metabolic rate:
  - For example, weight gain, cold intolerance, tiredness, reduced appetite, mental slowness, bradycardia, and 'peaches and cream' appearance

6.4.3 Hyperthyroidism

- Commonest cause is Grave's disease:
  - Serum IgG antibodies bind to the TSH receptors
  - This causes excessive thyroid hormone production
- The symptoms and signs are of an increased metabolic rate, such as:
  - Increased appetite, weight loss, palpitations, tachycardia, AF, and restlessness
  - These patients often develop a goitre and exophthalmos

6.5 Calcium and bone physiology

6.5.1 Functions of calcium in health

- Intracellular calcium is important in:
  - Muscle contraction
  - Release of neurotransmitters
  - Hormone response
  - Secretion from exocrine glands
  - Activation of many intracellular enzymes
- Extracellular calcium:
  - Clotting cascade
  - Function of sodium channels
- Because this free intracellular calcium needs to be kept at very low levels, most is stored in the ER or mitochondria. 99% of calcium is stored in bone, 1% intracellularly, and 0.1% extracellularly.

- Calcium is transported through the bloodstream in ionized form or bound to proteins such as albumin. Only ionized calcium exerts a biological effect.

6.5.2 Factors affecting calcium handling

- The total amount of calcium in the body depends on the amount of calcium absorbed from the GI tract vs the amount excreted renally.
- Vitamin D3 (which is metabolized to its active metabolite calcitriol in the proximal tubule of the kidney) and PTH play a pivotal role in intestinal calcium absorption through carrier-mediated transport.
- Vitamin D deficiency leads to rickets in children and osteomalacia in adults.
- Parathyroid hormone (PTH) is the main factor that controls the distribution of free calcium in ECF and ICF:
  - Acts on bone, gut (as previously mentioned), and kidneys
  - Secreted from chief cells in the parathyroid gland when plasma levels of free calcium decrease
  - When free calcium levels are high the release of PTH is inhibited
- PTH initially increases free calcium:
  - Stimulates osteocytic osteolysis of bone
  - Osteoclast activity is increased over a longer time period
  - Almost all calcium is reabsorbed by the nephron, mostly in the proximal tubule
  - PTH, however, acts on the thick ascending limb of the LoH and the distal tubule to increase calcium re-absorption

6.5.3 Calcitonin

- When plasma free calcium levels are high, calcitonin is produced by the parafollicular cells (C cells) in the thyroid gland.
- Calcitonin reduces bone resorption by osteocytes.
- Does not have a pivotal physiological role as calcitonin deficiency does not cause disease of calcium metabolism.

6.5.4 Effects of disordered calcium physiology

- Osteomalacia:
  - Caused by a vitamin D deficiency
  - Characterized by:
    - Reduced bone density
    - Increase osteoid volume
    - Unmineralized osteoid
  - Osteomalacia is distinguished from hypoparathyroidism by a low phosphate
- Osteoporosis:
  - Chronic disease of reduced bone density (2.5SD below the young adult mean). It is commonest in postmenopausal women. There is a gradual imbalance of osteoclastic vs osteoblastic activity leading to reduced bone density
  - Oestrogens, glucocorticoids, thyroid hormones, and calcium metabolism play a multifactorial role in the development of this disease:
    - Oestrogens act on osteoblasts increasing bone formation
    - Glucocorticoids inhibit calcium and phosphate absorption therefore reducing bone density
    - Thyroid hormones also reduce mineral density
- Reduced bone density disposes patients to fractures even with minimal trauma.

PHARMACOLOGY

Gastrointestinal system

CONTENTS

Drug management is based upon symptom severity and often requires patient lifestyle changes in order to achieve maximal success.

1.1 Antacids

- Neutralize gastric acidity.
- Relieve symptoms of dyspepsia and gastro-oesophageal reflux disease (GORD).
- Promote ulcer healing (less well than antisecretory drugs).
- Can bind to other drugs reducing absorption.

1.1.1 Aluminium- and magnesium-containing antacids (common)

- Relatively unabsorbed by the gut.
- Low water solubility therefore slow onset but long acting if retained in stomach.
- Aluminium salts (e.g. hydroxide) predispose to constipation.
- Magnesium salts (e.g. carbonate) predispose to diarrhoea.
- Combination preparations reduce colonic side effects.

1.1.2 Sodium bicarbonate

- Ingredient in some antacid preparations.
- Water-soluble hence fast acting.
- Increases pH rapidly, which liberates carbon dioxide. This stimulates gastrin release, which in turn stimulates acid secretion, thus producing 'acid rebound' and belching.
- Absorbed by gut therefore can cause metabolic alkalosis (avoid long-term use).
- Avoid in sodium-restricted diet.

1.2 Alginates

- Form a viscous raft on top of the gastric contents.
- Reduce symptoms of acid reflux.
- Often combined with antacids.
- For example, Gaviscon™.

1.3 Antispasmodics (antimuscarinics)

- Antimuscarinics (anticholinergics) block muscarinic receptors:
  - Reduces intestinal motility
  - Relaxes intestinal smooth muscle
- Used for treatment of irritable bowel syndrome (IBS) and diverticular disease.
- Cautions:
  - Down's syndrome
  - GORD
  - Ulcerative colitis (UC)
  - Acute myocardial infarction (MI)
  - Hypertension
  - Pregnancy
  - Closed-angle glaucoma
- Contraindications:
  - Myasthenia gravis
  - Paralytic ileus
  - Pyloric stenosis
  - Prostatic enlargement
- Side effects:
  - Constipation
  - Urinary retention
  - Blurred vision
  - Dry mouth, dry skin, reduced bronchial secretions
  - Transient bradycardia followed by tachycardia
  - Confusion
- Hyoscine butylbromide (Buscopan®) is poorly absorbed from the gut, limiting its utility as an oral medication:
  - It is more effective when given IV

1.4 Ulcer-healing drugs

- Non-steroidal anti-inflammatory drugs (NSAIDs) and *Helicobacter pylori* (*H. pylori*) are independent risk factors and cause the majority of gastric/duodenal ulcers:
  - NSAID use should be withdrawn
  - High risk:
    - Age >65 years
    - Previous peptic ulcer or serious gastrointestinal (GI) disease
  - Proton pump inhibitors (PPIs), H_2 receptor antagonists, and misoprostol can heal NSAID-associated ulcers
  - *H. pylori* infection requires triple therapy (antibiotics ×2 + PPI)

- In patients already taking an NSAID, eradication of *H. pylori* is unlikely to reduce the risk of NSAID-induced bleeding or ulceration
- However, in patients with dyspepsia or a history of gastric or duodenal ulcer who are *H. pylori* positive and who are about to start treatment with NSAIDs, eradication of *H. pylori* may reduce the overall risk of ulceration

1.4.1 Proton pump inhibitors

- Block the proton pump (H^+/K^+-ATPase) on the parietal cell luminal membrane.
- Produce virtually total acid suppression.
- Can be used to prevent or treat NSAID-related ulcers.
- Other indications include:
  - Any peptic ulcer disease
  - Reflux oesophagitis
  - Zollinger–Ellison syndrome
  - Preoperative acid suppression
- More effective than H_2 receptor antagonists.
- Side effects include:
  - GI disturbance—nausea, vomiting, abdominal pain, diarrhoea, constipation
  - Headache
  - Rashes
- Potentiates some drugs via inhibition of hepatic cytochrome p450 (e.g. warfarin, phenytoin, diazepam, aminophylline)
- Caution in liver disease—can cause derangement of LFTs
- For example, omeprazole:
  - Doses vary depending on indication:
    - Typically 10–40mg orally (PO) or 40mg intravenous (IV)
    - Higher in Zollinger–Ellison syndrome
- Single dose reduces acid secretion but has an increasing antisecretory effect for 5 days until plateau reached.

1.4.2 H_2 receptor antagonists

- Competitively block histamine (H_2) receptors at the parietal cell.
- Produce ~90% acid suppression (less effective than PPIs).
- Similar uses to PPIs—2nd line.
- Ranitidine has fewer side effects than cimetidine, which inhibits cytochrome p450.

1.4.3 Misoprostol

- Synthetic prostaglandin E_1 analogue.
- Protective and antisecretory effects.

1.5 Acute diarrhoea

- Rather than attempting to treat acute diarrhoea using drugs, management should focus on accurate assessment of hydration status and correction of fluid and electrolyte imbalance.
- Children and the elderly are at particular risk from dehydration and electrolyte disturbance.
- Antimotility drugs, antispasmodics, and antiemetics should be avoided in young children because they are rarely effective and have troublesome side effects.

1.5.1 Antimotility drugs

- Can relieve the symptoms of diarrhoea in adults.
- Usually opiates (loperamide, codeine phosphate).
- Reduce motility by μ-receptor activation, which results in reduced acetylcholine (Ach) release at the myenteric plexus, thus reducing motility.

1.5.2 Loperamide

- Pethidine congener but relatively GI selective (doesn't cross blood–brain barrier (BBB), therefore no central effects/dependence).
- Side effects:
  - Abdominal cramps
  - Nausea and vomiting

1.6 Chronic bowel disorders: inflammatory bowel disease

- UC and Crohn's disease are inflammatory disorders with uncertain aetiology.
- Treatment comprises a combination of drug therapy, effective nutrition, and selective surgery.
- Drug therapy includes:
  - Corticosteroids (hydrocortisone, budesonide, prednisolone):
    - Main agents used for acute attacks
    - Local, via suppository/enema, or systemic
    - Side effects limit use for maintenance treatment
  - Aminosalicylates (balsalazide, mesalazine, sulfasalazine):
    - Main agents for maintenance therapy
    - Reduce relapse rates
    - More effective in UC than Crohn's disease
  - Immunosuppressive medications (ciclosporin, azathioprine, mercaptopurine, methotrexate) and cytokine modulators (infliximab, adalimumab):
    - Reserved for acute attacks unresponsive to steroids or those with frequently relapsing disease
    - Require specialist supervision

1.7 Laxatives

- Main uses:
  - Constipation
  - Bowel clearance prior to surgery/examination
- Act in a variety of ways.
- Bowel cleansing solutions often contain combinations of laxatives, can cause significant electrolyte disturbance, and are not treatments for constipation.
- Laxatives should be prescribed for children by a healthcare professional experienced in the management of constipation in children.
- Laxatives should generally be avoided except where straining will exacerbate a condition (such as angina) or increase the risk of rectal bleeding as in haemorrhoids:
  - Thus have a very limited role in the emergency department

1.7.1 Bulk-forming laxatives

- Form a bulky hydrated mass that stimulates peristalsis.
- Examples: ispaghula husk (Fybogel®), methcellulose, bran.

1.7.2 Osmotic laxatives

- Retain or draw water into the bowel, speeding up small bowel transit and delivering a large volume to the colon.
- Examples: lactulose, macrogols (Movicol®), magnesium salts, phosphates (PR).

1.7.3 Stimulant laxatives

- Increase intestinal motility by stimulating mucosal secretion and possibly stimulating enteric nerves.
- Often cause abdominal cramps.
- Examples: sodium docusate (also a faecal softener), dantron, glycerol (PR), senna, sodium picosulphate.

1.7.4 Faecal softeners

- Soften and lubricate.
- Examples: sodium docusate, liquid paraffin, arachis oil.

Cardiovascular system

CONTENTS

2.1 Cardiac glycosides (digoxin)

- Comes from foxglove plant (*Digitalis* spp.).
- Foxgloves contain a number of glycosides of which digoxin is the most important.
- Used in treatment of supraventricular tachyarrhythmias (e.g. AF/atrial flutter) and heart failure.

2.1.1 Mechanism

- Binds to and inhibits the Na^+/K^+ pump on the myocyte cell membrane (competes with the K^+ ion).
- Increases intracellular Na^+ concentration.
- Reduces the extrusion of intracellular Ca^{2+} via the Na^+/Ca^{2+} exchange transporter.
- Increased Ca^{2+} is stored in the sarcoplasmic reticulum.
- Increased amounts of Ca^{2+} released during each action potential.
- Force of contraction increased.
- Digoxin also increases vagal tone by enhancing Ach release at muscarinic receptors, thus slowing the heart rate, atrioventricular (AV) conduction, and the AV nodal refractory period.

2.1.2 Side effects

- Cardiac arrhythmias: ectopics, bigeminy, heart block, ventricular tachycardia (VT), ventricular fibrillation (VF).
- Gut: nausea, vomiting, diarrhoea.
- Visual disturbance: blurred/yellow vision.
- Rash.
- Confusion/psychosis.

2.1.3 Toxicity

- Relatively common due to narrow therapeutic window.

- Precipitated by hypokalaemia (less completion at Na^+/K^+ pump), hypercalcaemia, acidosis, renal failure.
- Can cause hyperkalaemia.
- Treatment involves:
  - Supportive management
  - Withdrawal of digoxin and correction of electrolyte abnormalities
  - Digoxin-specific antibody fragments (Digibind®):
    - Severe cases only
    - Binds digoxin more favourably than its receptor, removing it from its site of action
    - The digoxin–antibody complex is then excreted by the kidneys

2.2 Diuretics

- Salt and water re-absorption is controlled by aldosterone and antidiuretic hormone (ADH, vasopressin).
- Diuretics act on the kidney to increase the excretion of Na^+ and H_2O.

2.2.1 Thiazides

- Used in treatment of hypertension, oedema, and mild chronic heart failure.
- Weak diuretic action.
- Examples:
  - Bendroflumethiazide: common
  - Metolazone: used in combination with loop diuretics (powerful synergistic action) in severe resistant oedema
- Mechanism:
  - Inhibits Na^+/Cl^- co-transporter in the proximal distal tubule
  - Increases Na^+, Cl^-, and H_2O excretion
- Side effects:
  - Hypokalaemia: increased Na^+ load delivered to distal tubule exchanged for K^+ and H^+
  - Hyponatraemia
  - Hypochloraemic alkalosis
  - Hypomagnesaemia
  - Hyperuricaemia and gout
  - Hypercalcaemia
  - Hyperglycaemia
  - Postural hypotension
  - Weakness
  - Impotence

2.2.2 Loop diuretics

- Used in treatment of acute pulmonary oedema, chronic heart failure, peripheral oedema, and hypertension.
- Effective in renal failure.
- Produce a powerful diuresis due to their site of action.
- Examples:
  - Furosemide
  - Bumetanide
- Mechanism:
  - Inhibit the $Na/K/2Cl$ co-transporter in the thick ascending loop of Henle
  - Also have a poorly understood vasodilator effect when given IV

- Side effects:
  - Hypokalaemia
  - Hyponatraemia
  - Hypochloraemic alkalosis
  - Hypomagnesaemia
  - Hypocalcaemia
  - Hyperuricaemia and gout
  - Hyperglycaemia (less so than thiazides)
  - Hypotension and hypovolaemia
  - Deafness (high doses): due to changes in the endolymph of the middle ear

2.2.3 Potassium-sparing diuretics

- Spironolactone:
  - Aldosterone antagonist
  - Increases Na^+ and H_2O excretion but reduces K^+ excretion
  - Weak diuretic
  - Used in ascites secondary to liver cirrhosis, Conn's syndrome, severe heart failure, and with other diuretics to prevent hypokalaemia (e.g. with digoxin therapy)
  - Can cause hyperkalaemia (more likely in renal failure and with concomitant ACE inhibitor use)
- Amiloride:
  - Blocks luminal Na^+ channels in distal tubule/collecting duct
  - Similar indications to spironolactone

2.2.4 Osmotic diuretics

- Mannitol:
  - Carbohydrate derivative (polyhydric alcohol)
  - Pharmacologically inert, it creates an osmotic gradient and is freely filtered by the glomerulus and not reabsorbed
  - Requires IV administration
  - *Within plasma*: doesn't cross an intact BBB or enter the eye, therefore can be used to reduce raised intracranial or intraocular pressure (transient effect only)
  - *Within the nephron*: reduces passive water re-absorption
  - Used in cerebral oedema, acute glaucoma, and perioperatively to maintain a diuresis

2.2.5 Carbonic anhydrase inhibitors

- Acetazolamide:
  - Inhibits carbonic anhydrase, reducing bicarbonate absorption in the proximal tubule
  - Increases HCO_3^-, Na^+, and H_2O excretion
  - Weak diuretic action
  - Used in treatment of glaucoma (reduced HCO_3^- secretion into aqueous humour) and to prevent mountain sickness (causes metabolic acidosis counteracting the respiratory alkalosis associated with mountain sickness)

2.3 Antiarrhythmics

The Resuscitation Council guidelines for the management of bradyarrhythmias, tachyarrhythmias, and cardiac arrest are extremely relevant to this section and will help put the following information into context.

2.3.1 Adenosine

- Naturally occurring purine nucleoside produced endogenously and present in all cells:
- Uses:
  - Stable regular narrow-complex tachycardias:
    - Terminates supraventricular tachycardia (SVT) due to AV node re-entrant circuits
    - Can help reveal the underlying rhythm (e.g. atrial flutter) in other cases
  - Broad complex tachycardias known to be SVT with bundle branch block
- Mechanism:
  - Stimulates A1-adenosine receptors in the AV node → opens K channels → hyperpolarizes the cell membrane → rapid slowing of AV nodal transmission
  - Rapidly inactivated—actions and side effects short lived ($t_{1/2}$ 8–10s)
- Side effects:
  - Chest discomfort
  - Facial flushing
  - Bronchospasm/dyspnoea
  - Nausea
  - Transient rhythm disturbances
- Contraindicated:
  - Asthma
  - Sick sinus syndrome
  - 2nd/3rd-degree heart block
- Interactions:
  - Effects potentiated by dipyridamole and carbamazepine
  - Effects reduced by theophylline
- Dose:
  - 6mg rapid IV injection into proximal vein followed by large flush
  - Follow with 12mg then 12mg if unsuccessful

2.3.2 Amiodarone

- Despite multiple side effects it is often safer than many of the other antiarrhythmics in the acute setting.
- Uses:
  - Shock refractory VF/pulseless VT
  - Shock refractory unstable tachycardias
  - Stable VT/pre-excited arrhythmias including WPW/broad complex tachycardias
  - AF <48 hours onset
- Mechanism:
  - Blocks K^+ channels → prolongs the cardiac action potential (seen clinically as prolonged QT_c)
- Side effects:
  - Acute:
    - Prolongs the QT interval hence potentially arrhythmogenic (notably torsades)
    - Hypotension and bradycardia (reduced if given slowly)
    - IV preparation extremely irritant if extravasates—use central vein except in emergency
  - Chronic (mnemonic—HATPEN):
    - Hepatic dysfunction
    - Alveolitis/pulmonary fibrosis
    - Thyroid disorders—hyper and hypo (contains iodine)
    - Photosensitivity—slate grey colour skin (advise the use of sunscreen)

- Eye problems—corneal deposits
- Neuropathy
- Interactions:
  - Avoid use with other drugs that prolong the QT_c: tricyclic antidepressants, phenothiazines, thiazides (hypokalaemia that prolongs the QT_c)
  - Increases concentration of warfarin, phenytoin, digoxin (all protein bound)

2.3.3 Flecainide

- Use has declined in the emergency department:
  - Alternative drug for cardioversion of AF and AV nodal re-entrant tachycardias in patients with *no* LV dysfunction
  - Prophylaxis in paroxysmal AF
- Increased risk of VF and death if used post-MI.
- Negatively inotropic.
- Acts by binding to Na^+ channels and dissociating slowly, therefore prolonging phase 0 of the action potential.

2.3.4 Lidocaine

- Use has declined as an antiarrhythmic:
  - 2nd-line agent in ventricular arrhythmias now only used when amiodarone unavailable
- Binds to inactivated Na^+ channels, especially in areas of ischaemia.

2.4 Beta-adrenoceptor blockers

Knowledge of the physiological effects of adrenoceptor stimulation on different tissues is important for the understanding of this section.

- Competitively antagonize β-receptors (compete with norepinephrine).
- Differ in a number of ways that affect their use (see Table E.2.1):
  - Receptor selectivity:
    - Cardioselective β-blockers block β_1-receptors preferentially over β_2 receptors, hence avoid many unwanted side effects of β_2-blockade
    - No β-blocker is cardiospecific, hence all produce β_2 effects at high doses and can have enough β_2 activity at low dose to cause bronchospasm in patients with asthma

Table E.2.1 Differences between β-blockers

	β_1 selectivity	Lipid solubility	ISA	α_1 blockade
Atenolol	Yes	+	–	–
Metoprolol	Yes	+++	–	–
Esmolol	Yes	+++	–	–
Propranolol	–	+++	–	–
Labetalol	–	+++	Yes	Yes
Sotalol	–	+	–	–
Carvedilol	–	+	–	Yes

- Lipid solubility:
  - More lipid-soluble—better absorbed from gut, more extensively metabolized in liver hence shorter $t_{1/2}$, cross BBB therefore cause CNS side effects
  - Less lipid-soluble—opposite of previous bullet point, excreted unchanged by kidneys hence dose reduction required in renal failure
- Intrinsic sympathomimetic activity (ISA):
  - Some β-blockers also act as partial agonists at β-receptors
- Membrane-stabilizing activity:
  - Little clinical significance at doses used clinically
- Additional α-receptor blockade:
  - Some β-blockers also block α_1-receptors hence cause vasodilation

2.4.1 Effects

- Cardiac:
  - Negatively inotropic and chronotropic:
    - β_1-blockade reduces workload and lengthens diastole hence increases coronary artery perfusion time
    - Cardiac output (CO) reduced
  - Antiarrhythmic:
    - Primarily attenuate effects of the sympathetic system
- Circulatory:
  - Antihypertensive:
    - Probably by combination of reduced CO, reduced renin secretion (β_1-blockade at juxtaglomerular apparatus), and a central effect reducing sympathetic activity
  - Poor peripheral circulation and cold extremities (peripheral β_2-blockade causes vasoconstriction but doesn't appear to affect BP)
- Respiratory:
  - Bronchospasm (β_2-blockade):
    - Not significant in normal subjects, highly significant in asthmatics
- CNS:
  - Nightmares, fatigue, sleep disturbance
- Metabolic:
  - Increase risk of exercise-induced hypoglycaemia in diabetics
- Ocular:
  - Reduce intraocular pressure

2.4.2 Main uses of β-blockers

See Table E.2.2.

- Hypertension
- Angina
- MI
- Arrhythmias
- Heart failure (stable)
- Thyrotoxicosis
- Phaeochromocytoma
- Glaucoma
- Migraine prophylaxis
- Essential tremor
- Anxiety

Table E.2.2 Examples of specific β-blockers and their indications and properties

	Main indication	Properties
Propranolol	All indications listed in Chapter E2, Section 2.4.2 except glaucoma	
Atenolol	Hypertension, angina, post MI, arrhythmias	Poor lipid solubility therefore reduced CNS side effects
Esmolol	Supraventricular arrhythmias, tachycardia/hypertension perioperatively	Very short $t_{1/2}$ therefore effects short lived, requires IV administration
Labetalol	Hypertensive crisis, hypertension in pregnancy/angina/post MI	Additional α1 blockade produces vasodilation
Sotalol	Ventricular arrhythmias, prophylaxis supraventricular arrhythmias	Additional antiarrhythmic activity, torsades de points potential side effect

2.4.3 Cautions and contraindications

- Contraindicated in patients with 2nd- or 3rd-degree heart block.
- Should be avoided in patients with:
  - Worsening unstable heart failure
  - History of asthma or bronchospasm
- In patients with diabetes can lead to a small deterioration of glucose tolerance and interfere with metabolic and autonomic responses to hypoglycaemia.

2.5 Hypertension and heart failure

- Lowering raised BP decreases the risk of stroke, coronary events, heart failure, and renal impairment.
  - Patients should be given advice on lifestyle changes to reduce BP or cardiovascular risk; these include smoking cessation, weight reduction, reduction of excessive intake of alcohol, reduction of dietary salt, reduction of total and saturated fat, increasing exercise, and increasing fruit and vegetable intake.
- However, hypertension rarely requires treatment in the emergency department.
  - Even in malignant hypertension with evidence of encephalopathy (headaches, vomiting, retinal changes, confusion, ↓ Glasgow Coma Score (GCS)) oral therapy can usually be instigated rather than risking the dangerous acute falls in BP (risk of cerebral infarction, blindness, renal failure, cardiac ischaemia) that are more common with IV medication.
- The following thresholds for treatment are recommended:
  - Accelerated (malignant) hypertension or acute cardiovascular complications: admit for immediate treatment
  - Systolic ≥220mmHg or diastolic ≥120mmHg: *treat immediately*
  - Systolic 180–219mmHg or diastolic 110–119mmHg: confirm over 1–2 weeks then treat if these values are sustained
  - Systolic 160–179mmHg or diastolic 100–109mmHg:
    - Cardiovascular complications, target-organ damage (e.g. left ventricular hypertrophy, renal impairment), or diabetes mellitus—confirm over 3–4 weeks then treat if these values are sustained

- No cardiovascular complications, no target-organ damage, or no diabetes—advise lifestyle changes, reassess weekly, and treat if these values are sustained on repeat measurements over 4–12 weeks
- Systolic 140–159mmHg or diastolic 90–99mmHg:
  - Cardiovascular complications, target-organ damage, or diabetes—confirm within 12 weeks and treat if these values are sustained
  - No cardiovascular complications, no target-organ damage, or no diabetes—advise lifestyle changes and reassess monthly
  - A target systolic BP <140mmHg *and* diastolic BP <90mmHg is suggested.
  - A lower target systolic BP <130mmHg *and* diastolic BP <80mmHg should be considered for those with established atherosclerotic cardiovascular disease, diabetes, or chronic renal failure.

2.5.1 Implications of hypertension in other disease states

- Hypertension in diabetes:
  - Maintain systolic BP <130mmHg and diastolic BP <80mmHg
  - Most patients require a combination of antihypertensive drugs
  - Hypertension is common in type 2 diabetes (T2DM) and antihypertensive treatment prevents macrovascular and microvascular complications
  - In type 1 diabetes (T1DM), hypertension usually indicates the presence of diabetic nephropathy
  - In patients with T2DM, an ACE inhibitor (or an angiotensin-II receptor antagonist) can delay progression of microalbuminuria to nephropathy
- Hypertension in renal disease:
  - The threshold for treatment is a systolic BP ≥140mmHg *or* a diastolic BP ≥90mmHg
  - Optimal BP is a systolic BP <130mmHg and a diastolic pressure <80mmHg, or lower if proteinuria exceeds 1g in 24 hours
  - An ACE inhibitor (or an angiotensin-II receptor antagonist) should be considered for patients with proteinuria
- Hypertension in pregnancy:
  - High BP in pregnancy may usually be due to pre-existing essential hypertension or to pre-eclampsia
  - Methyldopa is safe in pregnancy
  - Beta-blockers are effective and safe in the 3RD trimester
  - Modified-release preparations of nifedipine (unlicensed) are also used for hypertension in pregnancy
  - IV administration of labetalol can be used to control hypertensive crises; alternatively, hydralazine may be used by the IV route

2.5.2 Vasodilators

- Sodium nitroprusside is an IV drug with short $t_{1/2}$ used occasionally in malignant hypertension and perioperatively.
- Decomposes to nitric oxide in the blood and thus vasodilates (arteries and veins).
- Also produces cyanide:
  - Can result in poisoning if accumulates (inhibition of cytochrome oxidase causes impairment in aerobic metabolism, which leads to metabolic acidosis, tachycardia, tachypnoea, sweating, arrhythmias)
  - More likely in renal/hepatic failure, hypothermia, vitamin B12 deficiency
- Treatment for cyanide poisoning:
  - Oxygen

- Antidotes—3 options:
  - Dicobalt edetate (best but potentially fatal if cyanide poisoning not present)
  - Sodium nitrite followed by sodium thiosulphate
  - Hydroxocobalamin
- Avoid self-contamination

2.5.3 Alpha-adrenoceptor blockers

- Vasodilate arteries and veins.
- Used in:
  - Phaeochromocytoma
    - α-blockers (e.g. phenoxybenzamine) used to vasodilate and control BP before β-blockers started to control tachycardia
    - If β-blockers given 1st it can worsen hypertensive crisis

2.5.4 Heart failure

- Treatment aims to relieve symptoms, improve exercise tolerance, reduce the incidence of acute exacerbations, and reduce mortality. An ACE inhibitor, titrated to a 'target dose' (or the maximum tolerated dose if lower), and a β-blocker is recommended to achieve these aims. A diuretic is also necessary in most patients to reduce symptoms of fluid overload.
- An angiotensin-II receptor antagonist may be a useful alternative for patients who, because of side effects such as cough, cannot tolerate ACE inhibitors.
- Spironolactone can be considered for patients with moderate to severe heart failure who are already taking an ACE inhibitor and a β-blocker.
- Digoxin improves symptoms of heart failure and exercise tolerance and reduces hospitalization due to acute exacerbations, but it does not reduce mortality. Digoxin is reserved for patients with atrial fibrillation (AF).

2.5.5 Angiotensin-converting enzyme (ACE) inhibitors

- Actions:
  - Vasodilate by preventing conversion of angiotensin I to angiotensin II
  - Decrease aldosterone secretion thereby increasing Na^+ and H_2O excretion
- Uses:
  - Chronic heart failure:
    - Used in combination with β-blockers and diuretics (+ digoxin if in AF)
    - Very useful as increased levels of angiotensin II in heart failure
    - Vasodilation + H_2O excretion causes decreased preload and afterload, which results in increased CO
  - Hypertension
  - Post-MI (especially in LV dysfunction)
  - Diabetic nephropathy
- Side effects:
  - Hypotension (especially 1st dose)
  - Hyperkalaemia
  - Hyponatraemia
  - Cough—increased levels of bradykinin normally broken down by ACE
  - Renal failure in the presence of:
    - Renal artery stenosis
    - Poor perfusion
    - Concurrent NSAID use

- Angio-oedema
- Rash and pruritus
- Taste disturbance
- Rarely agranulocytosis and thrombocytopenia
- Contraindications:
  - Pregnancy
  - Bilateral renal artery stenosis
  - Hypersensitivity to ACE inhibitors
- Examples:
  - Captopril:
    - 1st ACE inhibitor developed
    - An active drug metabolized to active metabolites
    - Competitive blocker of ACE
  - Others now include enalapril, ramipril, lisinopril, perindopril

2.5.6 Angiotensin II receptor antagonists

- Similar effects to ACE inhibitors but don't inhibit the breakdown of bradykinin hence don't cause persistent cough.
- Useful alternative when cough is a problem.
- Examples: losartan, candesartan, irbesartan, valsartan

2.6 Nitrates and antianginal drugs

- Stable angina:
  - Acute attacks should be managed with sublingual glyceryl trinitrate (GTN)
  - Patients with mild or moderate stable angina should be given a β-blocker
  - For those patients in whom β-blockers are not tolerated or are contraindicated, a long-acting nitrate or a rate-limiting calcium-channel blocker can be used
  - When a single drug fails to control symptoms, combination treatment can be used
- Unstable angina:
  - Oxygen should be administered if there is evidence of hypoxia, pulmonary oedema, or continuing myocardial ischaemia
  - Nitrates are used to relieve ischaemic pain. If pain continues, diamorphine or morphine can be given by slow IV injection; an antiemetic should also be given
  - Aspirin is given for its antiplatelet effect
  - Clopidogrel in a dose of 300mg and a low-molecular-weight heparin should also be given
  - Patients without contraindications should receive β-blockers
  - Revascularization procedures are often appropriate for patients with unstable angina

2.6.1 Nitrates

- Actions:
  - Mediated by the production of nitric oxide
  - Venodilate thereby reducing venous return, which reduces left ventricular (LV) work and O_2 demand
  - Vasodilate arteries including coronary arteries
- Uses:
  - Angina and acute coronary syndromes:
    - Prophylaxis and symptomatic relief of pain

- Heart failure:
  - Especially useful acute left ventricular failure (LVF)
- Anal fissure:
  - Topically—smooth muscle relaxant
- Side effects:
  - Headache
  - Flushing
  - Syncope
  - Hypotension
  - Methaemoglobinaemia (prolonged high dose)
- Common preparations and typical uses:
  - GTN:
    - Sublingual (SL) spray—delivers 400 micrograms for acute relief of angina pain
    - Buccal tablets (longer acting than spray)—2, 3, or 5mg tablets used in angina/acute coronary syndrome (ACS)
    - IV (titrated to BP)—acute LVF or intractable cardiac pain
    - Transdermal patch—prophylaxis angina
  - Isosorbide dinitrate:
    - IV—LVF or intractable cardiac pain
  - Isosorbide mononitrate:
    - Tablets—prophylaxis angina
    - Tolerance can develop therefore a nitrate-free period is required each day (hence take twice daily (bd) tablets in morning and at lunchtime rather than in evening)

2.6.2 Calcium channel antagonists

- Block L-type voltage-sensitive Ca^{2+} channels:
  - Arteries:
    - Smooth muscle relaxation causes vasodilation and thus decreases afterload
  - Heart:
    - Negatively inotropic and chronotropic
- Differ in their main site of action (see Table E.2.3).
- Uses:
  - Amlodipine, nifedipine:
    - Hypertension
    - Angina
  - Nimodipine:
    - Prevents/reduces vasospasm associated with subarachnoid haemorrhage
  - Verapamil:
    - Arrhythmias
    - Angina
    - Hypertension
    - NB Contraindicated use with β-blockers—risk of asystole
  - Diltiazem:
    - Angina (especially if β-blockers contraindicated)
    - Hypertension
    - NB Caution with β-blockers

Table E.2.3 Differences between calcium channel blockers

Chemical classification	Drug	Action	Main effect	Common side effects
Dihydropyridines	Nifedipine, amlodipine	Relatively smooth muscle-selective, peripheral and coronary arteries	Vasodilation	Headache Flushing Ankle swelling GI disturbance Palpitations Lethargy
	Nimodipine	Increased lipid solubility hence crosses BBB and affects cerebral arteries		
Phenylalkylamines	Verapamil	Relatively cardioselective	$\downarrow\downarrow$ myocardial contractility $\downarrow$ heart rate (via slowing of action potential at SA and AV node)	Constipation (in addition those listed for dihydropyridines) Risk of: hypotension, heart failure, heart block (high doses)
Benzothiazepines	Diltiazem	Intermediate between the previous 2 drug groups	Intermediate effects Less negatively inotropic and chronotropic than verapamil	Risk of bradycardia, heart block (in addition to the list in Chapter E2, Section 2.6.2)

2.7 Sympathomimetics

- Sympathomimetics are agonists and act via adrenoceptors or dopamine receptors in 2 ways:
  - Directly—attach to receptors themselves
  - Indirectly—cause release of endogenous norepinephrine to produce their effect
- Characteristics of different sympathomimetics depend on their receptor specificity.
- Most sympathomimetics are potentially arrhythmogenic and their effects are exaggerated and prolonged by the concurrent use of MAOI (monoamine oxidase inhibitor) antidepressants.

Knowledge of the physiological effects of adrenoceptor stimulation on different tissues is important for the understanding of this section—see Chapter D3, Section 3.8.

2.7.1 Dobutamine

- Acts directly at:
  - β_1 receptors (main effect)
  - β_2 receptors (small effect)
- Effects:
  - Increased heart rate, contractility, and O_2 demand (β_1 effects)
  - Decreased SVR (β_2—mild effect):
    - Overall increase in BP and CO

- Primary indications:
  - Low CO states in:
    - MI
    - Cardiac surgery
    - Cardiogenic shock
    - Septic shock

2.7.2 Dopamine

- Acts directly and indirectly via α, β, and δ receptors.
- Effects:
  - At low dose, β_1 effects predominate:
    - Increased heart rate, contractility, coronary blood flow, and O_2 demand, resulting in increased BP and CO
  - At high dose, α effects predominate:
    - Vasoconstriction causing increased SVR and venous return
  - Vasodilation of splanchnic blood vessels via δ_1 receptors, increasing blood flow to splanchnic circulation:
    - Increased urine output (may also be secondary to increased BP and CO)
  - Nausea and vomiting via stimulation of CTZ (chemoreceptor trigger zone)
- Uses:
  - Cardiogenic shock post-infarction
  - Cardiac surgery

2.7.3 Norepinephrine (noradrenaline)

- Acts directly via:
  - α_1 receptors (main effect)
  - β receptors (small effect)
    - Effects differ from endogenous norepinephrine
- Effects:
  - Potent vasoconstriction (α_1 effects):
    - Increased SVR, BP, myocardial O_2 demand, and venous return
    - Reflex bradycardia
    - Decreased CO and splanchnic blood flow
    - Decreased peripheral blood flow resulting in peripheral ischaemia at high dose
    - Decreased uterine blood flow causing foetal asphyxia
- Uses:
  - Septic shock
  - Hypotension

2.7.4 Epinephrine (adrenaline)

- Acts directly at α and β receptors.
- Effects:
  - At low dose, β effects predominate:
    - Increased heart rate, contractility, coronary blood flow, and O_2 demand causing increased CO (SVR may fall due to secondary β_2 effects)
  - At high dose, α_1 effects predominate:
    - Increased SVR
  - Bronchodilatation
  - Raised blood glucose via increasing glycogenolysis, gluconeogenesis, and lipolysis
  - Increased pain threshold

- Uses:
  - Cardiac arrest—IV bolus
  - Anaphylaxis—IM bolus
  - Circulatory failure—IV infusion
  - Upper airway obstruction—nebulized
  - Combined with local anaesthetics (to produce vasoconstriction)—1:80 000 or 1:200 000 solutions

2.7.5 Other vasoconstrictors

- Other vasoconstrictors have a limited role in the emergency department as an emergency method of raising BP when other methods have failed. They can all be given peripherally and include:
  - Ephedrine:
    - α and β effects
    - Increased heart rate, BP, CO, myocardial O_2 demand, and bronchodilatation
    - Doesn't constrict uterine vessels, hence useful in obstetric patients
  - Metaraminol:
    - Mainly α_1 effects
    - Increased SVR and BP
  - Phenylephrine:
    - Pure α_1 agonist
    - Raised SVR and BP

2.8 Anticholinergics (antimuscarinics)

- Blocks muscarinic receptors.
- Effects:
  - Elevated heart rate
  - Bronchodilatation and decreased bronchial secretions
  - Antisialagogue (reduced saliva secretion)
  - Mydriasis
  - Antiemetic
  - Sedation

2.8.1 Atropine

- Uses:
  - Asystolic/PEA cardiac arrest
  - Bradycardia and bradyarrhythmias
  - Drying secretions (e.g. decreased hypersalivation associated with ketamine use)
  - Organophosphate poisoning

2.8.2 Glycopyrrolate

- Doesn't cross the BBB therefore devoid of central effects (only causes increased heart rate, bronchodilatation, and decreased saliva secretion).
- Uses:
  - Drying secretions
  - Bradycardia (alternative to atropine)

■ Given with neostigmine (reversal of non-depolarizing neuromuscular block) to offset bradycardic effects.

2.9 Anticoagulants

Knowledge of normal blood coagulation is important in understanding this section. See Chapter D1, Section 1.5.

2.9.1 Heparin

- Naturally occurring acidic mucopolysaccharide.
- Present in liver and with histamine in granules of mast cells.
- Extracted from bovine lung or porcine intestine.
- Initiates anticoagulation quickly.
- Used for short-term anticoagulation.
- Mechanism of action:
  - Requires antithrombin III
  - Heparin binds to and activates antithrombin III
  - 1000-fold increase in rate of formation of the inactive antithrombin III–thrombin complex
  - Heparin–antithrombin III complex also inhibits factors Xa, IXa, Xia, and XIIa
- Side effects:
  - Haemorrhage
  - HIT (heparin-induced thrombocytopenia)
    - Clinically important immune-mediated thrombocytopenia develops at 5–10 days
    - Can be complicated by venous thrombosis (50%) and arterial thrombosis (20%)
    - Treatment is to replace heparin with an alternative anticoagulant (lepirudin or danaparoid)
  - Hyperkalaemia
  - Osteoporosis
- Uses:
  - Prophylaxis and treatment of DVT and PE
  - Treatment:
    - Acute coronary syndromes
    - Acute peripheral arterial occlusion
  - Prophylaxis thromboembolism:
    - Atrial fibrillation
    - Prosthetic heart valves
  - Haemodialysis

2.9.2 Low-molecular-weight heparin (LMWH)

- LMWH (enoxaparin, dalteparin, tinzaparin):
  - Derived from heparin by chemical/enzymatic degradation
  - LMWH–antithrombin III complex only inhibits factor Xa
- Side effects:
  - Same as heparin but generally less marked
  - Haemorrhage is more problematic because of the longer $t_{1/2}$ and relative irreversibility
- Uses:
  - Same as heparin but is preferred for most indications due to ease of use and lower risk of HIT (see Table E.2.4)
  - Heparin preferred in patients with higher risk of bleeding and in situations when anticoagulation requires prompt discontinuation (e.g. preoperatively)

Table E.2.4 Contrasting properties of heparin and LMWH

	Heparin	LMWH
Molecular weight	5000–25 000Da (unfractionated)	2000–8000Da (different preparations have specific weights)
Factors inactivated	IIa, IXa, Xa, XI, XIIa	Xa
Administration	SC (bd) or IV infusion	SC (od or bd)
Duration of action	Short	Long
Monitoring required	Yes (APTT)	No
Reversible	Yes (protamine)	Partially reversible only
HIT	More likely (although uncommon)	Less likely

2.9.3 Protamine sulphate

- Made from fish sperm!
- Used to treat overdosage of heparin:
  - Forms an inactive complex with heparin
- Can cause hypotensive and allergic reactions.

2.9.4 Warfarin

- Coumarin derivative.
- Used for long-term oral anticoagulation.
- Requires monitoring of INR and regular dose adjustments to keep within therapeutic range.
- Highly protein-bound and metabolized in the liver.
- Mechanism of action:
  - Clotting factors II, VII, IX, and X are activated by vitamin K, which is oxidized in the process
  - Vitamin K is then converted back to its reduced form by vitamin K reductase in order to activate more clotting factors
  - Warfarin is similar in structure to vitamin K therefore competitively inhibits vitamin K reductase, preventing the return of vitamin K to the reduced form
- Side effects:
  - Haemorrhage:
    - Increased risk when INR is elevated above therapeutic levels
    - Can occur at therapeutic levels
    - Major bleeding requires: reversal of warfarin: IV vitamin K1; IV dried prothrombin complex (Beriplex®)—contains factors II, VII, IX, and X; FFP if dried prothrombin complex unavailable
    - Minor bleeding/high INR requires: omission of warfarin; PO/IV vitamin K1 as required
  - Teratogenic
- Interactions:
  - Many drugs can potentiate the effects of warfarin:
    - Hepatic enzyme inhibitors (e.g. cimetidine, chloramphenicol, ciprofloxacin, metronidazole, amiodarone)
    - Platelet inhibitors (e.g. aspirin, NSAIDs, clopidogrel)
    - Drugs that displace warfarin from protein (e.g. chloral hydrate)
    - Drugs that inhibit reduction of vitamin K (e.g. cephalosporins)
  - Many drugs can lessen the effects of warfarin
    - Hepatic enzyme inducers (e.g. rifampicin, carbamazepine)
    - Drugs that reduce absorption (e.g. cholestyramine)

- Uses:
  - Prophylaxis thromboembolism:
    - Prosthetic heart valves
    - Rheumatic heart disease
    - AF
  - Prophylaxis and treatment:
    - DVT/PE
  - Transient ischaemic attacks (aspirin more effective at reducing risk)

2.10 Antiplatelet drugs

Knowledge of normal platelet function is important in understanding this section. See Chapter D1, Section 1.5.4.
- Antiplatelet drugs are more effective in preventing arterial thrombosis than anticoagulants because in faster-flowing vessels thrombus consists of mainly platelets with little fibrin.

2.10.1 Aspirin

- Mechanism of action:
  - Normally:
    - Activated platelets produce TXA2 resulting in vasoconstriction and platelet aggregation
    - Vascular endothelium produces PGI2 resulting in vasodilation and platelet disaggregation
  - Low-dose oral aspirin inhibits COX irreversibly in platelets, with vascular endothelium being relatively unaffected:
    - Marked reduced TXA2
    - Decreased PGI2
  - Vascular endothelium can resynthesize COX whilst platelets cannot and have to wait for new platelets to be made (lifespan 8–10 days):
    - Balance therefore shifts towards PGI2 and antithrombotic effects
- Uses:
  - MI
  - Acute coronary syndromes
  - Postcoronary bypass/stenting
  - Ischaemic stroke/TIAs
  - Prophylaxis cardiovascular events
  - AF
  - Mild to moderate pain
- Side effects:
  - GI ulceration and haemorrhage
  - Bronchospasm
  - Haemorrhage elsewhere
- Contraindicated:
  - Children <16 years old: link with Reye's syndrome: hepatic failure, encephalopathy, cerebral oedema, death 40%
  - Active peptic ulceration
  - Haemophilia
  - Hypersensitivity
  - Breastfeeding

2.10.2 Clopidogrel

- Mechanism of action:
  - Normal platelet aggregation involves:
    - Binding of ADP and TXA2 to platelets
    - Increased cytoplasmic Ca^{2+}
    - Activation of the glycoprotein IIb/IIIa receptor, which binds to fibrinogen
  - Clopidogrel inhibits ADP binding to platelets:
    - Decreased ADP-induced aggregation
  - Because clopidogrel inhibits a different pathway of platelet aggregation to aspirin, its effects are additive
- Uses:
  - With aspirin in:
    - MI
    - Acute coronary syndromes
  - Alternative to aspirin when aspirin contraindicated
  - Prevention of cardiovascular events in peripheral vascular disease
- Side effects:
  - Haemorrhage
  - Dyspepsia
  - Avoid if breastfeeding

2.10.3 Glycoprotein IIb/IIIa receptor antagonists (abciximab, eptifibatide, tirofiban)

- Mechanism of action:
  - Blocks the glycoprotein IIb/IIIa receptor
  - Inhibits platelet aggregation by preventing binding to fibrinogen
- Uses (NICE guidance):
  - Preventing ischaemic complications in high-risk patients with acute coronary syndromes or those undergoing percutaneous intervention that is delayed (requires specialist supervision)
- Side effects:
  - Haemorrhage
  - Thrombocytopenia

2.11 Fibrinolytics (thrombolytics)

2.11.1 Mechanism of action
- Activate plasminogen to plasmin, which lyses fibrin and therefore dissolves thrombi.

2.11.2 Uses
- Acute MI:
  - NB Emergency PCI now preferred as 1st-line treatment
- Pulmonary embolism with shock or cardiac arrest.
- Ischaemic stroke (acute):
  - Within 4.5 hours of onset of symptoms

2.11.3 Contraindications
- These vary with indication.
- Absolute:
  - Active internal bleeding

- ■ Haemorrhagic stroke or ischaemic stroke in last 6 months
- ■ Cerebral neoplasm
- ■ Aortic dissection
- ■ GI haemorrhage within 1 month
- ■ Major surgery, head injury, or trauma within 3 weeks
- Relative:
  - ■ Acute pancreatitis
  - ■ Active peptic ulcer disease
  - ■ Severe liver disease
  - ■ Severe hypertension (systolic BP >180mmHg)
  - ■ Anticoagulant therapy
  - ■ Pregnancy
  - ■ Traumatic CPR
  - ■ Known intracardiac thrombus/endocarditis
  - ■ Non-compressible vascular puncture

2.11.4 Side effects

- Haemorrhage (including acute haemorrhagic stroke).
- Nausea and vomiting.
- Hypotension and bradycardia.
- Reperfusion arrhythmias (in MI).

2.11.5 Examples

- Streptokinase:
  - ■ IV infusion over ≥1 hour
  - ■ Once given the body forms antibodies against it—cannot be given again within 4 days
  - ■ More likely to cause allergic reactions and hypotension/bradycardia
  - ■ Cheap
  - ■ Slightly less effective at producing thrombolysis than other fibinolytics
- Reteplase:
  - ■ Double-bolus regimen
  - ■ Requires heparin for 48 hours as short acting
- Tenecteplase:
  - ■ Single weight related dose
  - ■ Requires heparin for 48 hours as short acting

2.12 Lipid-regulating drugs

- Statins are 3-hydroxy-3-methylglutaryl coenzyme A (HMG CoA) reductase inhibitors.
- HMG CoA reductase is an enzyme involved in cholesterol synthesis.

2.12.1 Mechanism

- Inhibit HMG CoA reductase:
  - ■ Reduced hepatic cholesterol synthesis causes compensatory increase in hepatic LDL receptors
  - ■ This causes a decrease in plasma LDL and therefore cholesterol (LDL particles are rich in cholesterol)
- Statins have been found to reduce cardiovascular events and total mortality irrespective of the initial cholesterol concentration.

2.12.2 Indications

- Hypercholesterolaemia.
- Symptomatic cardiovascular disease:
  - Ischaemic heart disease
  - Peripheral vascular disease
  - Stroke/TIA
- Diabetics >40 years old.
- Diabetics ≤40 years old with high-risk features:
  - Target organ damage, poor glycaemic control, raised BP, FH of premature CV disease, low HDL and high cholesterol concentration
- Total cholesterol to HDL-cholesterol ratio >6.
- Asymptomatic patients at increased risk.

2.12.3 Contraindications

- Acute liver disease (or persistently abnormal LFTs).
- Pregnancy.
- Breastfeeding.

2.12.4 Cautions

- History of liver disease.
- Alcohol excess.
- Myopathy (or high risk of).
- Acute porphyria.

2.12.5 Side effects

- Myositis and rhabdomyolysis:
  - Discontinue if severe muscle aches or CK >5× upper limit normal
- Abnormal LFTs, hepatitis, jaundice, hepatic failure:
  - Require LFT monitoring at 0, 3, and 12 months
- Rarely:
  - Pancreatitis
  - GI disturbance

2.12.6 Examples

- Simvastatin.
- Atorvastatin.

Respiratory system

CONTENTS

3.1 Bronchodilators

The curriculum assumes you know the BTS/SIGN Guidelines in relation to emergency clinical management of asthma.

3.1.1 Beta-2 agonists

- Act mainly at β_2-receptors although affects β_1-receptors at high doses:
  - Bronchodilatation
  - Vasodilation ± hypotension (low dose has β_2 effects)
  - Tachycardia (high dose has β_1 effects)
  - Hypokalaemia—stimulates Na^+/K^+-ATPase transporting K^+ into cells
  - Tremor—direct effect on skeletal muscle
  - Relaxes uterus—used occasionally in premature labour
- 2 types:
  - Short acting (salbutamol/terbutaline)—relief of bronchospasm in acute asthma and other diseases with reversible airways obstruction (e.g. COPD)
  - Long acting (salmeterol/formoterol)—added to corticosteroids for long-term relief
- Salbutamol can be delivered via metered dose inhalers, in nebulized solutions, orally (although little clinical use for this), and intravenously:
  - Doses of salbutamol vary greatly depending on the severity of asthma:
    - 100-microgram inhaler in mild adult asthma
    - Continuous nebulized solutions plus IV infusions titrated to pulse in life-threatening asthma
- Side effects (in addition to those already listed):
  - Arrhythmias and palpitations
  - Headache
  - Nervous tension
  - Muscle cramps

3.1.2 Antimuscarinics

- Blocks vagally mediated bronchoconstriction secondary to histamine stimulation of airway irritant receptors.
- Slower and less effective than β_2 agonists but useful in addition to them.
- 2 types:
  - Ipratropium bromide:
    - Short-term relief in asthma/COPD
    - Maximal effect at 30–60min
    - Duration of action 3–6 hours
  - Tiotropium:
    - Long-acting antimuscarinic used in COPD
- Delivered via inhaler or nebulizer.
- Side effects:
  - Similar to other antimuscarinics (e.g. hyoscine, atropine):
    - Dry mouth
    - Constipation
    - Urinary retention
    - Blurred vision
    - Dry skin
    - Reduced bronchial secretions
    - Tachycardia
    - Confusion
  - Acute closed-angle glaucoma:
    - Care needed to protect eyes from nebulized drug

3.1.3 Theophylline

- Bronchodilator.
- Not generally effective in exacerbations of COPD.
- Possible additive effect to β_2 agonists.
- Therapeutic plasma level is 10–20mg/L.
- Side effects include:
  - Palpitations and tachycardia
  - Headache
  - Insomnia
  - Hypokalaemia (additive to β_2 agonists)
- Levels above 20mg/L can produce toxicity:
  - Cardiac arrhythmias including VF
  - Tremor and seizures
  - Nausea and vomiting
  - Rhabdomyolysis
- Metabolized by hepatic cytochrome p450:
  - Drugs that induce liver enzymes reduce plasma concentration
  - Drugs that inhibit liver enzymes increase plasma concentration
- Plasma concentration is also decreased in:
  - Smokers
  - Chronic alcoholism
- Plasma concentration is also increased in:
  - Heart failure
  - Cirrhosis
  - Elderly

- Aminophylline:
  - 2nd-line medication in acute severe asthma and controlled COPD
  - 80% theophylline, 20% ethylenediamine (confers 20 times greater water solubility than theophylline alone, allowing IV administration)
  - Requires slow IV infusion
  - Avoid in patients already on theophylline unless plasma concentration known, as could precipitate toxicity

3.2 Corticosteroids

Corticosteroids are covered in more detail in Chapter E6, Section 6.3. The following information is relevant to the respiratory system only.
- Reduce airway inflammation:
  - Decrease oedema
  - Reduce mucus secretion
  - Down-modify allergic reactions

3.2.1 Inhaled steroids (beclomethasone, budesonide, fluticasone)

- Uses:
  - Prophylaxis in chronic asthma if:
    - β_2 agonists used more than twice per week
    - Symptoms disturb sleep more than twice per week
    - Exacerbations in last 2 years requiring systemic corticosteroid or a nebulized bronchodilator
  - COPD
  - Hay fever (nasal spray)
- Side effects:
  - Inhalation avoids most of the side effects associated with oral steroids but in high doses adverse effects can occur:
    - Adrenal suppression
    - Osteoporosis
    - Glaucoma
    - Hoarseness
    - Oral candidiasis—rinsing mouth after use and using a spacer ↓ risk

3.2.2 Oral and intravenous steroids (prednisolone, dexamethasone, hydrocortisone)

- Used during periods of stress or when airway obstruction or mucus production prevents delivery of inhaled steroids to small airways.
- IV use reserved for severely compromised patients.
- Uses:
  - Acute asthma
  - Difficult to control chronic asthma
  - Acute exacerbation of COPD
  - Croup
  - Anaphylaxis
- Side effects—see Chapter E6, Section 6.3.2.

3.3 Antihistamines

- Block H_1-histamine receptors.
- Divided into 2 groups:
  - Sedating antihistamines (promethazine, alimemazine, chlorphenamine, cyclizine):
    - Older drugs
    - Additional antimuscarinic effects: urinary retention, dry mouth, blurred vision, GI disturbance
    - Caution with prostatic hypertrophy, urinary retention, acute-angle glaucoma, pyloroduodenal obstruction
    - Cross BBB—cause drowsiness and psychomotor impairment
    - This sedating effect can be useful in pruritus and insomnia
  - Non-sedating antihistamines (loratadine, cetirizine):
    - Newer drugs
    - No antimuscarinic effects
    - Do not cross BBB to any extent—drowsiness and psychomotor impairment rare
- Uses:
  - Allergic rhinitis
  - Urticaria
  - Pruritus
  - Insect bites and stings
  - Anaphylaxis
  - Angio-oedema
  - Nausea and vomiting
  - Motion sickness and vertigo
  - Premedication
  - Insomnia

3.3.1 Allergic emergencies

The Resuscitation Council guidelines for the management of anaphylaxis are extremely relevant to this section and should be memorized.

- Epinephrine (adrenaline):
  - For mechanism of action see Chapter E2, Section 2.7
  - Give immediately in cases of anaphylaxis
  - IM route
  - 1:1000 (1mg/mL) epinephrine solution
  - Dose as seen in Table E.3.1

Table E.3.1 Epinephrine (adrenaline) dosages

Age	Dose	Volume epinephrine 1:1000 (1mg/mL)
Child <6 years	150 micrograms	0.15mL
Child 6–12 years	300 micrograms	0.3mL
Adult and child >12 years	500 micrograms	0.5mL

- Doses can be repeated at 5min intervals.
- NB Only in extreme cases where there is doubt about the circulation should IV epinephrine be used. In this instance use 1:10 000 (100 micrograms/1mL) solution and give small 50-microgram (0.5mL) boluses.
- Epinephrine comes in prefilled 'auto-injectors' for patients with known anaphylaxis for self-administration:
  - Epipen®—delivers 300 micrograms per dose
  - Epipen Jr®—delivers 150 micrograms per dose
- Side effects:
  - Nausea and vomiting
  - Tachycardia, arrhythmias, palpitations
  - Anxiety, tremor, restlessness, headache, dizziness
  - Sweating
  - Dyspnoea, pulmonary oedema (excessive dose)
  - Hyperglycaemia
  - Urinary retention
  - Acute closed-angle glaucoma

3.4 Oxygen

- Most frequently given drug in emergency departments:
  - Increases alveolar O_2 tension
  - Decreases work of breathing
- Should be given to all acutely ill patients to achieve O_2 saturations of normal or near normal (94–98%)
- Should be used with caution in those at risk of developing type 2 respiratory failure (hypoxia and hypercapnia), aiming for O_2 saturations of 88–92%:
  - Repeated blood gas analysis required to achieve optimal concentration
  - Conditions at risk of type 2 respiratory failure:
    - COPD
    - Cystic fibrosis (CF)
    - Bronchiectasis
    - Severe kyphoscoliosis/ankylosing spondylitis
    - Musculoskeletal disorders with respiratory weakness
    - Overdose causing respiratory depression (e.g. opiate, benzodiazepine)
- In certain conditions it is appropriate to aim for O_2 saturations of as high as possible (e.g. cardiac arrest, carbon monoxide poisoning)
- Long-term O_2 therapy prolongs survival in some patients with COPD
- Should only be prescribed by respiratory experts
- Assessment for long-term therapy:
  - Requires measurement of PaO_2 on 2 occasions, at least 3 weeks apart, to demonstrate stability, and not sooner than 4 weeks after acute exacerbation of disease
- Short-burst (intermittent) O_2 therapy is sometimes used:
  - To improve exercise capacity and recovery
  - To relieve episodes of breathlessness not relieved by other treatments in COPD, interstitial disease, heart failure, and palliative care

Central nervous system

CONTENTS

4.1 Hypnotics and anxiolytics

- Hypnotics: used to treat sleeping disorders (sleeping tablets).
- Anxiolytics: used to treat anxiety states (sedatives).

4.1.1 Benzodiazepines

- Most commonly used hypnotics and anxiolytics.
- Also have muscle relaxant, anticonvulsant, and amnesic actions.
- Indicated only for the *short-term* relief of anxiety that is severe or disabling.
- Mechanism:
  - Facilitate action of γ-aminobutyric acid (GABA), the main inhibitory neurotransmitter within the CNS
  - $GABA_A$ receptors are ligand-gated chloride ion (Cl^-) channels
  - Binding of GABA to $GABA_A$ receptors increases Cl^- conductance, hyperpolarizing the neuronal membrane
  - Benzodiazepines bind to $GABA_A$ receptors at a different site and potentiate this action
- Effects/side effects:
  - Drowsiness and light-headedness (e.g. following day)—can impair motor skills such as driving
  - Confusion and ataxia (especially elderly)
  - Amnesia
  - Dependence
  - Muscle weakness
  - Respiratory depression, apnoea, and hypotension (IV use)
  - Paradoxical increase in excitement and aggression
- Interactions:
  - Effects, especially respiratory depression, markedly increased by other CNS depressants (opiates, alcohol, antihistamines)

Table E.4.1 Characteristics of benzodiazepines

Drug	Half-life (hours)	Active metabolites	Overall duration of action (hours)	Main usage
Midazolam	1–4	Yes	<6	Procedural sedation Anaesthesia Anticonvulsant
Lorazepam	8–12	No	12–18	Hypnotic Anxiolytic Anticonvulsant
Diazepam	20–40	Yes	24–48	Anxiolytic Muscle relaxant Anticonvulsant
Chlordiazepoxide	20–40	Yes	24–48	Alcohol withdrawal

- Dependence and withdrawal:
  - Dependence can occur quickly
  - Should only be given for short periods (2–4 weeks)
  - Sudden withdrawal after prolonged treatment can result in withdrawal syndrome:
    - Anxiety, insomnia, tremor, sweating, loss of appetite, perceptual disturbance
    - Occasionally confusion, psychosis, convulsions
    - Features can occur up to 3 weeks after stopping benzodiazepine
    - Requires gradual reduction in dose to try and avoid
    - Withdrawal features can persist for weeks to months
- Overdose:
  - The effects of benzodiazepines can be reversed by the benzodiazepine antagonist flumazenil:
    - Can result in seizures and arrhythmias and is especially dangerous if tricyclics have been taken where it can cause cardiac arrest, hence its use should be avoided if at all possible
    - Has a short duration of action therefore sedation can reoccur
- To understand the different characteristics of various benzodiazepines, and how their use is primarily governed by the duration of action, please see Table E.4.1.

4.2 Antipsychotics

- Also known as neuroleptics.
- Generally tranquillize without impairing consciousness.

4.2.1 Mechanism

- Block dopamine D_2 receptors in different parts of the brain:
  - Cortex and limbic system → antipsychotic effects:
    - Impaired performance
    - Sedation
  - Basal ganglia → extrapyramidal side effects:
    - Parkinsonian symptoms (including tremor)
    - Dystonia (abnormal face and body movements)

- Akathisia (restlessness)
- Tardive dyskinesia (rhythmic abnormal movements of tongue, face, and jaw)
- Pituitary gland → hyperprolactinaemia:
  - Gynaecomastia
  - Menstrual irregularities
  - Impotence
  - Weight gain
- Chemoreceptor trigger zone → antiemetic
- May also block:
  - Muscarinic receptors → anticholinergic effects (dry mouth, blurred vision, urinary retention, constipation)
  - α receptors → postural hypotension, hypothermia
  - Histamine receptors
  - 5HT (serotonin) receptors
- Dystonic reactions can be rapidly abolished with IV procyclidine.

4.2.2 Classification

- Phenothiazines:
  - Can be split into 3 groups—please see Table E.4.2
- Other, older antipsychotics resemble the group 3 phenothiazines:
  - Butyrophenones (haloperidol)
  - Thioxanthenes (flupentixol)
  - Substituted benzamides (sulpiride)
  - Diphenylbutylpiperidines (pimozide)
- Newer antipsychotics are termed 'atypical antipsychotics':
  - Fewer extrapyramidal side effects
  - Include olanzapine, quetiapine, risperidone

4.2.3 Neuroleptic malignant syndrome

- Serious potential side effect of treatment.
- Features include:
  - Hyperthermia
  - Muscle rigidity
  - Extrapyramidal signs
  - Fluctuating conscious level
  - Autonomic dysfunction (pallor, sweating, labile BP, tachycardia, incontinence)
- Treatment:
  - Withdraw antipsychotic
  - IV dantrolene

Table E.4.2 Classification of phenothiazines

	Group 1	Group 2	Group 3
Sedation	+++	++	+
Anticholinergic effects	++	+++	+
Extrapyramidal effects	++	+	+++
Example	Chlorpromazine	Thioridazine	Prochlorperazine

4.3 Antimania drugs

4.3.1 Lithium

- Uses:
  - Mania
  - Bipolar disorder
  - Recurrent depression
- *Narrow* therapeutic window:
  - Plasma level 0.4–1.0mmol/L at 12 hours post dose
- Side effects include:
  - GI disturbance
  - Fine tremor
  - Polyuria and polydipsia (ADH antagonism—nephrogenic diabetes insipidus)
  - Thyroid enlargement ± hypothyroidism
  - Weight gain
- Requires monitoring of lithium levels, U&Es, and TFTs.
- Toxicity:
  - Occurs at levels >1.5mmol/L
  - Complication of long-term therapy (decrease excretion secondary to dehydration/renal failure/infections/NSAIDs/diuretics—Na^+ depletion)
  - Acute overdose
- Toxic features:
  - Nausea, vomiting, and diarrhoea
  - Ataxia, dysarthria, nystagmus, weakness, coarse tremor
  - Coma and convulsions
  - Renal failure
  - Electrolyte imbalance
  - ECG changes and arrhythmias
  - Circulatory failure
  - Death
- Treatment:
  - Supportive
  - Withdraw drug, increase urine output with generous fluid administration, avoid diuretics
  - Correct electrolyte disturbance, control seizures
  - Haemodialysis/filtration in severe cases
- Lithium cards:
  - Available from pharmacies
  - Provide information for users about how to take lithium, what to do if a dose missed, side effects, reasons for regular blood tests, and drug interactions/illnesses that affect levels

4.4 Tricyclic antidepressants

4.4.1 Amitriptyline

- Uses:
  - Depression
  - Neuropathic pain
  - Nocturnal enuresis

- Mechanism:
  - Blocks neuronal uptake of 5HT and norepinephrine:
    - Antidepressant action
  - Blocks muscarinic, histamine, and α receptors and has non-specific sedative effects:
    - Hence similar side effects to antipsychotics (see Chapter E4, Section 4.2)
- Toxic in overdose:
  - Cardiovascular effects:
    - Tachycardia, arrhythmias, hypotension
    - ECG changes: sinus tachycardia; PR and QT_c prolongation; QRS widening; ventricular arrhythmias
  - CNS effects:
    - Agitation, convulsions
    - Coma, divergent squint, extensor planters, myoclonus
    - Hallucinations
  - Anticholinergic effects:
    - Dry mouth, urinary retention, dilated pupils
  - Metabolic acidosis
- Treatment overdose:
  - Supportive, close observation, monitor ECG/ABGs
  - Airway control—intubation/mechanical ventilation if necessary
  - Activated charcoal
  - Arrhythmias/QRS widening → sodium bicarbonate 8.4%
  - Prolonged seizures → lorazepam
  - Hypotension → IV fluids, raising foot of bed, glucagon in severe cases

4.5 Nausea and vomiting (N&V)

- Normal vomiting:
  - Complex process coordinated by the vomiting centre (VmC) in the medulla
  - VC receives afferents from:
    - CTZ: located in area postrema on floor of 4th ventricle outside BBB. Stimulated by circulating toxins/drugs
    - Vestibular apparatus: N&V related to vestibular disease/disorders
    - Vagal afferents (cardiovascular and GI): stimulated by direct irritants or local release of 5HT (cytotoxic drugs in the gut)
    - Spinal cord: N&V related to peripheral pain
    - Limbic cortex: N&V related to unpleasant odours/sights
    - Nucleus solitaries: gag reflex
  - Receptors involved:
    - D_2 and $5HT_3$ receptors involved in transmission at the CTZ
    - Muscarinic (cholinergic) and histamine receptors involved in transmission at the VmC
  - VmC projects efferents to the vagus, phrenic, and spinal motor neurons, which coordinate reverse peristalsis, glottis closure, breath holding, sphincter relaxation, muscle contraction, and ejection of vomitus
  - Antiemetics should be chosen with the aetiology of vomiting in mind

4.5.1 Antiemetics

- Antihistamines (cyclizine):
  - Block H_1 receptors and have anticholinergic effects (see Chapter E3, Section 3.3)
  - Uses:
    - N&V secondary to many conditions including vestibular diseases and motion sickness

- Side effects include:
  - Anticholinergic effects including tachycardia
  - Occasionally acute confusion and hypotension (sometimes seen when given IV in the elderly)
- Phenothiazines (prochlorperazine):
  - Block D_2 receptors at the CTZ
  - Also block muscarinic, histamine, 5HT, and α receptors (see Chapter E4, Section 4.2)
  - Uses include:
    - N&V secondary to drugs, neoplastic disease, radiation sickness, and anaesthesia
    - Vertigo and labyrinthine disorders
  - Side effects: see Chapter E4, Section 4.2
- Metoclopramide:
  - Antiemetic and prokinetic
  - Blocks D_2 (primarily) and $5HT_3$ receptors
  - Uses:
    - Similar to phenothiazines
    - May be superior in emesis related to gastroduodenal, hepatic, or biliary disease
  - Side effects:
    - Similar to phenothiazines
    - Acute dystonic reactions and oculogyric crisis more common in young females
- Domperidone:
  - Blocks D_2 receptors
  - Doesn't cross the BBB hence unlikely to cause central effects like metoclopramide and the phenothiazines
  - Not available IV
- $5HT_3$ antagonists (ondansetron):
  - Block $5HT_3$ receptors at the CTZ and gut
  - Uses:
    - N&V secondary to cytotoxics, drugs, and anaesthesia
  - Side effects:
    - Headache, flushing, constipation, and bradycardia (on fast injection)

4.6 Analgesics

- The choice of analgesic should be made according to the origin and severity of pain.
- Certain analgesics are more suitable than others for some types of pain:
  - Musculoskeletal pain—NSAID/paracetamol
  - Visceral pain—opioid
  - Neuropathic pain—gabapentin/amitriptyline
- The 'analgesic ladder' should be used to titrate medication to severity of pain and effect.

4.7 Non-opioid analgesics

4.7.1 Aspirin

- Now used primarily for its antiplatelet properties (see Chapter E2, Section 2.10.1).
- Still present in many over-the-counter preparations for headaches, musculoskeletal pain, dysmenorrhoea, and fever.
- Other NSAIDs preferred in inflammatory conditions as better tolerated.

- Mechanism (NSAIDs and aspirin):
  - Irreversibly inhibit COX:
    - ↓ TXA2—antiplatelet effect
    - ↓ PGE2 and PGF2α—anti-inflammatory and analgesic effect
    - ↓ prostaglandins in stomach—normally protect gastric mucosa hence results in gastric irritation/ulceration
    - ↓ prostaglandins in brain (which stimulate pyrexia produced as a result of IL-1 released from leucocytes)—antipyretic effect
    - ↓ prostaglandins in kidney—nephrotoxicity
    - ↑ leukotrienes—bronchospasm
  - Other side effects:
    - Skin rash
- Contraindications:
  - See Chapter E2, Section 2.10.1

4.7.2 NSAIDs

- See Chapter E8, Section 8.2.

4.7.3 Paracetamol

- Uses:
  - Mild to moderate pain
  - Pyrexia
- Mechanism is unclear.
- Side effects are rare (rashes, blood disorders).
- Metabolism:
  - Normally:
    - Paracetamol metabolized to mainly glucuronide conjugates
    - Small amount converted to the toxic NAPQI (*N*-acetyl P-amino-benzoquinoneimine), which is quickly made safe by conjugation with glutathione
  - Overdose:
    - Glucuronide pathway becomes saturated
    - More NAPQI produced → cell death and hepatic necrosis
  - Antidotes:
    - Methionine (PO): increase glutathione synthesis
    - *N*-acetylcysteine (IV): hydrolysed to cysteine, glutathione precursor

---

4.8 Opioid analgesics

- Opiate: naturally occurring substance with morphine-like properties.
- Opioid: compounds with an affinity for opioid receptors and whose effects are antagonized by naloxone.
- Opioid receptors—found in the CNS, spinal cord, and periphery:
  - There are 3 types of opioid receptor that are then further subdivided—see Table E.4.3

4.8.1 Morphine salts

- Morphine remains the most valuable opioid analgesic for severe pain.
- PO, IM, IV, IN, PR, epidural, and intrathecal administration available.
- Preferred analgesia for oral treatment in palliative care.
- Peak effect when given IV reached after 10min, duration 3–4 hours.
- Renal excretion hence accumulates in renal failure.

Table E.4.3 Types of opioid receptor

Receptor type	Effect
μ	Analgesia, respiratory depression, meiosis, constipation, euphoria, sedation, physical dependence
κ	Analgesia, papillary constriction, dysphoria, sedation
δ	Analgesia, respiratory depression, constipation

- Tolerance develops rapidly (few days) requiring dose escalation.
- Main effects:
  - Analgesia
  - Euphoria, sedation, and dysphoria: euphoria and the relief of agitation is an important component of its analgesic effect
  - Respiratory depression: brainstem sensitivity to CO_2 reduced more than sensitivity to O_2 → supplemental O_2 can potentiate respiratory depression
  - N&V
  - Miosis (constricted pupils)
  - Cough suppression
  - Constipation (reduced gut motility)
  - Bronchospasm and hypotension (histamine release)
- Overdose:
  - Acute overdose (IV drug users):
    - Coma
    - Respiratory depression and apnoea
    - Constricted pupils
  - Treatment—naloxone:
    - Pure opioid antagonist
    - Reverses coma and respiratory depression when given in appropriate dose
    - Duration of action 30–40min—less than morphine/diamorphine hence coma and respiratory depression can recur. Repeated doses often required
    - Can cause hypertension, pulmonary oedema, ventricular arrhythmias, and cardiac arrest
    - Can precipitate withdrawal syndrome in addicts—abdominal pain, vomiting, diarrhoea, aggression
- Opioid toxicity (palliative care):
  - Symptoms:
    - Vivid dreams
    - Hallucinations
    - Agitation and confusion
    - Sedation
    - Myoclonic jerks
  - Treatment:
    - Rehydrate
    - Reduce dose of opioid
    - Haloperidol sometimes required to manage altered sensorium
    - Naloxone rarely required

4.8.2 Codeine phosphate

- 10 times less potent than morphine (10% is metabolized to morphine, which is responsible for its analgesic effects).

- PO or IM formulations (IV avoided because of histamine release).
- Uses:
  - Mild to moderate pain
  - Cough suppression
  - Diarrhoea
- Main side effects:
  - Constipation
  - Nausea and vomiting
  - Sedation
- Effects reversed by naloxone.

4.8.3 Tramadol

- 5–10 times less potent than morphine.
- Produces analgesia by blocking opioid receptors and enhancing 5HT and norepinephrine pathways.
- PO, IM, and IV administration available.
- Uses: moderate to severe pain.
- Side effects:
  - Less respiratory depression and constipation than typical opioids
  - Occasional psychiatric reactions
- Interactions:
  - TCAs and SSRIs (blocks 5HT and norepinephrine uptake): can result in seizures, therefore avoid in epilepsy
- Respiratory depression and analgesia reversed by naloxone

4.9 Antiepileptics

4.9.1 Phenytoin

- Mechanism:
  - Binds to inactivated neuronal Na^+ channels, preventing them from returning to the resting state (which they must return to before they can fire again)
  - High-frequency repetitive firing (during a seizure) increases the number of channels in the resting state, hence these cells are preferentially blocked
- Uses:
  - All seizures except absence type
  - Trigeminal neuralgia (if carbamazepine inappropriate)
  - Status epilepticus
- Toxicity:
  - *Narrow* therapeutic index—plasma concentration 40–80 micromol/L
  - Therapeutic index difficult to maintain (blood monitoring useful)
  - Relationship between dose and plasma concentration non-linear
  - Many interactions:
    - Hepatic enzyme inducer: ↑ metabolism of warfarin, OCP, paracetamol to NAPQI in overdose
    - Metabolized by liver: its metabolism ↑ by other inducers (carbamazepine, alcohol, rifampicin, and itself!). Its metabolism ↓ by inhibitors (metronidazole, chloramphenicol)
    - Individual variability
    - Missed doses

- Features of toxicity:
  - Ataxia, diplopia, dysarthria, nystagmus, vertigo, confusion (cerebellar signs)
- Side effects:
  - Acne, gum hypertrophy, coarse facies, and hirsutism
  - Serious:
    - Blood disorders (aplastic anaemia, leucopenia, megaloblastic anaemia)
    - Skin rashes (Stevens–Johnson syndrome, toxic epidermal necrolysis)
  - Teratogenicity

4.9.2 Carbamazepine

- Mechanism:
  - Similar to phenytoin
- Uses:
  - Partial and generalized seizures
  - Trigeminal neuralgia
  - Bipolar disorder (unresponsive to lithium)
- Interactions:
  - Powerful hepatic enzyme inducer and metabolized by liver (see Chapter E4, Section 4.9.1)
- Side effects:
  - Mild neurotoxic effects can limit use (nausea, dizziness, blurred vision, ataxia)
  - Serious:
    - Blood disorders (see Chapter E4, Section 4.9.1)
    - Rashes (see Chapter E4, Section 4.9.1)
    - Hepatic disorders (hepatitis, cholestatic jaundice)
  - Teratogenicity

4.9.3 Sodium valproate

- Mechanism:
  - Similar action to phenytoin at Na^+ channels
  - Increases GABA-mediated central neuronal inhibition, possibly by reducing GABA inactivation (for action of GABA see Chapter E4, Section 4.1.1)
- Uses:
  - All forms of epilepsy
- Side effects:
  - Adverse effects are generally mild compared with most antiepileptic drugs:
    - Nausea
    - Weight gain
    - Transient hair thinning—regrowth may be curly!
    - Thrombocytopenia
  - Serious (rare):
    - Hepatitis/liver failure
    - Pancreatitis
  - Teratogenicity

4.10 Status epilepticus

- Continuous generalized seizures lasting ≥30min *or* recurrent seizures where consciousness is not regained lasting ≥30min

- Requires urgent management to prevent cerebral damage:
  - ABC, secure airway, O_2 monitoring, IV access
  - Check BM and temperature—correct hypoglycaemia
  - Consider:
    - IV thiamine (Pabrinex®)—alcoholics
    - IV magnesium—pregnancy-related seizures (eclampsia)
    - Paracetamol—febrile seizures
  - Terminate seizures: drug delivery usually follows the following sequence with ≤10min between each drug until seizures are terminated:
    - IV lorazepam
    - IV lorazepam
    - IV phenytoin/fosphenytoin infusion
    - Rapid sequence intubation with thiopentone/propofol
  - PR paraldehyde can be given after the 2nd dose of lorazepam in certain circumstances (usually in children):
    - No IV access
    - Poor resuscitation facilities
  - Other options if no IV access available:
    - PR diazepam
    - Buccal midazolam

4.10.1 Lorazepam, diazepam, midazolam

- See Chapter E4, Section 4.1.1.
- NB Buccal midazolam is given by drawing up the desired dose (0.4mg/kg children <10 years, 10mg adults/children >10 years) of IV preparation and delivering it into the buccal region with a syringe.

4.10.2 Phenytoin

- See Chapter E4, Section 4.9.1.
- NB Fosphenytoin is a prodrug of phenytoin.

4.10.3 Paraldehyde

- Useful when no resuscitation facilities as causes little respiratory depression.
- Requires mixing with olive oil or saline to produce an enema—avoid arachis oil because of patients with peanut allergy.
- Avoid contact with plastic/rubber—reacts with it (once made up in plastic syringe must use immediately).
- Side effects:
  - Rectal irritation
  - Rashes

CHAPTER E5

Infections

CONTENTS

5.1 Notifiable diseases

- The following are all notifiable diseases:
  - Anthrax
  - Cholera
  - Diphtheria
  - Dysentery (amoebic/bacillary)
  - Encephalitis (acute)
  - Food poisoning
  - Haemorrhagic fever (viral)
  - Hepatitis (viral)
  - Leprosy
  - Leptospirosis
  - Malaria
  - Measles
  - Meningitis (acute)
  - Meningococcal septicaemia
  - Mumps
  - Ophthalmia neonatorum
  - Paratyphoid fever
  - Plague
  - Poliomyelitis (acute)
  - Rabies
  - Relapsing fever
  - Rubella
  - Scarlet fever
  - Small pox
  - Tetanus

- Typhoid fever
- Typhus
- Whooping cough
- Yellow fever

5.2 Antibacterial drugs

The following antibiotics are the recommended 1st-line therapeutic agents for the conditions listed.

5.2.1 Gastrointestinal system

- Gastroenteritis
- Antibiotics not usually indicated
- *Campylobacter* enteritis:
  - Treat severe infection with ciprofloxacin or erythromycin
- *Salmonella*:
  - Ciprofloxacin or cefotaxime
  - Treat severe infection or those at high risk (e.g. immunocompromised)
- Shigellosis:
  - Ciprofloxacin or azithromycin
- Typhoid fever:
  - Ciprofloxacin or cefotaxime
  - Sensitivity should be tested and antibiotics prescribed accordingly due to high resistance
- *Clostridium difficile*:
  - Oral metronidazole or oral vancomycin
  - Treat for 10–14 days
- Biliary tract infection:
  - Ciprofloxacin or gentamicin or a cephalosporin
- Peritonitis:
  - A cephalosporin plus metronidazole

5.2.2 Cardiovascular system

- Endocarditis: usually requires at least 4 weeks of antibiotics (6 weeks if prosthetic valve). Treatment depends on the organism isolated:
  - 'Blind' therapy:
    - Flucloxacillin (benzylpenicillin can be used in mild infections) plus gentamicin
    - If cardiac prosthesis or penicillin-allergic or possible MRSA: vancomycin plus rifampicin
  - Staphylococci:
    - Flucloxacillin (vancomycin + rifampicin if penicillin-allergic or if MRSA)
  - Streptococci (e.g. viridans streptococci):
    - Benzylpenicillin (vancomycin if penicillin-allergic) plus gentamicin
  - Enterococci:
    - Amoxicillin (vancomycin if penicillin-allergic/resistant) plus gentamicin
  - 'HACEK' organisms (*Haemophilus, Actinobacillus, Cardiobacterium, Eikenella*, and *Kingella* spp.):
    - Amoxicillin (ceftriaxone if amoxicillin resistant) plus low-dose gentamicin

5.2.3 Respiratory system

- *Haemophilus influenzae* epiglottitis:
  - IV cefotaxime or chloramphenicol

- Acute exacerbations of chronic bronchitis:
  - Amoxicillin or tetracycline
  - Treat for 5 days
- Low-to-moderate severity community-acquired pneumonia
  - Amoxicillin
  - Add clarithromycin if infection of moderate severity or if atypical pathogens suspected
  - Add flucloxacillin if staphylococci suspected (e.g. in influenza or measles)
  - Vancomycin if MRSA suspected
  - Treat for 7 days (14–21 days for staphylococcal infections)
- High-severity community-acquired pneumonia:
  - Co-amoxiclav/cefuroxime/cefotaxime plus clarithromycin
  - Add vancomycin if MRSA suspected
  - Treat for 7–10 days (longer if staphylococci or Gram-negative enteric bacilli suspected)
- Pneumonia possibly caused by atypical pathogens:
  - Clarithromycin
  - Doxycycline for *Chlamydia* and *Mycoplasma* infections
  - A quinolone if *Legionella* infection suspected
  - Treat for 14 days (7–10 days for *Legionella*)
- Hospital-acquired pneumonia:
  - Early onset less than 5 days after admission:
    - Co-amoxiclav or cefuroxime
    - Treat for 7 days
    - If severe, treat as for late onset hospital-acquired pneumonia
  - Late onset >5 days after admission to hospital:
    - Antipseudomonal penicillin (e.g. piperacillin with tazobactam)
    - Or a broad-spectrum cephalosporin
    - Or another antipseudomonal beta-lactam
    - Or a quinolone (e.g. ciprofloxacin)
    - Consider an aminoglycoside if severe illness caused by *Pseudomonas aeruginosa*
    - Add vancomycin if MRSA suspected
    - Treat for 7 days

5.2.4 Central nervous system

- Meningitis:
  - GPs should give benzylpenicillin before urgent transfer to hospital
  - Consider dexamethasone (particularly if pneumococcal meningitis suspected in adults); avoid in septic shock, meningococcal septicaemia, if immunocompromised, or in meningitis following surgery
- Meningococcal meningitis:
  - Benzylpenicillin or cefotaxime
  - Chloramphenicol if history of immediate hypersensitivity reaction to penicillin or cephalosporins
  - Treat for 7 days
  - Rifampicin for 2 days to eliminate nasopharyngeal carriage
- Pneumococcal meningitis:
  - Cefotaxime (if highly penicillin sensitive use benzylpenicillin)
  - If resistant use vancomycin
  - Treat for 10–14 days
  - Consider adjunctive treatment with dexamethasone starting before or with 1st dose of antibacterial (may reduce penetration of vancomycin into CSF)

- *Haemophilus influenzae* meningitis:
  - Cefotaxime
  - Chloramphenicol if immediate hypersensitivity reaction to penicillin/cephalosporins
  - Treat for at least 10 days
  - Consider adjunctive treatment with dexamethasone starting before or with 1st dose of antibacterial
- Meningitis caused by *Listeria*:
  - Amoxicillin plus gentamicin
  - Treat for 10–14 days

5.2.5 Urinary tract

- Acute pyelonephritis:
  - Broad-spectrum cephalosporin or a quinolone
  - Treat for 10–14 days
- Acute prostatitis:
  - Ciprofloxacin or ofloxacin or trimethoprim
  - Treat for 28 days
- 'Lower' urinary tract infection:
  - Trimethoprim or nitrofurantoin or amoxicillin or cephalosporin
  - 3 days in uncomplicated infections in women
  - Otherwise treat for 7 days

5.2.6 Genital system

- Syphilis:
  - Benzathine benzylpenicillin or doxycycline or erythromycin
- Uncomplicated gonorrhoea:
  - Ciprofloxacin
  - Single-dose treatment in uncomplicated infection
- Uncomplicated genital *Chlamydia* infection, non-gonococcal urethritis, and non-specific genital infection:
  - Azithromycin (14 days) or doxycycline (7 days)
- Pelvic inflammatory disease:
  - Doxycycline plus metronidazole (14 days) plus IM ceftriaxone (single dose)
- Bacterial vaginosis:
  - Oral or topical metronidazole (5–7 days)

5.2.7 Blood

- Community-acquired septicaemia:
  - A broad-spectrum antipseudomonal penicillin or a broad-spectrum cephalosporin (e.g. cefuroxime)
- Hospital-acquired septicaemia:
  - A broad-spectrum antipseudomonal beta-lactam antibiotic (e.g. piperacillin with tazobactam)
- Septicaemia related to vascular catheter:
  - Vancomycin
- Meningococcal septicaemia:
  - Benzylpenicillin *or* cefotaxime

5.2.8 Musculoskeletal system

- Osteomyelitis:
  - Flucloxacillin

- Clindamycin if penicillin-allergic
- Treat acute infection for 4–6 weeks and chronic infection for at least 12 weeks
- Septic arthritis:
  - Flucloxacillin
  - Clindamycin if penicillin-allergic
  - Treat for 6 weeks

5.2.9 Eye

- Purulent conjunctivitis:
  - Chloramphenicol or gentamicin eye-drops

5.2.10 Ear, nose, and oropharynx

Consider carefully the need for antibiotics. Most upper respiratory tract infections are caused by viruses. Antibiotics are indicated if the patient is systemically unwell, has a severe infection, or there is evidence of bacterial infection.

- Pericoronitis:
  - If systemic features present, metronidazole or amoxicillin
- Acute necrotizing ulcerative gingivitis:
  - If systemic features present, metronidazole or amoxicillin
- Periapical or periodontal abscess:
  - Amoxicillin or metronidazole
- Periodontitis:
  - Metronidazole or doxycycline
- Throat infections:
  - Phenoxymethylpenicillin
  - Clindamycin if penicillin-allergic
  - Avoid amoxicillin if possibility of glandular fever
- Sinusitis:
  - Amoxicillin or doxycycline or clarithromycin
  - Treat for 7 days
  - Oral co-amoxiclav is an alternative if no improvement after 48 hours
- Otitis externa:
  - Flucloxacillin
  - Clarithromycin if penicillin-allergic
- Otitis media:
  - Amoxicillin
  - Clarithromycin if penicillin-allergic

5.2.11 Skin

- Impetigo:
  - Topical fusidic acid
- Erysipelas:
  - Phenoxymethylpenicillin
  - Clarithromycin if penicillin-allergic
  - Treat for at least 7 days
- Cellulitis:
  - Benzylpenicillin plus flucloxacillin
  - Clarithromycin if penicillin-allergic
- Animal and human bites:
  - Co-amoxiclav
  - Doxycycline plus metronidazole if penicillin-allergic

5.2.12 Prophylaxis

- Recurrence of rheumatic fever:
  - Phenoxymethylpenicillin or sulfadiazine
- Secondary case of invasive group A streptococcal infection:
  - Phenoxymethylpenicillin
  - Erythromycin in penicillin allergy
- Secondary case of meningococcal meningitis:
  - Rifampicin or ciprofloxacin
- Secondary case of *Haemophilus influenzae* type b:
  - Rifampicin
- Secondary case of diphtheria (non-immune patient):
  - Erythromycin
- Secondary case of pertussis (non-immune patient):
  - Erythromycin
- Pneumococcal infection (patients with asplenia or sickle-cell disease):
  - Phenoxymethylpenicillin
- Gas-gangrene in high lower-limb amputations or following major trauma:
  - Benzylpenicillin
  - Metronidazole if penicillin-allergic
- Tuberculosis in susceptible close contacts or those who have become tuberculin positive:
  - Isoniazid (6 months) or isoniazid plus rifampicin (3 months)
- Infection in GI tract:
  - This is not relevant to emergency medicine; please refer to the BNF for further information
- Infective endocarditis undergoing interventional procedures:
  - NICE recommends prophylaxis is not required for procedures of the following:
    - Dental
    - Upper and lower respiratory tract
    - Genitourinary tract
    - Upper and lower GI tract
  - In patients at high risk of endocarditis:
    - Treat any infections promptly to reduce the risk
    - Should receive appropriate antibiotics that include cover against organisms that cause endocarditis if undergoing a GI or genitourinary tract procedure where infection is suspected
    - Advise to maintain good oral hygiene
    - Advise of the signs of endocarditis
- Joint prostheses and dental treatment:
  - No benefit of prophylaxis

5.3 Penicillins

- Mechanism of action:
  - Bactericidal, mostly against Gram-positive organisms
  - Contains a beta-lactam ring that interferes with cell wall synthesis by inhibiting peptidoglycan cross-links
  - Water then enters the cell and causes it to burst
- Resistance:
  - Due to the production of beta-lactamase by the bacteria
  - Co-amoxiclav contains clavulanic acid that inactivates beta-lactamases

- Penicillins have good penetration into body tissues, fluids, and CSF (when meninges inflamed)
- Implications of allergy or atopy in the prescribing of penicillins:
  - Hypersensitivity in 1–10% of individuals
  - Asthma or hay fever at higher risk
  - Caution prescribing other beta-lactam antibiotics in patients with immediate hypersensitivity to penicillins
  - Other beta-lactam agents can be used in patients with a history of minor reaction

5.3.1 Benzylpenicillin

- Inactivated by bacterial beta-lactamases.
- Effective for use against streptococcal, gonococcal, and meningococcal infections.
- Indications:
  - Throat infections
  - Otitis media
  - Endocarditis
  - Meningococcal disease
  - Pneumonia
  - Cellulitis
  - Anthrax
- Contraindicated in penicillin hypersensitivity.
- Reduce dose in renal impairment.
- Side effects:
  - Hypersensitivity
  - Other rare side effects (see BNF)
- Dose: 2.4–4.8g qds IM/IV.

5.3.2 Phenoxymethylpenicillin (penicillin V)

- Similar to benzylpenicillin but less active.
- Indications:
  - Oral infections
  - Tonsillitis
  - Otitis media
  - Erysipelas
  - Cellulitis
  - Group A streptococcal infection
  - Rheumatic fever
  - Pneumococcal prophylaxis
- Cautions and side effects as for benzylpenicillin.
- Dose: 500–1000mg qds PO.

5.3.3 Flucloxacillin

- Not inactivated by penicillinases, which makes most staphylococci resistant to benzylpenicillin.
- Indications—infections caused by penicillin-resistant staphylococci:
  - Otitis externa
  - Adjunct in pneumonia
  - Impetigo
  - Cellulitis
  - Osteomyelitis
  - Staphylococcal endocarditis
- Well absorbed from the gut.

- MRSA resistant to flucloxacillin is difficult to treat and antibiotics such as vancomycin, linezolid, and daptomycin could be used following discussion with the microbiologist.
- Contraindication is penicillin hypersensitivity and hepatic dysfunction from flucloxacillin.
- Caution in hepatic impairment.
- Side effects: cholestatic jaundice and hepatitis may occur; very rare.
- Dose: may need to reduce in renal impairment; 250–500mg qds PO, 0.25–2g qds IV

5.3.4 Ampicillin

- Active against certain Gram-positive and Gram-negative organisms.
- Inactivated by penicillinases; resistance likely.
- Excreted in the bile and urine.
- Indications:
  - Urinary tract infections
  - Otitis media
  - Sinusitis
  - Oral infections
  - Bronchitis
  - Uncomplicated community-acquired pneumonia
  - *Haemophilus influenzae* infections
  - Invasive salmonellosis
  - Listerial meningitis
- Contraindication: penicillin hypersensitivity.
- Side effects:
  - GI disturbance
  - See Chapter E5, Section 5.3.1
- Dose: 0.25–1g qds PO, 500mg qds IV/IM.

5.3.5 Amoxicillin

- Derivative of ampicillin.
- Better absorbed than ampicillin when given by mouth.
- Indications:
  - See Chapter E5, Section 5.3.4
  - Oral infections
  - Endocarditis
  - Anthrax
  - Adjunct in *Listeria* meningitis
- Contraindications: see Chapter E5, Section 5.3.4.
- Reduce dose in severe renal impairment.
- Dose 250–500mg tds PO, 500mg–1g tds IV/IM.

5.3.6 Co-amoxiclav

- Amoxicillin and clavulanic acid.
- Clavulanic acid inactivates beta-lactamases.
- More active against beta-lactamase-producing bacteria.
- Co-amoxiclav should be reserved for infections likely, or known, to be caused by amoxicillin-resistant beta-lactamase-producing strains.
- Indications:
  - Respiratory tract infections
  - Genitourinary infection
  - Abdominal infections

- Cellulitis
- Animal bites
- Severe dental infection with spreading cellulitis
- Dental infection not responding to 1st-line antibacterial

5.4 Cephalosporins

Cephalosporins have a beta-lactam ring. They are broad-spectrum and excreted by the kidneys.

5.4.1 Cefalexin

- Indications:
  - Infections due to sensitive Gram-positive and Gram-negative bacteria
- Contraindications:
  - Cephalosporin hypersensitivity
  - Avoid in beta-lactam immediate hypersensitivity
- Side effects:
  - Rarely antibiotic-associated colitis
  - GI upset
  - Headache
  - Allergic reactions
  - Stevens–Johnson syndrome and toxic epidermal necrolysis reported
  - Disturbances in liver enzymes, transient hepatitis, and cholestatic jaundice
- Dose: 250–500mg tds PO.

5.4.2 Cefotaxime

- Indications:
  - See Chapter E5, Section 5.4.1
  - Gonorrhoea
  - Surgical prophylaxis
  - *Haemophilus* epiglottitis
  - Meningitis
- Contraindication: see Chapter E5, Section 5.4.1.
- Side effects:
  - See Chapter E5, Section 5.4.1
  - Rarely arrhythmias following rapid IV injection
- Dose: 1–2g bd up to 8g a day IV/IM.
- 500mg single dose for gonorrhoea.

5.4.3 Ceftriaxone

- Indications:
  - See Chapter E5, Section 5.4.1
  - Surgical prophylaxis
- Cautions:
  - May displace bilirubin from serum albumin
- Contraindications:
  - See Chapter E5, Section 5.4.1
  - Neonates <41 weeks
  - Neonates >41 weeks with jaundice, hypoalbuminaemia, or acidosis
  - Concomitant treatment with IV calcium in neonates >41 weeks—risk of precipitation in urine and lungs

- Dose may need to be reduced in hepatic and renal impairment.
- Side effects:
  - See Chapter E5, Section 5.4.1
  - Calcium ceftriaxone precipitates in urine or in gallbladder—consider discontinuation if symptomatic
  - Rarely prolongation of prothrombin time and pancreatitis
- Dose IV/IM 1g up to 4g daily.

5.4.4 Cefuroxime

- Indications:
  - See Chapter E5, Section 5.4.1
  - Surgical prophylaxis
  - Increased activity against *Haemophilus influenzae* and *Neisseria gonorrhoeae*
  - Lyme disease
- Contraindications: see Chapter E5, Section 5.4.1
- Side effects: see Chapter E5, Section 5.4.1
- Dose (reduce in renal impairment): 750mg–1.5g tds IV/IM.

5.5 Tetracyclines

Bacteriostatic drugs that act by interfering with protein synthesis. They are poorly absorbed and excreted mostly renally. Patients should be advised to avoid taking with foods as they bind to heavy metal ions, which reduces absorption. They have a broad spectrum but their use is becoming limited due to increasing bacterial resistance.

5.5.1 Doxycycline

- Indications:
  - *Chlamydia*
  - *Rickettsia*
  - *Brucella*
  - Lyme disease
  - Respiratory and genital mycoplasma infections
  - Acne
  - Destructive (refractory) periodontal disease
  - Exacerbations of chronic bronchitis
  - Chronic prostatitis
  - Sinusitis
  - Syphilis
  - Malaria treatment and prophylaxis
- Cautions:
  - May increase muscle weakness in myasthenia gravis
  - May exacerbate systemic lupus erythematosus
  - Aluminium, calcium, iron, magnesium, and zinc salts decrease the absorption of tetracyclines, as do antacids
  - Hepatic impairment
- Contraindications:
  - Affects bone and teeth growth, therefore avoid in:
    - Children <12 years
    - Pregnant or breastfeeding women

- Side effects:
  - GI upset
  - Dysphagia and oesophageal irritation
  - Other rare side effects in BNF
  - Dose: 200mg PO on day 1, then 100mg daily

5.6 Aminoglycosides

- Aminoglycosides are bactericidal and work by inhibiting protein synthesis, although their true mechanism is unclear.
- They enter the cell by active transport and anaerobes are therefore resistant as they have little energy for this process.
- Lipid-soluble and therefore parenteral administration is required.
- They are not metabolized and are renally excreted, therefore caution in renal failure.
- Side effects:
  - Dose related
  - Important side effects are ototoxicity and nephrotoxicity
  - Occur most frequently in the elderly and in patients with renal failure

5.6.1 Gentamicin

- Indications:
  - Septicaemia
  - Meningitis and other CNS infections
  - Biliary tract infection
  - Acute pyelonephritis or prostatitis
  - Endocarditis
  - Pneumonia in hospital patients
  - Adjunct in listerial meningitis
- Cautions:
  - Very young and very old
- Contraindications:
  - Myasthenia gravis
- Side effects:
  - Vestibular and auditory damage
  - Nephrotoxicity (rarely)
  - Hypomagnesaemia on prolonged therapy
  - Antibiotic-associated colitis
  - Stomatitis
- Dose: usually 3–5mg/kg daily IV/IM (in 3 divided doses).
- Monitor serum gentamicin levels (predose trough):
  - Prevents subtherapy and toxic side effects

5.7 Macrolides

- Macrolides inhibit protein synthesis.
- They are bacteriostatic but can be bacteriocidal in high doses.

5.7.1 Erythromycin

- Indications:
  - Susceptible infections in patients with penicillin hypersensitivity

- Oral infections
- Syphilis
- Non-gonococcal urethritis
- Respiratory tract infections
- Skin infections
- Whooping cough
- Legionnaires' disease
- *Campylobacter* enteritis
- Acne vulgaris and rosacea
- Prophylaxis of diphtheria and group A streptococcal infection
- Cautions:
  - Neonates <2 weeks
  - Predisposition to QT prolongation
  - Acute porphyria
- Side effects:
  - Nausea, vomiting, and diarrhoea are the commonest side effects
  - Allergic reactions
  - Rarer:
    - Reversible hearing loss after high doses
    - Cholestatic jaundice
    - Pancreatitis
    - Chest pain and arrhythmias
    - Myasthenia-like syndrome
    - Stevens–Johnson syndrome and toxic epidermal necrolysis
- Dose (reduce in renal impairment): 500mg qds PO.

5.8 Other antibiotic agents

5.8.1 Chloramphenicol eye preparations

- Inhibit protein synthesis.
- Broad spectrum.
- Indicated in superficial eye infections.
- Well tolerated.
- Side effect—transient stinging.
- Either drops or ointment:
  - Eye drops: apply 1 drop at least every 2 hours
  - Eye ointment:
    - At night (if eye drops used during the day)
    - Otherwise 3–4 times daily (if eye ointment used alone)

5.8.2 Fusidic acid

- Protein synthesis inhibitor.
- Used topically in creams and eye drops.
- Used for staphylococcal infections.

5.8.3 Vancomycin

- Glycopeptide that inhibits bacterial cell wall synthesis.
- Highly active against Gram-positive organisms.
- Long duration of action.
- Poorly absorbed orally therefore given IV for systemic infection (PO for *Clostridium difficile*).

- Indications:
  - Endocarditis
  - Peritonitis associated with peritoneal dialysis
  - *C. difficile*
- Cautions:
  - Avoid rapid infusion
  - History of deafness
  - Elderly
  - Pregnancy (okay if breastfeeding)
- Side effects:
  - Nephrotoxicity
  - Ototoxicity (discontinue if tinnitus occurs)
  - Blood disorders including neutropenia
  - Nausea
  - Chills
  - Fever
  - Eosinophilia
  - Anaphylaxis
  - Rashes
  - Stevens–Johnson syndrome, toxic epidermal necrolysis, and vasculitis
  - Further details on side effects in BNF
  - Dose (reduce in renal impairment): 125mg qds PO, IV 1–1.5g bd
  - Plasma trough monitoring required

5.8.4 Metronidazole

- Inhibits DNA replication.
- Indications:
  - Anaerobic infections
  - Protozoal infections
  - *Helicobacter pylori* eradication
  - Skin infection
- Cautions:
  - Disulfiram-like reaction with alcohol
  - Avoid in acute porphyria
  - Avoid high doses in pregnancy and if breastfeeding
  - Hepatic encephalopathy
- Side effects:
  - GI disturbances (including N&V)
  - Taste disturbances
  - Furred tongue
  - Oral mucositis
  - Anorexia
  - Rarer side effects in BNF
- Dose (reduce in hepatic impairment): 400mg tds PO, 500mg tds IV.

5.9 Management of tuberculosis

Because *Mycobacterium tuberculosis* is an intracellular organism that has a varying drug resistance, it is very difficult to eradicate. Therefore, we use a multiple drug regimen over 6 months. Management is in 2 phases, an initial phase followed by a continuation phase.

5.9.1 Initial phase

- 4 drugs for 2 months.
- Reduces the bacterial population.
- Prevents the emergence of drug resistance.
- Usually isoniazid, rifampicin, pyrazinamide, and ethambutol.
- Started without waiting for culture results.
- Streptomycin is rarely used in the UK but it may be used in the initial phase of treatment if resistance to isoniazid has been established before therapy is commenced.

5.9.2 Continuation phase

- After the initial phase.
- Treatment for a further 4 months.
- Isoniazid and rifampicin.
- Longer treatment for:
  - Meningitis
  - Direct spinal cord involvement
  - Resistant organisms

5.9.3 Pregnancy and breastfeeding

- The standard regimen may be used during pregnancy and breastfeeding.
- Streptomycin should not be given in pregnancy.

5.9.4 Monitoring

- Isoniazid, rifampicin, and pyrazinamide:
  - Associated with liver toxicity
  - Hepatic function should be checked before treatment with these drugs
  - Those with pre-existing liver disease or alcohol dependence should have frequent checks, particularly in the 1st 2 months
- Renal function should also be checked before treatment:
  - Streptomycin or ethambutol should preferably be avoided in patients with renal impairment, but if used the dose should be reduced and the plasma-drug concentration monitored

5.10 Quinolones

You should be aware of the risks of tendon damage in patients prescribed a quinolone.

5.10.1 Ciprofloxacin

- Particularly active against Gram-negative bacteria.
- Indication:
  - *Salmonella*
  - *Shigella*
  - *Campylobacter*
  - *Neisseria*
  - *Pseudomonas*
  - Respiratory tract infections (but not for pneumococcal pneumonia)
  - Urinary tract infections
  - Infections of the GI system (including typhoid fever)
  - Bone and joint infections
  - Gonorrhoea and septicaemia caused by sensitive organisms

- Caution:
  - History of epilepsy/seizures
  - G6PD deficiency
  - Myasthenia gravis (risk of exacerbation)
  - Children or adolescents
  - Exposure to excessive sunlight should be avoided (discontinue if photosensitivity occurs)
- Contraindications:
  - Quinolone hypersensitivity
  - Tendon disorders
- Side effects:
  - Tendon damage:
    - Reported rarely
    - Rupture may occur within 48 hours of starting treatment
    - Has been reported several months after
    - Patients >60 years of age are more prone to tendon damage
    - Risk is increased by age >60 years and concomitant use of corticosteroids
    - Stop immediately if tendonitis suspected
  - Flatulence
  - Pain and phlebitis at injection site
- Dose:
  - UTI: 500–750mg bd PO, 400mg bd/tds IV
  - Gonorrhoea: 500mg PO single dose

5.11 Urinary tract infections

- More common in women than in men.
- In men, there may be an abnormality of the renal tract.
- Recurrent episodes of infection are an indication for further investigation.
- Organisms:
  - Commonest is *Escherichia coli*
  - *Staphylococcus saprophyticus* common in sexually active young women
- Urine should be sent for culture and sensitivity before starting antibacterial therapy.
- Uncomplicated infections respond well to trimethoprim, nitrofurantoin, amoxicillin, or nalidixic acid for 7 days (3 days in women).
- Acute pyelonephritis:
  - Can lead to septicaemia
  - IV broad-spectrum antibiotic (e.g. cefuroxime or a quinolone)
  - Gentamicin if patient very unwell
- Prostatitis:
  - Difficult to cure
  - Several weeks' treatment with trimethoprim or some quinolones
- Children:
  - Require prompt antibacterial treatment to reduce risk of renal scarring

5.11.1 Trimethoprim

- Bacteriostatic; inhibits folic acid synthesis.
- Indications:
  - Urinary tract infections
  - Acute and chronic bronchitis
  - Pneumocystis pneumonia

- Cautions:
  - Predisposition to folate deficiency
  - Elderly
  - Neonates
  - Blood disorders on long-term treatment
- Contraindications:
  - Blood dyscrasias
  - Pregnancy—teratogenic risk in 1st trimester
- Side effects:
  - GI disturbances
  - Rashes
  - Hyperkalaemia
  - Depression of haematopoiesis
- Dose (reduce in renal impairment): 200mg bd PO.

5.12 Antifungal preparations

5.12.1 Candidiasis

- Fungal infection commonly caused by *Candida albicans*.
- Usually superficial (e.g. oral thrush) or systemic.
- Life-threatening infections found in immunocompromised.
- Management is usually topical but systemic therapy is available for severe infections.

5.12.2 Nystatin

- Indications—candidiasis:
  - Oral infection
  - Skin infection
- Side effects:
  - GI disturbance
  - Oral irritation and sensitization
  - Rash (including urticaria)
  - Rarely Stevens–Johnson syndrome reported
- Dose (intestinal candidiasis): 500 000 units qds.

5.13 Herpes virus infections

Herpes simplex virus (HSV; herpes virus hominis) and varicella zoster virus are the 2 most important herpes viruses.

5.13.1 Herpes simplex infections

- Commonly mouth and lips and in the eye associated with HSV-1.
- Genital infection most often associated with HSV-2.
- Treatment should be started within 5 days of the appearance of the infection.
- Topical antiviral drug in patients with normal immune function.
- Systemic antivirals required for:
  - Severe infection
  - Neonatal herpes infection
  - Immunocompromised patients
  - Primary or recurrent genital herpes simplex infection is treated with oral antivirals
- Specialist advice in pregnancy.

5.13.2 Chicken pox (varicella zoster)

- Neonates require parenteral antiviral to avoid severe disease.
- Children aged 1 month to 12 years usually do not require treatment.
- More severe in adolescents and adults:
  - Antiviral treatment within 24 hours of the onset of rash may reduce severity and symptoms
- Parenteral antiviral treatment is generally recommended in immunocompromised patients and those at special risk.
- In pregnancy (before 28 weeks) it can lead to foetal varicella syndrome ($\rightarrow$ various foetal malformations):
  - Specialist advice should be sought

5.13.3 Shingles (herpes zoster)

- Systemic antiviral treatment may reduce severity and symptoms.
- Treatment should be started within 72 hours of the onset of rash.
- Immunocompromised patients at high risk of severe infection should be treated with a parenteral antiviral therapy.

5.13.4 Aciclovir

- Active but does not eradicate.
- Indications:
  - Herpes simplex
  - Varicella zoster
- Cautions:
  - Ensure patient well hydrated
  - Elderly
  - Renal impairment
- Side effects:
  - Abdominal disturbance
  - Headache
  - Fatigue
  - Rash, urticaria, pruritus
  - Photosensitivity
  - IV—severe local inflammation
- Dose (reduce dose in renal impairment): 200mg 5 times a day PO, 5mg/kg (ideal body weight) tds IV.

5.14 Antimalarials

5.14.1 Malaria

- Caused by the *Plasmodium* parasite, which is spread by mosquitoes.
- The most serious form of malaria is caused by *Plasmodium falciparum*.
- Important to consider malaria in travellers with fever returning from a malaria region.
- Treat for falciparum malaria (if suspected), even if organism is unknown.
- Falciparum malaria is especially dangerous in pregnancy (worst in the last trimester); treatment is challenging due to the lack of agents licensed for use in pregnancy.

5.14.2 Treatment of falciparum malaria

- Resistant to chloroquine.
- Quinine or malarone orally are 1st-line agents if no serious signs
- Quinine (can be given in pregnancy) IV if the patient is seriously ill or unable to take tablets.

Endocrine system

CONTENTS

6.1 Diabetes

- Diabetes mellitus (DM) is characterized by persistent hyperglycaemia. This can be caused by the body's failure to produce insulin (T1DM) or by increased insulin resistance (T2DM).
- T1DM usually presents in younger people with polyuria, polydipsia, and weight loss. Long-term treatment of T2DM is with insulin, the preferred regimen being a long-acting insulin, with a short-acting insulin being given with meals (basal-bolus regimen). Initial management can be difficult due to 'honeymoon' period where the pancreas still produces small amounts of insulin.
- T2DM is usually in older patients who are overweight and usually has an insidious onset. It may have features of polyuria and polydipsia, or may present with either macrovascular or microvascular complications.
- There are 3 potentially life-threatening emergencies in diabetes: diabetic ketoacidosis (DKA), hyperosmolar hyperglycaemic non-ketotic coma (HONK), and hypoglycaemia.
- DKA:
  - The hallmark of T1DM
  - May be initial presentation, secondary to concurrent illness or poor blood sugar control
  - Presentation:
    - Acidosis
    - Ketones in urine
    - Hyperventilation (Kussmaul respiration)
    - Nausea, vomiting, and abdominal pain
  - Management: see Chapter E6, Section 6.1.3
- HONK:
  - T2DM
  - Severe hyperglycaemia, hyperosmolality without significant ketosis
  - Intercurrent illness, drug induced, or poor control of DM
  - Investigate for cause
  - Management:
    - ABCDE

- Aggressive fluid resuscitation (careful not to correct hypernatraemia too quickly due to risk of cerebral oedema)
  - Insulin infusion
  - Monitor electrolytes (especially potassium and sodium) and correct as appropriate
- Hypoglycaemia:
  - Usually caused by medications

6.1.1 Insulin

- Polypeptide hormone produced in the islet cells of pancreas:
  - Facilitates the uptake of glucose into muscle and fat cells
  - Stimulates glyconeogenesis and protein synthesis
  - Inhibits gluconeogenesis and lipolysis
- Animal-derived/synthetic/recombinant DNA technology
- Types of insulin preparations:
  - Very short acting
    - Peak effect 15min
    - For example, insulin aspart (Novorapid®), glulisine, and lispro
    - Preferred for those who are prone to hypoglycaemia before meals and nocturnal hypoglycaemia
  - Short acting:
    - Peak effect 1–2 hours (SC) and duration of 4–8 hours
    - When given IV, $t_{1/2}$ of 5min
    - For example, Actrapid®
  - Biphasic
    - For example, Mixtard 30®
    - Has short-acting and intermediate/long-acting insulin
  - Long acting:
    - SC onset of action 1–2 hours
    - Peak effect 4–12 hours
    - Duration 16–35 hours
    - For example, Lantus®
- There are various regimens for insulin, which are very dependent on the individual patient:
  - Once-a-day long-acting insulin and very short-acting insulin before meals is the preferred regimen for tight sugar control and allows patient to be more flexible with meal times
  - SC: normal route of administration
  - SC continuous infusion: for tight control; requires frequent monitoring
  - IV: emergency, perioperative

6.1.2 Notification of DVLA

- Drivers are required to notify the DVLA if:
  - They are insulin-dependent diabetics
  - They are on oral antidiabetic drugs with complications
- Driving is not permitted if there are:
  - Recurrent hypoglycaemic episodes
  - Lack of hypoglycaemic awareness

6.1.3 Use of insulin in management of diabetic ketoacidosis

- ABC initially.
- Key priority is fluid resuscitation:
  - 2L normal saline 1st 2 hours

■ If the patient is shocked, then more aggressive fluid resuscitation is required
■ If profoundly acidotic, comatose, or not responding well to fluid therapy, consider escalation of care
● Begin insulin (Actrapid®) infusion usually 6 units/hour (depends on local protocol).
● Can be stopped when patient has had 2 meals and maintains blood sugars.
● Long-acting insulin should be continued.
● Replace potassium depending on levels. If potassium <5mmol/L add ~20mmol potassium chloride (KCl) to each litre. If <4mmol/L add ~30mmol KCl, and if <3mmol/L add ~40mmol.

6.1.4 Oral antidiabetic drugs

● NICE guidance on management of T2DM is initially with diet and lifestyle advice to maintain an HBa1C <6.5.
● If this is unsuccessful then usually tablets are initiated in a stepwise fashion with metformin, followed by a sulphonylurea, and if still unable to control blood sugars then a thiazolidinedione or insulin therapy should be considered.
● The 2 main classes of drugs are:
   ■ Sulphonylureas:
      ● Augment existing insulin secretion
      ● Can cause persistent hypoglycaemia and patients must be treated in hospital
   ■ Biguanides (i.e. metformin):
      ● Reduces gluconeogenesis
      ● Enhances peripheral utilization of glucose
      ● Very unusual to cause hypoglycaemia

6.1.5 Treatment of hypoglycaemia

● Treat BM <3.0mmol/L (do not wait for venous lab glucose level to return).
● Management:
   ■ ABCDE approach
   ■ Give sugary drinks/GlucoGel© (formerly known as Hypostop®) if patient can take oral preparations
   ■ Glucagon is the next option
   ■ IV dextrose 10%; can give 50% but is very hyperosmolar and can cause local necrosis
● Glucagon:
   ■ Can be given SC/IM/IV at a dose of 1mg given stat
   ■ Polypeptide hormone; mobilizes glycogen from liver
   ■ Not to be used in hypoglycaemia if:
      ● Chronic hypoglycaemia
      ● Associated with liver failure
      ● Patient on sulphonylurea drugs
      ● Associated with chronic alcoholism

6.2 Thyroid disease

6.2.1 Hypothyroid management

● Most cases are managed with levothyroxine through primary care and referral for further investigation.
● In the acute setting, long-term untreated hypothyroidism can present as a myxoedema coma:
   ■ Typically in elderly women
   ■ Progressive symptoms of hypothyroidism

- Comatose/reduced mentation
- History of hypothyroidism or treated hyperthyroidism
- Management:
  - ABCDE approach
  - IV fluids and ventilation may be required
  - IV liothyronine:
    - More rapidly metabolized and more rapid onset than levothyroxine
    - 5–20 micrograms every 4–12 hours as necessary
    - Can be given orally: 10–20 micrograms tds
    - Expert advice required as IV therapy controversial and may increase mortality
  - Hydrocortisone:
    - Stress dose 100 micrograms IV
  - Treat any precipitating infection

6.2.2 Thyrotoxic storm management

- Life-threatening complication of hyperthyroidism:
  - Poorly-treated hyperthyroidism or 1st presentation
  - Hyperthermia >40°C
  - Tachycardia
  - Delirium
  - Diaphoresis
  - Clinical signs of hyperthyroidism
- Management:
  - ABCDE approach
  - Supportive management includes:
    - IV fluids with dextrose
    - O_2
    - Investigate for precipitating cause (i.e. infection) and treat
  - Further management:
    - Carbimazole oral 15–40mg daily followed by Lugol's solution (5% iodine and 10% potassium iodide) 0.1–0.3mL tds
    - Propranolol 5mg IV
    - IV hydrocortisone 100 micrograms qds (as sodium succinate)

6.3 Corticosteroids

- Corticosteroids are produced in the adrenal glands. Can be classified as mineralocorticoids and glucocorticoids.
- The main mineralocorticoid is aldosterone (not used therapeutically) and the main glucocorticoid is hydrocortisone (cortisol), although this does exhibit some mineralocorticoid effect.
- Mineralocorticoids:
  - Cause sodium retention and hence passive retention of water
  - Increase sodium reuptake and secretion of potassium in the distal tubule of the kidney
  - Fludrocortisone (no glucocorticoid activity) is used in adrenal insufficiency
- Glucocorticoids:
  - Reduce immune response:
    - Inhibit proinflammatory mediators
    - Stimulate anti-inflammatory mediators

- Maintain blood glucose:
  - Stimulate gluconeogenesis in the liver
  - Inhibit uptake of glucose into muscle mediated by insulin
  - Increases appetite and truncal fat distribution
- Inhibits collagen synthesis (→ thin skin and osteoporosis in long-term steroid use)

6.3.1 Side effects and complications

- Patients on long-term steroid use are at risk of the following:
  - Adrenal suppression:
    - In long-term use (e.g. prednisolone >7.5mg a day), → adrenal atrophy due to corticotrophin suppression
    - Therefore withdraw steroid slowly to prevent Addisonian crisis
    - Steroids should be doubled in times of stress/illness (unless on high dose) because the body cannot respond to increased requirements, to prevent Addisonian crisis
  - Infections:
    - Due to the suppression of the inflammatory response patients are more susceptible to infection. Reactivation of dormant infections (e.g. TB) may occur
    - Patients may present atypically, with a longer duration of symptoms, as they will not produce the usual inflammatory response to infection
    - Patients who are not immune to chicken pox (not previously infected) are at risk of severe chicken pox, with complications such as encephalitis, pneumonia, and hepatitis.
    - Varicella zoster immunoglobulin is required for post-exposure prophylaxis; this provides passive immunity
    - Increase steroid dose if infected
    - Patients should also be advised to avoid exposure to measles and should receive post-exposure immunoglobulin within 72 hours if they are exposed
- All patients on long-term steroids should carry a 'steroid card' to inform medical practitioners that they are on steroids or have been on steroids (for up to a year as adrenal suppression can be prolonged).

6.3.2 Specific steroids

- Prednisolone:
  - PO, 2.5–15mg, daily (maintenance)
  - PO, 10–60mg, daily (inflammation/allergy)
  - Mainly glucocorticoid action (5 times more potent than hydrocortisone)
  - Primarily used for disease suppression
  - Indications:
    - Rheumatological/autoimmune conditions
    - Asthma
    - Temporal arteritis
    - Adrenal insufficiency (acute)
- Hydrocortisone:
  - IV/IM, 100–500mg, 3–4 times daily
  - PO, 20–30mg, divided doses
  - Topical, as ointment
  - Glucocorticoid and weak mineralocorticoid action
  - Short-term treatment of emergency conditions
  - Mineralocorticoid effect and resulting fluid retention means unsuitable for long-term treatment for disease suppression
  - Is used long-term with fludrocortisone in adrenal suppression

- Indications:
  - Adrenal insufficiency
  - Addison's disease
  - Anaphylaxis
  - Acute allergy
  - Asthma
  - Shock
  - Angio-oedema
  - Hypersensitivity reactions
  - Severe inflammatory bowel disease
  - Rheumatic disease
- Dexamethasone:
  - PO, 0.5–10mg, daily
  - IM/IV, 0.5–24mg
  - Very high glucocorticoid activity
  - Long duration of action
  - Very little fluid retention
  - Particularly used in cerebral oedema
  - Indications:
    - Cerebral oedema
    - Perioperatively
    - Inflammatory disorders
    - Croup
    - Intractable nausea
    - Diagnosis of Cushing's
    - Temporal arteritis

Fluids and electrolytes

CONTENTS

7.1 Oral preparations

- Oral potassium may be required in:
  - Patients taking certain antiarrhythmics (e.g. digoxin), where hypokalaemia may lead to arrhythmias
  - Patients with secondary hyperaldosteronism
  - Excessive potassium loss (e.g. chronic diarrhoea or malnutrition in elderly)
- Use of potassium-sparing diuretic is recommended in diuretic-induced hypokalaemia.

7.1.1 Oral rehydration therapy

- Oral rehydration should be designed to:
  - Replace water and electrolytes efficiently (increased absorption) and safely
  - Counter acidosis
  - Prevent induction of diarrhoea, therefore should be hypo-osmolar
  - Be easy to access, easy to use, and palatable
- Dioralyte™:
  - Electrolyte replacement when 5 sachets mixed with 1L water:
    - 60mmol sodium
    - 20mmol potassium
    - 60mmol chloride
    - 90mmol glucose
    - 10mmol citrate
  - Infants: 1–1.5 × normal feed volume (after each loose motion)

7.2 Parenteral preparations

- IV fluid should be given to patients who:
  - Are unable to tolerate oral fluids
  - Require fluid maintenance (e.g. if nil by mouth)
  - Require fluid replacement

- Are in shock
- Require emergency electrolyte replacement (e.g. hyponatraemia)
- Fluid choice and rate is patient dependent (e.g. care should be taken not to replace sodium too quickly as risk of causing cerebral oedema).
- Colloids vs crystalloids:
  - Colloids:
    - Have high osmotic pressure
    - Will expand extracellular volume
    - Used in intravascular volume depletion to rapidly improve blood pressure
  - Crystalloids:
    - Isotonic and therefore more equally distributed across the cell membrane; will expand intracellular compartment as well as intravascular compartment
    - Used as maintenance and rehydration fluid
    - Cheaper than colloids
- There has been much debate about whether to use colloids and crystalloids in a shocked patient. In reality there is little difference between them and you should choose the fluid most readily available.

7.2.1 Crystalloids

- Sodium chloride (0.9%):
  - 154mmol/L Na^+, 154mmol/L Cl^-
- Hartmann's:
  - 150mmol/L Na^+, 111mmol/L Cl^-, 5mmol/L K^+, 29mmol/L lactate, 2mmol/L calcium, 5mmol/L K^+, 29mmol/L HCO_3^-
- Glucose (5%, 10%, 25%, 50%):
  - 5%: 50mg/mL glucose
  - 10%: 100mg/mL glucose etc.
  - Inappropriate for aggressive fluid resuscitation as 5% dextrose is hypotonic
- Potassium chloride mixtures:
  - Preparations:
    - Preformed infusion solutions
    - Ampoules (to be added to NaCl solutions—*not* glucose)
  - Caution:
    - Renal impairment
- Sodium bicarbonate:
  - Treatment of severe metabolic acidosis (pH <7.1)
  - Correct hypovolaemia and anoxia before administration
  - Bicarbonate not routinely indicated during CPR
- For maintenance fluids the body's daily requirement is ~2–3L of water, 140mmol sodium, and 60mmol potassium. Therefore an appropriate regimen would be 1L of 0.9% sodium chloride and 2L of 5% dextrose, with appropriate potassium addition (no more than 40mmol KCl per 8 hours) over 24 hours.

7.2.2 Colloids

- Albumin (isotonic 4–5% or concentrated 20–25%):
  - Colloid—contains electrolytes and soluble proteins
  - Treatment of oedematous states (liver failure, cirrhosis) and subacute plasma loss
- Gelatin:
  - Colloid—used for rapid replacement of intravascular depletion (e.g. burns):
    - Volplex®
    - Haemaccel®
    - Gelofusine®

7.3 Vitamin B

- The B vitamins play an important role in cell metabolism and growth, as well as enhancing immune and neurological function.
- In total there are 8 B vitamins.
- Vitamin B deficiency is rare in the UK.
- A deficiency of thiamine, the first B vitamin, leads to:
  - Wernicke's encephalopathy: triad of ataxia, acute confusion, ophthalmoplegia
  - Korsakoff's syndrome: memory loss, confabulation (late)
- Wernicke's and Korsakoff's very often lead to irreversible neurological deficit. Alcoholics are at particular risk because they are malnourished.
- Alcohol inhibits thiamine absorption from the gut and its metabolism. It is therefore essential to give thiamine replacement to chronic alcoholics and rapid thiamine replacement to any patient with signs and symptoms suggestive of Wernicke's/Korsakoff's.

7.3.1 Thiamine

- Thiamine (PO, 10–300mg/day) for chronic depletion.
- Pabrinex® (IV/IM, 1 pair of vials over 30min) for severe depletion:
  - Most effective way of replacing thiamine
  - Potentially life-threatening allergic reactions, therefore:
    - Should only be given when essential
    - Given slowly >10min
    - Anaphylaxis equipment nearby
- Indications:
  - Malnutrition
  - Hyperemesis gravidarum
  - Alcoholism
  - Haemodialysis
- Give *before* glucose administration (may precipitate Wernicke's encephalopathy)

Musculoskeletal system

CONTENTS

8.1 Non-pharmacological measures

- Management of musculoskeletal injuries and diseases involves more than just pharmacological intervention.
- Consideration of splinting, physiotherapy, and early mobilization can be the most effective way to ease pain and improve long-term outcome.
- Simple advice to rest, ice, compress, and elevate (RICE) injuries, along with simple analgesics, may all be that is required to manage a high percentage of soft tissue injuries.

8.2 Non-steroidal anti-inflammatory drugs (NSAIDs)

- Single dose—analgesia comparable to paracetamol.
- Analgesic full effect up to 7 days.
- Anti-inflammatory full effect up to 21 days.
- Antipyretic.
- Variable action and tolerance to different NSAIDs.

8.2.1 Pharmacology

- Cyclooxygenase (COX) catalyses the production of prostaglandins through the intermediate arachidonic acid.
- Prostaglandins regulate the body's inflammatory response.
- COX has 2 isoenzymes:
  - COX-I regulates many physiological processes including protection of gastric mucosa
  - COX-II is expressed in inflammatory cells
- Most NSAIDs inhibit both COX-I and COX-II.
- Some newer drugs inhibit just COX-II, therefore reducing gastric side effects.
- Recent studies have shown that NSAIDs increase the risk of cardiovascular complications in at risk patients, including MI.
- Cautions:
  - Pregnancy
  - Lactation

- Cardiac impairment
- Renal impairment
- Hepatic impairment
- Side effects:
  - GI effects
  - Hypersensitivity reactions
  - Renal failure (dehydration, ACE inhibitors)
  - Heart failure
  - Tinnitus
  - Hypertension
  - Thrombotic events
  - Fluid retention
- Risk of GI side effects:
  - High: indometacin, piroxicam, ketorolac
  - Medium: aspirin, naproxen, sulindac
  - Low: ibuprofen, diclofenac
- NSAIDs should be chosen based on risk of GI and other side effects and the underlying disease (e.g. diclofenac in gout):
  - Ibuprofen is the safest NSAID but has low anti-inflammatory properties
  - Indometacin has the best efficacy but highest incident of side effects
  - Naproxen is a popular choice because it has a high efficacy and relatively low side effect profile

8.2.2 Ibuprofen

- Has fewest side effects.
- Good analgesic and antipyretic properties.
- Minimal anti-inflammatory properties, therefore unsuitable for inflammatory conditions such as gout.
- Used in mild to moderate pain.
- High doses may be used in rheumatoid arthritis and migraine.
- PO 400mg tds; max. 2.4g/daily.

8.2.3 Naproxen

- Good efficacy.
- Low incidence of side effects but more than ibuprofen.
- Can be used in musculoskeletal disorders, rheumatological disorders, acute gout, and dysmenorrhoea.
- PO 250mg–1.25g in 1–4 divided doses.

8.2.4 Diclofenac

- Similar to naproxen.
- Indicated in musculoskeletal conditions, postoperative pain, ureteric colic, and acute gout.
- PO/PR/IM/IV 75–150mg daily.
- Extra contraindications include:
  - Porphyria
  - In IV use:
    - Concomitant NSAID or anticoagulant use
    - Haemorrhagic diathesis
    - Suspected/confirmed cerebrovascular bleeding
    - Asthma
    - Moderate/severe renal impairment
    - Hypovolaemia/dehydration

8.2.5 Mefenamic acid

- Low anti-inflammatory properties.
- PO 500mg tds.
- Indicated in mild to moderate pain, dysmenorrhoea, and osteoarthritis.
- Side effects:
  - Aplastic anaemia
  - Thrombocytopenia
  - Haemolytic anaemia (+ve Coombes)

8.3 Corticosteroids

Please note, these drugs also appear in Chapter E6, Section 6.3.

8.3.1 Systemic

- Pharmacology:
  - Glucocorticoids are important in management of musculoskeletal disorders.
  - They downregulate COX and lipooxygenase, which leads to reduced production of inflammatory mediators.
  - Given in high doses to reduce inflammation in diseases such as rheumatoid arthritis and temporal arteritis. Steroids are then reduced down to the lowest level where the disease remains suppressed.

8.3.2 Local

- Local treatment of steroids is always preferable to systemic wherever possible, to minimize adverse effects.
- Administration can be with creams, intra-articular injections, inhalations, eye drops, or enemas.
- Striae and skin thinning can be a particular problem with topical use.

8.4 Drugs used in gout and hyperuricaemia

8.4.1 Management of acute gout

- High-dose NSAIDs.
- Colchicine if NSAID intolerance.
- Avoid aspirin and allopurinol.
- Corticosteroids as alternative to NSAIDs.

8.4.2 Colchicine

- Probably as effective as NSAIDs.
- Preferred in patients with heart failure as does not induce fluid retention and can be given to patients on anticoagulants.
- PO 500 micrograms, 2–4 divided doses, max. 6mg per course.
- Side effects:
  - GI upset
  - Haematological disorders (prolonged courses)
  - Less risk of fluid retention compared to NSAIDs
  - Caution with clarithromycin and erythromycin

Immunological products and vaccines

CONTENTS

9.1 Active immunity

Vaccines stimulate production of antibodies and other components of the immune mechanism.

9.1.1 Types of vaccine

- Inactivated:
  - Heat/chemically inactivated virulent microorganism (virus or bacteria)
  - May require a primary series of injections of vaccine to produce an adequate antibody response, and in most cases booster (reinforcing) injections are required; the duration of immunity varies from months to many years. Some inactivated vaccines are adsorbed onto an adjuvant (such as aluminium hydroxide) to enhance the antibody response
  - Examples:
    - Polio
    - Hepatitis A
    - Plague
    - Cholera
    - Flu
    - BCG
- Live attenuated:
  - Live microorganism; virulence attenuated in lab
  - Better immunological response (but less than natural immunity)
  - Avoid in immunosuppressed/pregnant
  - Examples:
    - Yellow fever
    - Measles
    - Mumps
    - Rubella
- Detoxified exotoxin:
  - Intact/extract of exotoxins
  - High efficacy

- Examples:
  - Tetanus
  - Diphtheria
- Subunit:
  - Protein subunits of specific pathogen
  - Immune system will recognize on exposure
  - Examples:
    - Hepatitis B (surface protein)
    - HPV (capsid protein)
- Conjugate:
  - Polysaccharide coat + protein
  - Examples:
    - HIB

9.1.2 Contraindications

- Acute febrile illness.
- Anaphylaxis to components.
- Egg allergy (MMR, yellow fever, encephalitis, flu).
- Pregnancy and immunosuppression (live vaccines).
- NB Stable neurological conditions are not a contraindication to vaccination

9.1.3 Side effects

- Discomfort at site of injection.
- Abscess.
- Mild fever and malaise.
- Hypersensitivity reactions.

9.1.4 Postimmunization infant pyrexia

- Use paracetamol or ibuprofen PRN.
- Seek medical advice if pyrexia persists after 2 doses of paracetamol:
  - Keep infant cool
  - Maintain hydration
  - Investigate for alternative cause
  - Don't give aspirin as risk of Reye's syndrome

9.1.5 The United Kingdom immunization schedule

Table E.9.1 UK immunization schedule

At-risk neonates	BCG Hep B
2 months	DTP, Polio, Hib, Pneumococcal
3 months	DTP, Polio, Hib, Meningococcal C
4 months	DTP, Polio, Hib, Meningococcal C, Pneumococcal
12 months	Hib, Meningococcal C
13 months	MMR, Pneumococcal
3 years 4 months to 5 years	DTP + Polio or DTP + Polio + Hib +MMR (2nd dose)

Table E.9.1 Continued

At-risk neonates	BCG Hep B
12–13 years	HPV (3 doses)—females only
13–18 years	DT, Polio
Childbearing-aged women (if at risk)	MMR
>65 years	Pneumococcal + Flu

9.2 Passive immunity

- The transfer of antibody-mediated immunity from one individual to another individual.
- Readymade antibodies:
  - Antibodies from human origin are termed 'immunoglobulins'
- Confers immediate immunity against specific organism.
- Short-lasting protection (weeks).
- Use:
  - Mostly for post-exposure prophylaxis
  - Can be used as pre-exposure prophylaxis
  - To attenuate disease
- Can be repeated to give longer immunity.

9.3 Specific vaccines and preparations

9.3.1 BCG

- Live attenuated vaccine from *Mycobacterium bovis*:
  - Hypersensitivity to *M. tuberculosis*
- Skin test first to check hypersensitivity (>6years age)
- Intradermal injection:
  - Causes induration (>2 weeks post injection and scar formation if successful)
- Serious reaction uncommon but can lead to:
  - Anaphylaxis
  - Abscess
  - Disseminated BCG → osteitis/osteomyelitis
- Recommended for:
  - Infants and neonates in TB-prone areas
  - Immigrants (from TB-prone areas)
  - Healthcare workers, lab workers, and vets
  - Homeless people
  - Travellers to TB-prone areas for >1 month
- May be given simultaneously with a live vaccine; otherwise there should be an interval of 4 weeks between them.

9.3.2 Diphtheria

- Toxin of *Corynebacterium diphtheriae*.
- Stimulates the production of antitoxin.
- For children 2 months to 10 years:

- ■ 3 primary doses
- ■ Booster 3 years after finishing course
- ■ Final booster 10 years when finished course
- Staff working directly with *C. diphtheriae* or *C. ulcerans* should receive a booster, then at 10-year intervals if still at risk.
- Travellers: DTP booster if >10 years since last immunization.
- Contacts: booster if fully immunized, 10-year intervals thereafter.

9.3.3 Haemophilus influenzae type B (Hib)

- Capsulated polysaccharide, conjugated with a protein such as tetanus toxoid to increase immunogenicity.
- Combined with diphtheria, tetanus, pertussis, and poliomyelitis vaccines
- 3 primary doses, 1 booster in infants.
- Not required if >10 years of age (unless high risk, e.g. sickle-cell disease, post-splenectomy).

9.3.4 Hepatitis A

- Recommended for:
  - ■ Lab workers
  - ■ Care workers
  - ■ Travellers to endemic areas
  - ■ Primate handlers
  - ■ IV drug users
  - ■ Liver disease
  - ■ Haemophiliacs
  - ■ High-risk sexual behaviour
- Single dose, 1–2 boosters.
- Mild side effects include induration, erythema, and pain.

9.3.5 Hepatitis B

- Inactive HbsAg, made using recombinant DNA technology.
- Recommended for:
  - ■ Healthcare workers
  - ■ IV drug users
  - ■ Sexual partners of infected people
  - ■ Haemodialysis
  - ■ Haemophiliacs
  - ■ Prisoners
- 3–4 primary doses, further booster at 5 years.
- Immunization may take up to 6 months.
- 'Accelerated schedule' for high risk.
- Immunoglobulin (HBIG) for inoculation injuries.

9.3.6 Measles, mumps, rubella (MMR)

- Aim is to eliminate.
- Live vaccine (avoid in immunosuppressed).
- 2 doses preschool:
  - ■ 1st dose aged 13 months
  - ■ 2nd dose 3–5 years
- Offer to sero-negative women (rubella protection).
- Not suitable as post-exposure prophylaxis to mumps or rubella.

- Should be given to children >6 months within 3 days of contact with a case of measles.
- Malaise, fever, and rash may occur.
- Contraindications:
  - Immunosuppression
  - Live vaccine within 4 weeks
  - Anaphylaxis to gelatin and neomycin
  - Avoid pregnancy within 1 month

9.3.7 Meningococcal vaccines

- Almost all childhood meningitis is caused by *Neisseria meningitides* B and C.
- Conjugate vaccine: serotype C protection only.
- 2 primary doses, 1 booster.
- Single dose for university students.
- Asplenic patients require immunization.
- Travellers to countries at risk should be immunized.
- Side effects include:
  - Local: redness, swelling, and pain
  - Systemic: fever, irritability, malaise, dizziness, nausea, vomiting, diarrhoea, anorexia, rash, lymphadenopathy, hypotonia, and paraesthesia
  - Anaphylaxis
  - Rarely seizures

9.3.8 Pertussis

- Usually given in combination (DTP)
- Acellular
- 3 primary doses, 1 booster
- Vaccine should still be given even if preceding dose caused:
  - Fever
  - Persistent crying
  - Severe local reaction

9.3.9 Poliomyelitis

- 2 types:
  - Live (oral, Salk)
  - Inactivated (IM, Sabin)
- 3 primary doses, 2 boosters.
- Booster doses not required for adults unless high risk.
- Inactivated vaccine usually used.
- Live vaccine used in outbreaks only as risk of vaccine-associated paralytic polio.

9.3.10 Rabies

- Following exposure to rabies:
  - Clean and irrigate wound for several minutes
  - Disinfectant and simple dressing
  - Avoid suturing (may increase risk)
  - Advice should be sought from your national health protection agency
  - In immunized patients, 2 doses of cell-derived vaccine 3 days apart
  - In unimmunized patients, 5 doses of vaccine given over a month (day 0, 3, 7, 14, and 30) and immunoglobulin given at day 0

9.3.11 Tetanus

- Exotoxin.
- 3 primary doses, 2 boosters.
- Unimmunized adults: 3 doses of DTP.
- Tetanus-prone wound/burn:
  - Delayed presentation >6 hours
  - Highly devitalized tissue
  - Puncture wounds
  - Contact with soil or manure
  - Compound fractures
  - Evidence of sepsis
- Management:
  - Basic wound care
  - Consider need for antibiotics and delayed closure
  - Clean wounds:
    - Fully immunized (5 doses) do not require further immunization
    - Partially immunized require booster
    - Unimmunized (or unknown status) require immediate vaccination followed by a completed course
  - Prone wounds:
    - Same as for clean wounds with the addition of immunoglobulin
    - Only give immunoglobulin in fully immunized if they are at especially high risk

9.4 Immunoglobulins (Igs)

9.4.1 Normal Ig

- Normal human Ig comprises preformed antibodies from pooled human plasma.
- Contains immunoglobulin G (IgG) and antibodies.
- Uses:
  - Hepatitis A:
    - Preferred in individuals at risk
    - Not recommended for routine prophylaxis
    - IM Ig may be used for prevention of infection in a close contact (especially at high risk or with delay in diagnosis)
  - Measles:
    - Given to patients without adequate immunity to prevent or treat
    - IM, best given within 72 hours but is effective up to 6 days
  - Rubella
  - Varicella
  - Other viruses currently prevalent in the general population
- Cautions:
  - Obese
  - Prothrombotic conditions
  - Hypersensitivity to Ig
  - Recent immunization with live vaccine, as may affect immune response to live vaccines
- Side effects:
  - Flu-like symptoms
  - Anaphylaxis (rare)

9.4.2 Specific Ig

- Hepatitis B (HBIG):
  - Used in conjunction with vaccine for high-risk inoculation injuries (e.g. healthcare workers and the newborn infants of high-risk mothers)
- Varicella zoster immunoglobulin (VZIG):
  - Recommended for individuals who are at increased risk of severe varicella *and* who have no antibodies to varicella zoster virus *and* who have significant exposure to chicken pox or herpes zoster
  - High-risk groups:
    - Pregnant women (any gestation)—within 10 days of exposure
    - Neonates of mothers who develop chicken pox (7 days before and after delivery)
    - Premature/Special Baby Care/ITU infants
    - Immunosuppressed
    - Course of steroids within the last 3 months
    - Diabetics
    - Exposed neonates (within 7 days of birth)
- Tetanus:
  - See Chapter E9, Section 9.3.11
- Anti-D Ig:
  - Individuals are either rhesus negative or positive (patient expresses rhesus D antigen). This is important in pregnancy in rhesus-negative women who have a rhesus positive foetus. Foeto-maternal haemorrhage may sensitize the mother to produce antibodies against rhesus D and will lead to haemolytic disease of the newborn
  - Routine for antenatal prophylaxis in rhesus-negative pregnant women (administer at 28 and 34 weeks)
  - Sensitized rhesus-negative women (miscarriage/abortion/abruption/birth): administer within 72 hours of event
  - Anti-D (Rh_0) Ig is also given when significant foeto-maternal haemorrhage occurs in rhesus-negative women during delivery
  - Dose depends on degree of exposure
  - Anti-D (Rh_0) Ig is given to women of childbearing potential after the inadvertent transfusion of rhesus-incompatible blood components and is used for the treatment of idiopathic thrombocytopenia purpura

Anaesthesia

CONTENTS

10.1 Intravenous agents

10.1.1 Thiopental sodium

- Induction profile:
  - Barbiturate enhances effect of GABA
  - Used for RSI (5mg/kg), status epilepticus
  - Potent hypnotic, poor analgesic
  - Potent anticonvulsant
  - Anaesthesia in <30sec (unless low CO)
  - High lipid solubility → rapid redistribution into muscle then fat, therefore rapid awakening
  - Sedative effects can persist for 24 hours
  - Liver metabolism, renal excretion
- Side effects:
  - Laryngeal spasm
  - Respiratory depression
  - Hypotension
  - Tissue necrosis if extravasated
  - Anaphylactoid reaction (1:20 000)
  - Arrhythmias
  - Myocardial depression
  - Cough
  - Sneezing
  - Rash
  - Hypersensitivity reactions
- Contraindications:
  - Porphyria
  - Hypersensitivity to constituents
  - Airway obstruction
  - Myotonic dystrophy
  - Breastfeeding

10.1.2 Etomidate

- Induction profile:
  - Carboxylated imidazole derivative
  - Acts on GABA type A receptors
  - Action: within 10–65sec
  - $t_{1/2}$ = 1–4 hours
  - Rapid recovery without a hangover effect
  - High incidence of extraneous muscle movement (which can be minimized by an opioid analgesic or a short-acting benzodiazepine given just before induction)
  - Metabolized by the liver and renal excretion
- Side effects:
  - Injection pain
  - Venous thrombosis
  - Myoclonus
  - Arrhythmias
  - Coughing
  - Shivering
  - Adrenocortical suppression
  - Allergic reaction
  - Bronchospasm
  - Anaphylaxis
  - Convulsions
- Contraindications:
  - Acute porphyria
  - Severe cardiac disease

10.1.3 Propofol

- Induction profile:
  - Phenol derivative
  - Extremely lipid-soluble
  - Rapid recovery and less hangover effect than other IV anaesthetics
  - CNS anaesthesia in 10–30sec (loss of verbal contact most reliable)
  - Antiemetic
  - Metabolized by conjugation in the liver, as well as extrahepatic metabolism
- Side effects:
  - Painful injection
  - Flushing
  - Tachycardia
  - Bradycardia
  - Cough
  - Hiccough
  - Hypotension
  - Convulsions
  - Anaphylaxis
  - Transient apnoea
  - Headache
- Contraindications:
  - Egg/soya bean allergy
  - Acute porphyria
  - Stroke

- Children under 17 in ICU—risk of potentially fatal effects including metabolic acidosis, cardiac failure, rhabdomyolysis, hyperlipidaemia, and hepatomegaly

10.1.4 Ketamine

- Induction profile:
  - Mainly used for paediatric sedation
  - Used to induce a dissociative anaesthesia
  - Anaesthetic of choice when ventilation equipment is not available because it does not cause respiratory depression
  - Sometimes used for emergency surgery, as it increases/maintains CO
  - Non-competitive antagonist of NMDA receptor Ca^{2+} channel pore
  - CNS anaesthesia in 30sec
  - Duration of action 10–20min
- Side effects:
  - Re-emergence phenomena (worse in adults)
  - Hallucinations and nightmares
  - Tachycardia
  - Hypertension
  - Raised ICP
  - Laryngospasm
  - Increased secretions
  - Transient rash (15%)
  - Arrhythmias
  - Hypotension
  - Bradycardia
  - Anxiety
  - Insomnia
  - Raised intraocular pressure
- Contraindications:
  - Acute porphyria
  - Stroke
  - Head trauma
  - Raised ICP
  - Hypertension
  - Pre-eclampsia or eclampsia
  - Severe cardiac disease

10.2 Inhalational agents

10.2.1 Nitrous oxide

- Entonox: 50% O_2, 50% N_2O
- Anaesthetic and analgesic effects
- Has a rapid onset of action and quick recovery because it has a low blood solubility
- Relative analgesia, where patient loses the sensibility to feel pain
- Used for maintenance of light anaesthesia
- Side effects:
  - Prolonged use may cause megaloblastic anaemia
  - Neurological effects

- Bone marrow suppression
- Hypoxia
- Contraindications:
  - Pneumothorax
  - Intracranial air (after head trauma)
  - Susceptibility to malignant hyperthermia

10.3 Sedatives and analgesics

10.3.1 Benzodiazepines

- Effects:
  - Anxiolytic
  - Anticonvulsant
  - Hypnotic
  - Sedative
  - Muscle relaxant
  - *No* analgesic effect
- Action:
  - Enhancement of GABA-mediated CNS inhibition

10.3.2 Diazepam (PO/IM/IV/PR)

- Effects:
  - Mild sedation and amnesia
  - $t_{1/2}$: 32 hours (long-acting, active metabolites)
  - 2nd period of drowsiness can occur several hours after administration
- Indications:
  - Acute anxiety
  - Insomnia
  - Status epilepticus
  - Alcohol withdrawal
  - Febrile convulsions
- Side effects:
  - Confusion
  - Dizziness
  - Ataxia
  - Dependency
  - Aggression
  - Respiratory depression

10.3.3 Temazepam

- Short anxiolytic effects (90min).
- Faster onset than oral diazepam.
- $t_{1/2}$: 6 hours.
- Side effects similar to diazepam.

10.3.4 Lorazepam (PO/IV/IM)

- More prolonged sedation than temazepam.
- Marked amnesic effects.

- Indications:
  - Status epilepticus
  - Short-term anxiety/insomnia
- $t_{1/2}$: 12 hours (no active metabolites).
- Side effects similar to diazepam.

10.3.5 Midazolam (IV/IM/PR/buccal)

- Water-soluble, rapid onset of action, rapid elimination.
- Mostly protein-bound and changes in plasma protein concentrations can greatly alter clinical response.
- Potent sedative and amnesic.
- Indications:
  - Status epilepticus
  - Dental and surgical procedures (profound sedative and amnesic effects)
  - Anaesthetic induction
- Side effects:
  - Ataxia
  - Confusion
  - Hallucinations
  - Bronchospasm
  - Laryngospasm
  - Apnoea
  - Respiratory depression/arrest
  - Hypotension

10.4 Muscle relaxants

10.4.1 Depolarizing agents

- For example, suxamethonium.
- Act at acetylcholine receptors.
- Cause ion channels to open → inactivation of Na^+ channels in muscle-fibre membrane → action potentials not generated.

10.4.2 Non-depolarizing agents

- For example, vecuronium, pancuronium, atracurium.
- Competitive antagonists of acetylcholine.
- Endplate depolarization is reduced → action potential not generated at motor endplate.

10.4.3 Atracurium

- Competitive antagonism of acetylcholine at postsynaptic N_2 receptors of neuromuscular junction → neuromuscular blockade.
- Facilitates ventilation and intubation.
- Action: 90sec
- Recovery: 20–35min.
- Caution:
  - Hypersensitivity
  - Prolonged action in myasthenia gravis and in hypothermia
  - Resistance may develop in patients with burns

- Side effects
  - Histamine release:
    - Skin flushing
    - Hypotension
    - Tachycardia
    - Bronchospasm
    - Anaphylactoid reactions

10.4.4 Suxamethonium

- Depolarizing agent (used for RSI).
- Brief neuromuscular blockade of skeletal muscle (2–6min).
- Mimics acetylcholine at NMJ.
- Avoid in hyperkalaemia (burns, crush injuries, renal failure, prolonged immobilization).
- Suxamethonium paralysis can occur in atypical/low plasma cholinesterases (may run in families).
- Postoperative muscular pains common.
- Rare cause of malignant hyperpyrexia.
- Contraindications:
  - FH of malignant hyperthermia
  - Low plasma cholinesterase activity (including severe liver disease)
  - Hyperkalaemia
  - Major trauma
  - Severe burns
  - Neurological disease involving acute wasting of major muscle
  - Prolonged immobilization
  - Personal or family history of congenital myotonic disease
  - Duchenne muscular dystrophy
- Side effects:
  - Postoperative muscle pain
  - Myoglobinuria/myoglobinaemia
  - Tachycardia
  - Arrhythmias
  - Cardiac arrest
  - Hypertension
  - Bronchospasm
  - Apnoea
  - Prolonged respiratory depression
  - Anaphylaxis
  - Hyperkalaemia
  - Hyperthermia
  - Increased gastric pressure
  - Rash
  - Flushing

10.5 Antagonist agents

10.5.1 Flumazenil (IM/IV)

- Competitive BDZ antagonist.
- Indication:
  - Reversal of BDZ sedation
  - Short duration of action so patients may become re-sedated

- Side effects:
  - Anxiogenic
  - May precipitate seizures
  - Flushing
  - Nausea
  - Vomiting
  - Agitation, anxiety, and fear if wakening too rapid
  - Hypersensitivity reaction
- Contraindications:
  - Life-threatening condition (e.g. raised intracranial pressure, status epilepticus) controlled by benzodiazepines
  - Mixed OD
  - TCA OD

10.5.2 Naloxone (IM/IV/SC)

- Specific antagonist at opioid receptors.
- Indication:
  - Reversal of opioid-induced respiratory depression
  - Short duration of action (may need repeated doses)
- Side effects:
  - Hypo/hypertension
  - Cardiac arrest
  - VF
  - VT
  - Pulmonary oedema
  - Nausea
  - Vomiting
  - Dyspnoea
  - Headache
  - Dizziness
  - Agitation
  - Tremor
  - Seizures
  - Hypersensitivity reactions
  - Acute withdrawal

10.6 Local anaesthesia

- Local anaesthetics reversibly block activated sodium channels preventing depolarization and hence the conduction of action potentials along axons.
- They are more active in rapidly firing neurons and small, non-myelinated neurons (i.e. those carrying pain signals).
- Local anaesthetics are bases and their action is reduced by acidosis (e.g. caused by wound inflammation).

10.6.1 Lidocaine

- Amide anaesthetic 0.5%, 1%, 2% (plain), and with epinephrine.
- Dose: 3mg/kg *plain*, 7mg/kg with *vasoconstrictor*.
- Equivalence: 1% solution = 10mg/mL.
- $t_{1/2}$ = 120min.
- Peak blood levels 10–25min.

- Effect 30–60min.
- Toxicity: numbness/paraesthesia, tinnitus, confusion, seizures, coma.

10.6.2 EMLA (lidocaine 2.5%, prilocaine 2.5%)

- Topical anaesthetic for cannulation, surgical procedures.

10.6.3 Bupivacaine

- Used for spinal and epidural anaesthesia, postoperative analgesia, nerve blocks.
- Slow onset (30min).
- Duration of action: 8 hours.

10.6.4 Prilocaine

- Similar onset and duration to lidocaine.
- Less toxicity in equipotent doses.

PATHOPHYSIOLOGY

CHAPTER F1

Respiratory

CONTENTS

1.1 Control of ventilation

- Respiratory centres in the brainstem are groups of neurons in the reticular formation rather than defined nuclei.
- These include:
  - Medullary centres
  - Pontine centres
  - Higher centres

1.1.1 Medullary centres

- 2 pools of ventilator control neurons:
  - Inspiratory and expiratory pool
- Function by a system of reciprocal innervations:
  - As activity increases in one centre, a rising level of inhibitory activity is relayed from the opposite centre
  - This results in a reversal of the ventilator phase
- Inspiratory pool:
  - Located in the dorsal medullary reticular formation
  - The source of basic ventilatory rhythm
  - Referred to as the pacemaker of the respiratory system
  - Rhythmic activity persists even when connections to the neurons are blocked
  - During inspiration, activity of the inspiratory pool leads to increased output to the muscles of inspiration—principally the diaphragm
  - At the same time increasing inhibitory activity from the expiratory centre is relayed to the inspiratory neurons until inspiratory activity ceases and expiration begins

- Expiratory pool:
  - Located in the ventral medullary reticular formation
  - During inspiration increasing activity from the expiratory pool inhibits the inspiratory pool until expiration begins
  - At the same time inhibitory activity is relayed to the expiratory neurons from the inspiratory pool until expiration ceases and inspiration begins

1.1.2 Pontine centres

- There are 2 respiratory centres in the pons:
  - The *pneumotaxic* centre in the upper pons:
    - Fine-tunes ventilator rate and tidal volume (V_T) to minimize respiratory work
    - Controls V_T by switching off the inspiratory centre during the inspiratory phase
    - This control of the inspiratory phase also varies the respiratory rate
  - The *apneustic* centre in the lower pons:
    - Thought to prolong the inspiratory phase by acting on the medullary inspiratory pool of neurons
    - Also provides some control over the ventilatory rate and pattern

1.1.3 Higher centres

- The cerebral cortex also affects breathing pattern.
- Precise neural pathways remain unknown, however.
- Voluntary hypo- and hyperventilation can be performed and maintained to the extent of producing a measurable change in the arterial pH.
- The hypothalamus and limbic systems can also affect respiration as seen in emotional states.

1.2 Reflexes in ventilatory control

- Primary goal of ventilation is to maintain homeostasis of PaO_2 and $PaCO_2$.
- Various reflexes are integrated to produce responses to disturbance in arterial blood gases or the increased demand of exercise.
- Other reflexes protect the airway by coordinating breathing around talking and eating while enabling coughing and sneezing.
- These reflexes are mediated by specialized receptors.

1.2.1 Specialized receptors

- Central chemoreceptors:
  - Situated bilaterally beneath the ventral surface of the medulla
  - Highly sensitive to changes in hydrogen ion concentration
- Peripheral chemoreceptors:
  - Found in the carotid bodies—located at the bifurcation of the common carotid artery and in the aortic bodies
  - Afferent nerve fibres of the carotid bodies pass through Hering's nerves to the glossopharyngeal nerves
  - Those of the aortic bodies pass through the vagi to the dorsal respiratory centre
  - The chemoreceptors have a very high oxygen consumption:
    - Respond to decreases in oxygen content of arterial blood and to decreases in blood flow
    - They therefore act as oxygen delivery sensors to the brain
  - The effect of CO_2 and hydrogen ion concentration on the peripheral receptors is much less than the direct effects of both these factors on the respiratory centre itself:
    - Peripheral stimulation occurs 5 times more rapidly than the central effect
    - Peripheral receptors therefore increase the response to CO_2 at the onset of exercise

1.3 Pressure, chemical, and irritant receptors

- In the mucosa of the upper airway:
  - Help protect the lungs from inhalation of noxious substances (e.g. gastric acid)
  - Reflexes initiate laryngeal closure, apnoea, hyperpnoea, and bronchoconstriction
- Within the smooth muscle of all airways: help to control depth of respiration.

1.4 J receptors

- Located in the alveolar walls near the capillaries.
- Stimulation causes rapid, shallow breathing or apnoea.
- Thought to be involved in the tachypnoea observed in pulmonary oedema and irritation of the lungs.

1.5 Pulmonary stretch receptors

- Lie in the smooth muscle of the airways.
- Inhibit inspiration in response to lung distension.
- Slow ventilator rate by increasing expiratory time.

1.6 Golgi tendon organs

- Particularly plentiful in the intercostal muscles.
- Involved in the pulmonary stretch reflex.
- When lungs distend, the chest wall is stretched.
- Golgi tendons inhibit further inspiration.

1.7 Muscle spindles

- Located in the inspiratory muscles and diaphragm.
- Contribute to control of depth and effort during inspiration.
- Thought to activate when particularly intense respiratory efforts are required (e.g. in airways obstruction).
- Also thought to be responsible for the sensation of dyspnoea.

1.8 Lung volumes

- The lung can be divided into various volumes.
- Identified by measurement or according to the function of the lung in gas exchange.

1.8.1 Volumes derived from spirometry

- Lung volumes vary with age, sex, and body height.
- The lung volumes are:
  - *Total lung capacity* (TLC): volume of gas present in the lungs at the end of maximal inspiration
  - *Tidal volume* (V_T): amount of gas inspired and expired during normal quiet breathing
  - *Inspiratory reserve volume* (IRV): extra volume of gas that can be inspired over and beyond the V_T

- *Expiratory reserve volume* (ERV): amount of gas that can be forcefully expired at the end of normal tidal expiration
- *Residual volume* (RV): amount of gas remaining in the lungs at the end of maximum forced expiration
- *Vital capacity* (VC): maximal volume of gas that can be expelled after a maximal inspiration
- *Functional residual capacity* (FRC): lung volume following expiration during quiet breathing

1.8.2 Measurement of lung volumes

- Spirometry does not give a value for TLC, FRC, or RV.
- These can be derived if FRC is measured.
- 2 methods of measuring FRC include:
  - Helium dilution:
    - Requires a spirometer and a helium concentration analyser
    - Subject is connected to a spirometer containing a known volume of fresh gas with a known initial concentration of helium
    - Normal breathing is conducted until the helium is diluted
    - FRC can be derived by measuring final helium concentration
  - Body plethysmograph:
    - FRC is measured by placing the subject in a closed chamber and measuring the pressure and volume changes occurring with an inspiratory effort
    - Boyle's gas law can be applied before and after the inspiratory effort to derive FRC

1.9 Pulmonary mechanics

- Movement of gas in the lungs is a mechanical process.
- Dependent on:
  - The respiratory muscles
  - Compliance of the chest wall and lungs
  - Gas flow in the airways

1.9.1 The respiratory muscles

- Divided into expiration and inspiration.
- Expiration—passive process.
- Inspiration—active process:
  - Lungs expanded within degrees of freedom
  - Involves displacement of the abdominal contents by the diaphragm:
    - Principal breathing muscle
    - Contraction moves abdominal viscera downward and forward
    - Predominantly slow-twitch muscle fibres, therefore making it relatively resistant to fatigue
  - Involves radial expansion of the thoracic cage by accessory musculature:
    - These comprise the external intercostals and strap muscles (sternocleidomastoid, serrati, and scalene)
    - During quiet breathing their contribution is minor
    - They act to stabilize the upper ribs and to prevent indrawing
    - As respiration deepens, the contribution of these muscles increases

1.9.2 Compliance of the chest wall and lungs

- Respiratory system comprises 2 main compartments:
  - The lungs and the thoracic cage
  - These move together as a unit

- Airway pressures in the lung can be approximated to atmospheric pressure.
- The lungs expand due to a pressure gradient produced along their surface—the *transpulmonary pressure*:
    - The transpulmonary pressure is equal to the difference between the airway pressure in the lungs and the pressure on the lung surface (the *intrapleural pressure*)
- Intrapleural pressure:
    - The resting position of the lungs and chest wall occurs at FRC
    - The chest wall is coupled to the lung surface by the thin layer of intrapleural fluid
    - This opposes chest wall recoil and forces are at equilibrium at FRC
    - Intrapleural pressure can be measured by an intrapleural catheter
- Lung and chest compliance:
    - The lungs expand due to the transpulmonary pressures generated by the respiratory muscles
    - The amount of expansion for a given transpulmonary pressure represents the ease with which the lungs expand
    - This is called the *lung compliance*
    - Compliance is reduced at high lung volumes because the elastic fibres are fully stretched and are close to their elastic limit
    - At low lung volumes compliance is reduced as airway and alveolar collapse occurs
    - Chest wall compliance can be reduced by disease as in ankylosing spondylitis where the chest wall can become almost rigid
    - This can give a very low compliance value

1.9.3 Gas flow in the airways

- Movement of gas in and out of the lungs is produced by the transpulmonary pressure.
- The ease of gas flow is dependent on airways resistance and pattern of gas flow.

1.10 Oxygen transport in the blood

- Most of the oxygen in blood is transported in combination with haemoglobin (Hb).
- Once Hb is saturated, only marginal increases in oxygen occur by dissolving of O_2 in blood.

1.10.1 Haemoglobin

- Please see Chapter F5, Section 5.1.5.

1.10.2 Oxyhaemoglobin dissociation curve (ODC)

- The percentage of Hb saturation with oxygen (SO_2) at different partial pressures of oxygen is known as the ODC.
- This is a sigmoid-shaped curve.
- Various factors can shift the ODC to the left or right, altering oxygen uptake and delivery.
- Sequential increase in oxygen affinity explains the sigmoid curve.
- Myoglobin is a single-chain molecule.
- It has a hyperbolic ODC.

1.10.3 Left shift of the ODC

- Represents an increase in the affinity of Hb for oxygen in the pulmonary capillaries.
- Requires lower tissue capillary PO_2 to achieve oxygen delivery.
- Factors that cause a left shift in the ODC:
    - Alkalosis
    - Decreased PCO_2

- Decreased concentration of 2,3-DPG
- Decreased temperature
- Presence of fetal haemoglobin (HbF)

1.10.4 Right shift of the ODC

- This represents an increase in the affinity of Hb for oxygen.
- Higher pulmonary capillary saturations are required to saturate Hb.
- Right shift enhances oxygen delivery to the tissues.
- Factors causing right shift of the ODC include:
  - Acidosis
  - Increased PCO_2
  - Increased concentration of 2,3-DPG
  - Increased temperature

1.10.5 The Bohr effect

- The shift in the position of ODC caused by CO_2 entering or leaving blood is known as the Bohr effect.
- Enhances unloading of oxygen in the tissues where PCO_2 levels are high compared to pulmonary capillaries.
- In the tissues, CO_2 enters the red cells and combines with water.
- This produces H^+ and HCO_3^-.
- The increased H^+ shifts the ODC to the right, facilitating release of oxygen from Hb.
- HCO_3^- diffuses out of the cells and chloride moves in.

1.11 Carbon dioxide transport

- CO_2 diffuses passively down its concentration gradient.
- Transfer is rapid due to the high solubility of CO_2.
- Partial pressures of CO_2 in the tissues equilibrate with capillary blood to produce a venoarterial PCO_2 difference of about 0.7kPa.
- This corresponds to a CO_2 content difference of about 4mL/100mL of blood.
- The 4mL CO_2 that is added to each 100mL arterial blood as it passes through the tissues consists of the following:
  - 2.8mL enters erythrocytes to form carbonic acid. This reaction is catalysed by carbonic anhydrase
  - 0.9mL is carried as carbamino compounds
  - 0.3mL is carried in solution

1.11.1 Haldane effect

- In the tissues, deoxygenation of Hb enhances carriage of CO_2.
- Conversely, oxygenation of Hb causes the reverse effect and displaces H^+ and CO_2 in the lungs.
- This dependency of CO_2-carrying capacity on the oxygenation state of Hb is known as the Haldane effect.

1.12 DO$_2$/VO$_2$ relationships

- Please also see Chapter F2, Section 2.10.
- The primary goal of the cardiorespiratory system is to deliver adequate oxygen to the tissues to meet their metabolic requirements:
  - This is a balance between oxygen delivery and oxygen uptake

- Oxygen delivery (DO_2) is the amount of oxygen delivered to the tissues:
  - Calculated by multiplying the arterial oxygen content by the cardiac output (CO)
- Oxygen uptake is the amount of oxygen taken up by the tissues:
  - It is calculated from the difference between oxygen delivery and the oxygen returned to the lungs in mixed venous blood

1.13 Carbon monoxide

- Consists of 1 carbon atom and 1 oxygen atom.
- Connected by a covalent double bond and a dative covalent bond.
- It is the simplest oxocarbon and is an anhydride of formic acid.
- 240 times greater affinity for Hb than oxygen.
- Combines with Hb to form carboxyhaemoglobin (COHb):
  - This reduces the total oxygen carrying capacity of the blood
  - This results in tissue hypoxia

1.14 Theory of pulse oximetry

1.14.1 Principles

- Non-invasive technique of calculating the percentage of Hb saturated with oxygen (O_2)—SpO_2.
- Probe is applied to extremity and pulses light at 2 different wavelengths. Ratio of how much light is absorbed at 650nm (by desaturated Hb) vs at 805nm (by HbO_2) enables circuitry to compute SpO_2.
- Reliant on pulsatile flow (circuitry relies on this to discriminate arterial from venous flow).
- This method is only reliable where SpO_2 >70%.

1.14.2 Pros

- Non-invasive.
- Cheap.
- Rapid and portable; minimal training required.
- Visual and audible representation of quality of pulse:
  - NB: ensure you understand the screen gain before being reassured by an apparently large pulse volume

1.14.3 Cons and contraindications

- Poor peripheral perfusion gives unreliable readings or sometimes causes device error message—repositioning may work.
- Venous congestion.
- Vulnerable to environmental electrical interference, especially theatre lighting and diathermy.
- Chemical composition of blood can affect reading—COHb seen in carbon monoxide poisoning gives falsely high readings:
  - NB: also transient reduced SpO_2 when using methylene blue
- Probe–tissue interface must be sound; most common problem is use of nail polish:
  - NB: neither dark skin nor jaundice causes problems in oximetry

1.14.4 Alternatives

- Arterial blood gases.
- Central venous saturation—via central venous catheter (CVC).

1.15 Effect of altitude

- The partial pressure of ambient and hence alveolar and arterial oxygen falls in a near linear relationship to altitude:
  - Below 3000m there are few clinical effects
  - Commercial aircraft are pressurized to 2750m
- Resultant hypoxia causes breathlessness in people with severe cardiorespiratory pathology.
- Above 3000–3500m hypoxia causes a spectrum of clinical syndromes:
  - Syndromes occur during acclimatization
  - This process takes several weeks

1.15.1 Acute mountain sickness

- Acute mountain sickness includes malaise, nausea, and lassitude.
- Usually has a latent interval of 6–36 hours.
- Treatment is rest with analgesics as required.

1.15.2 High-altitude pulmonary oedema

- Breathlessness with frothy sputum indicates oedema.
- Unless treated rapidly this causes cardiorespiratory failure and death.

1.15.3 High-altitude cerebral oedema

- This is another sequelae of hypoxia.
- Due to an abrupt increase in cerebral blood flow.
- Headache is usual.
- Accompanied by drowsiness and papilloedema.

1.16 Dysbarism

- Dysbarism refers to medical conditions resulting from changes in ambient pressure.
- Various activities are associated with pressure changes—scuba diving is the most frequently cited example.
- Different types of illness result from increases and decreases in pressure.

1.16.1 Decompression sickness (DCS)

- Decompression sickness, also called 'the bends', is the most well-known complication of scuba diving.
- It occurs as divers ascend, and often from ascending too fast or without doing decompression stops.
- Culminates in the release of bubbles of inert gas (nitrogen or helium).
- Bubbles are large enough and numerous enough to cause physical injury.
- When DCS occurs, bubbles disrupt tissues in the joints, brain, spinal cord, and lungs amongst other organs.
- DCS may be as subtle as unusual tiredness after a dive.
- It may present dramatically, with unconsciousness, seizures, paralysis, shortness of breath, or death.
- Paraplegia is not uncommon.

1.16.2 Arterial gas embolism (AGE)

- This phenomenon occurs when inert gases are produced in the arterial circulation during decompression.
- AGE can present in similar ways to arterial blockages seen in other medical situations:
  - Affected people may suffer acute neurological events
  - Myocardial ischaemia/infarction can also occur
  - Pulmonary embolism is not uncommon
- It is often difficult to distinguish AGE from DCS; however, treatment is the same.
- AGE and DCS can be referred to as *decompression illness* (DCI).

1.16.3 Nitrogen narcosis

- When compressed air is breathed below 30m, narcotic effects of nitrogen impair brain function.
- This can cause changes in mood and performance.
- This syndrome is avoided by replacing air with helium–oxygen mixtures.

1.16.4 Barotrauma

- Barotrauma is injury caused by pressure effects on air spaces.
- This may occur during ascent or descent.
- The ears are the most commonly affected body part.
- The most serious injury is lung barotrauma, which can result in pneumothorax, pneumomediastinum, and pneumopericardium.

Cardiovascular system

CONTENTS

2.1 Control of blood pressure and heart rate

- Central control of BP and heart rate is via the vasomotor centre located in the medulla oblongata.
- Sympathetic nerves, which constrict arterioles and veins and increase heart rate and stroke volume, act as efferents in the feedback control of rate and pressure.
- The efferent vagus nerve acts to slow the heart rate.
- Afferent nerves affecting the control of BP and heart rate include the arterial and venous baroreceptors—carotid sinus and aortic arch afferents.

2.1.1 Physiological mechanisms to maintain normal blood pressure

- BP is determined by the rate of blood flow produced by the heart (*cardiac output*—CO) and the resistance of the blood vessels to blood flow.
- This resistance is produced mainly in the arterioles and is known as the *systemic vascular resistance* (SVR) (or by the older term total peripheral resistance).
- $BP = CO \times SVR$.
- BP is controlled by several physiological mechanisms acting in combination. They ensure that the pressure is maintained within normal limits by adapting their responses both in the short and long term to provide an adequate perfusion to the body tissues.
- Other important mechanisms in the homeostasis of BP include:
  - Autonomic nervous system
  - Capillary shift mechanism
  - Hormonal responses
  - Kidney and fluid balance mechanisms
- Pulse pressure = systolic pressure − diastolic pressure.

2.1.2 Effect via the autonomic nervous system

- The autonomic nervous system is the most rapidly responding regulator of BP.
- It receives continuous afferent information from the baroreceptors situated in the carotid sinus and the aortic arch. This information is relayed to the brainstem and the vasomotor centre.
- A decrease in BP causes activation of the sympathetic nervous system resulting in increased contractility of the heart (beta receptors) and vasoconstriction of both the arterial and venous side of the circulation (alpha receptors).

2.1.3 The capillary fluid shift mechanism

- This refers to the exchange of fluid that occurs across the capillary membrane between the blood and the interstitial fluid.
- This fluid movement is controlled by:
  - Capillary BP
  - Interstitial fluid pressure
  - Colloid osmotic pressure of the plasma
- Low BP results in fluid moving from the interstitial space into the circulation, helping to restore blood volume and BP.

2.1.4 Hormonal control of blood pressure

- Hormones exist both for lowering and raising BP. They act in various ways including vasoconstriction, vasodilatation, and alteration of blood volume.
- The principal hormones raising BP are epinephrine (adrenaline) and norepinephrine (noradrenaline). These are secreted from the adrenal medulla in response to sympathetic nervous system stimulation:
  - Increase CO and cause vasoconstriction
  - Rapid onset of action
- Renin and angiotensin production is increased in the kidney when stimulated by hypotension due to the fall in renal perfusion.
- Circulating angiotensin in the plasma is converted in the lung to angiotensin II, which is a potent vasoconstrictor.
- In addition, these hormones stimulate the production of aldosterone from the adrenal cortex, which decreases urinary fluid and electrolyte loss
- See Chapter F4, Section 4.4.1 for further details.
- This system is responsible for the long-term maintenance of BP but is also activated very rapidly in the presence of hypotension.

2.1.5 Renal effects on blood pressure

- Regulate BP by increasing or decreasing the blood volume and also by the renin–angiotensin system described earlier in Chapter F2, Section 2.1.4.
- Most important organs for the long-term control of BP.

2.2 Control of heart rate

- The heart will beat independently of any nervous or hormonal influences—this is called intrinsic automaticity.
- This can be altered by nervous impulses or by circulatory hormones, such as epinephrine.
- Each cell in the heart will spontaneously contract at a regular rate.
- Muscle fibres from different parts of the heart have different rates of spontaneous depolarization.
- The cells from the ventricles are the slowest and those from the atria are faster.

2.2.1 Effects via the autonomic nervous system

- The automatic rhythm of the heart can be altered by the autonomic nervous system.
- Sympathetic nervous system supply to the heart leaves the spinal cord at the 1st 4 thoracic vertebrae, and supplies most of the muscle of the heart (efferent control).
- Stimulation via the cardiac beta-1 receptors causes the heart rate (HR) to increase and beat more forcefully.
- This is known as positive inotropic and chronotropic effect.
- The vagus nerve also supplies the atria, and stimulation causes bradycardia.
- Under normal circumstances the vagus nerve is the more important influence on the heart.

2.2.2 Central control of heart rate

- Afferents include nerves in the wall of the atria or aortic arch that respond to stretch (baroreceptors).
- The aorta contains high-pressure receptors:
  - When BP is high, these cause reflex slowing of the heart to reduce the CO and the BP
  - Similarly, when the BP is low, the heart rate increases, as in shock
- Similar pressure receptors are found in the atria:
  - When the atria distend there is a reflex increase in the heart rate to pump extra blood returning to the heart
  - When there is a sudden reduction in the pressure in the atria, the heart slows
  - This is called the *Bainbridge reflex*

2.2.3 Hormonal effects on heart rate

- Catecholamines, such as epinephrine, are released during stress, and will cause an increase in heart rate.
- Epinephrine acts on beta-receptors in the heart.
- Other hormones such as thyroxine can also affect the rate of the heart.

2.3 Cardiac output (CO)

- The result of myocardial contraction is ejection of blood. The volume of blood ejected by each ventricle per minute is the *CO*:
  - Average CO is ~5L/min
  - CO varies to meet the needs of the body
- *Stroke volume* (SV) is the volume of blood ejected by each ventricle per beat.
- CO = SV × HR.
- About two-thirds of blood in the ventricle at the end of diastole is ejected during systole—this is called the *ejection fraction*.
- The residual volume of blood in the ventricle is called the *end-systolic volume*.
- Decreasing ventricular function impairs ventricular emptying; this decreases SV and increases the end-systolic volume.

2.3.1 Determinants of CO

- Heart rate:
  - Under the extrinsic control of the autonomic nervous system
  - Parasympathetic and sympathetic fibres innervate the sinoatrial node (SAN) and atrioventricular node (AVN)
  - Parasympathetic stimulation decreases the heart rate
  - Sympathetic stimulation increases the heart rate

- At rest, parasympathetic stimulus prevails
- In the presence of heart disease sympathetic stimulus prevails
- Norepinephrine stored in cardiac sympathetic nerves adds to catecholamine supply
- This norepinephrine eventually depletes in chronic heart disease
- Stroke volume:
  - Dependent on preload, contractility, and afterload

2.3.2 Preload

- Starling's law of the heart states that stretching myocardial fibres during diastole increases the force of contraction.
- The degree of stretch is expressed as preload.
- The degree of preload is determined by ventricular volume.
- The degree of blood in the ventricles is dependent on venous return.
- Increasing venous return increases force of ventricular contraction.
- Starling's law is functional within limits determined by myocardial ultrastructure.
- This is seen as the hump in the ventricular function curve.
- Increased preload increases force of contraction and therefore the amount of blood ejected from the ventricles.

2.3.3 Frank–Starling curves

- As the heart fills with more blood, the force of the muscular contractions will increase.
- This is a result of an increase in the load experienced by each muscle fibre due to the increased blood entering the heart.
- The stretching of the muscle fibres increases the affinity of troponin C for calcium
- This causes a greater number of cross-bridges to form within the muscle fibres, ultimately increasing the contractile force of the cardiac muscle.
- The force that any single muscle fibre generates is proportional to the initial sarcomere length—*preload*.
- The stretch on the individual fibres is related to the end-diastolic volume of the ventricle.
- Maximal force is generated with an initial sarcomere length of 2.2 micrometres.
- Initial lengths larger or smaller than this optimal value will decrease the force the muscle can achieve (see Figure F.2.1).
- For larger sarcomere lengths, this is the result of less overlap of the thin and thick filaments.
- For smaller sarcomere lengths, the cause is the decreased sensitivity to calcium by the myofilaments.

2.3.4 Contractility

- Contractility is the force of myocardial contraction determining SV and CO, as well as myocardial oxygen demand.
- Extrinsic inotropic factors will affect contractility, that is, positive inotropic factors increase contractility.
  - Positive inotropic factors:
    - Increased sympathetic nervous system action
    - Circulating catecholamines
    - Inotropic drugs (such as digoxin, levothyroxine)
  - Negative inotropic factors:
    - Increased parasympathetic nervous system action (mild effect)
    - Hypoxia and hypercapnia
    - Acidosis and alkalosis

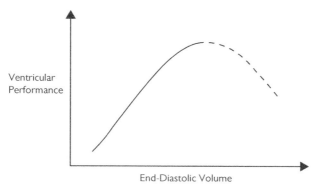

Figure F.2.1 Frank–Starling curve

- • Hyperkalaemia, hypocalcaemia (contractility is directly proportional to the amount of Ca^{2+} ions)
- • Drugs (such as most anaesthetic agents, antiarrhythmic agents)
- Intrinsic mechanisms also affect CO, such as cardiac filling (see Starling's law—Chapter F2, Section 2.3.3) or the presence of cardiac disease such as cardiomyopathy or ischaemic heart disease.

2.3.5 Afterload

- Afterload is the resistance to ventricular ejection from the systemic circulation.
- A function of intraventricular pressure, intraventricular size, and ventricular wall thickness.
- The relationship between wall tension, pressure, radius, and thickness is explained by the *Laplace equation*:
- $Pressure\ difference = wall\ tension \times \left(\dfrac{1}{radius_{(inner)}} + \dfrac{1}{radius_{(outer)}} \right)$

2.4 Measurement of cardiac output (CO)

- CO can be measured invasively or non-invasively.

2.4.1 Non-invasive measurements of CO

- Aorto-velography:
  - ▪ Use of a Doppler ultrasound probe in the suprasternal notch to measure blood velocity and acceleration in the ascending aorta
  - ▪ Generally an inaccurate method of measuring CO
- Oesophageal Doppler—portable devices:
  - ▪ Similar to concept for deriving CO as in the aorto-velography method
  - ▪ The velocity of blood in the ascending aorta is measured
  - ▪ This allows estimation of the length of a column of blood passing through the aorta in unit time
  - ▪ This is multiplied by the cross-sectional area of the aorta to give SV and, from this, CO
- Transthoracic impedance:
  - ▪ Measured across externally applied electrodes
  - ▪ Impedance changes with the cardiac cycle and specifically with changes in blood volume

- ■ The rate of change of impedance is a reflection of CO
- ■ It is useful for estimating changes but not for absolute measurements
- ● Echocardiography:
  - ■ 2-dimensional echocardiography can be used to measure the movement of the anterior and posterior ventricular walls
  - ■ The ejection fraction can be calculated with this data
- ● Transoesophageal echocardiography (TOE):
  - ■ An ultrasonic vibration is transmitted into the body and the change in frequency of the signal that is reflected off red blood cells is recorded
  - ■ Doppler techniques measure velocity and not flow
  - ■ The flow can be obtained by integrating the signal over the cross-sectional area of the vessel
  - ■ TOE can measure the length of blood in the ascending aorta in a unit time
  - ■ This is multiplied by the cross-sectional area of the aorta to give SV
  - ■ From this calculation CO can be calculated by multiplying by the heart rate
- ● Arterial pulse contour analysis:
  - ■ A technique combining transpulmonary thermodilution (see 'Pulmonary artery catheters' in Chapter F2, Section 2.4.2) and arterial pulse contour analysis
  - ■ The estimation of CO based on pulse contour analysis is indirect—CO is not measured directly but is computed from a pressure pulsation on the basis of a criterion or model

2.4.2 Invasive measurement of cardiac output

- ● Fick's principle:
  - ■ $Q = M/(V - A)$
    - ● Where Q is the volume of blood flowing through an organ per minute (e.g. CO)
    - ● M is the number of moles of a substance added to or removed from the blood by an organ in 1 minute (e.g. total oxygen consumption)
    - ● V and A are the venous and arterial concentrations of that substance (e.g. oxygen)
  - ■ This principle can be used to measure the blood flow through any organ that adds substances to, or removes substances from, the blood
  - ■ CO equals pulmonary blood flow
  - ■ The lungs add oxygen to the blood and remove carbon dioxide from it
  - ■ The concentration of oxygen in the blood in pulmonary veins is 200mL/L and in the pulmonary artery is 150mL/L
  - ■ Therefore, each litre of blood going through the lungs takes up 50mL of oxygen
  - ■ At rest, the blood takes up to 250mL/min of oxygen from the lungs
  - ■ 250mL must be carried away in 50mL portions; therefore, the CO must be 250/50 or 5L/min
  - ■ This method is difficult to perform:
    - ● Oxygen consumption is derived by measuring the expired gas volume over a known time
    - ● Accurate collection of the gas is difficult unless the patient has an endotracheal tube
    - ● Facemasks and mouthpieces inherently have leaks around the mouth
  - ■ Analysis of the gas is straightforward if the inspired gas is air. If it is oxygen-enriched air there are 2 problems:
    - ● The addition of oxygen can fluctuate and produce an error due to the non-constancy of the inspired oxygen concentration
    - ● Also it is difficult to measure small changes in oxygen concentration at the top end of the scale
  - ■ The arteriovenous oxygen content difference presents a further problem, in that the mixed venous oxygen content has to be measured and therefore a pulmonary artery catheter is needed to obtain the sample
  - ■ The Fick method is not practicable in routine clinical practice

- Dilutional techniques:
  - A known amount of dye is injected into the pulmonary artery, and its concentration is measured peripherally
  - Indocyanine green is suitable due to its low toxicity and short half-life
  - A curve is achieved, which is replotted semi-logarithmically to correct for recirculation of the dye
  - CO is calculated from the injected dose, the area under the curve (AUC), and its duration
  - Thermodilutional methods can also be used—see following bullet point on pulmonary artery catheters
- Pulmonary artery catheters:
  - Assessment of volume status where CVP is unreliable
  - Sampling of mixed venous blood to calculate shunt fraction
  - Measurement of CO using thermodilution
  - 5–10mL cold saline injected through the port of a pulmonary artery catheter
  - Temperature changes are measured by a distal thermistor
  - A plot of temperature change against time gives a similar curve to the dye method described in the earlier bullet point 'Dilutional techniques'
  - Calculation of CO is achieved through the Stewart–Hamilton equation
- Derivation of other cardiovascular indices, such as the pulmonary vascular resistance, oxygen delivery, and uptake.

2.5 Blood flow peripherally

- Blood flow depends on the pressure propelling the blood and the total resistance to flow.
- A pressure gradient must exist for blood to flow.
- The greater the gradient, the higher the flow.
- *Mean arterial pressure* (MAP) reflects blood volume and compliance in the arterial system:
  - ~100mmHg
  - ~0mmHg at the venous end of circulation
  - Pressure therefore decreases through the systemic circulation
  - MAP = diastolic pressure + 1/3 pulse pressure

2.5.1 Resistance

- Determined by the radius of the blood vessel:
  - Poiseuille's law shows that resistance (R) is inversely proportional to the 4th power of the radius of the vessel
  - Reduction of the radius by half increases the resistance by 16 times
- Blood viscosity and vascular length are also related to resistance.
- The arteriole is the major site of resistance.

2.5.2 Velocity of blood flow

- Velocity of blood flow through the vascular system depends on the area of the vessel.
- Velocity of flow decreases as the cross-sectional area increases.
- Velocity decreases in the peripheral arterial system due to progressive branching from arteries to the capillary bed.
- Vital for nutrient transfer.

2.5.3 Distribution of flow

- Distribution of blood according to metabolic needs and functional demands of tissues continuously changes.
- Dual control of CO is possible through extrinsic and intrinsic mechanisms.

2.5.4 Extrinsic control

- Blood flow to a given organ system can be increased by increasing CO or by shunting of blood from one organ system to another.
- Sympathetic tone can cause both the just-mentioned effects:
  - Sympathetic stimulus augments CO by increasing rate and force of contraction
  - Sympathetic effects on the arterioles preferentially constrict some arterioles and dilate others
  - This distributes blood flow according to demand

2.5.5 Intrinsic control

- Local control of blood flow is known as autoregulation.
- This permits blood flow relative to tissue metabolic activity.
- Vital organs such as the heart and brain utilize intrinsic mechanisms preferentially.

2.5.6 Cardiac reserve

- The heart can increase its resting activity according to demand.
- The heart can potentially increase output 5-fold.
- This is made possible through increases in heart rate and SV.
- Heart rate can increase from a rest level of 60–100 beats to 180 beats per minute.
- This occurs primarily through increased sympathetic tone.
- SV can increase either by increased ventricular emptying caused by increased contractility or by a rise in ejection volume.
- The effect of increased diastolic filling is limited by myocardial fibre stretch.

2.5.7 Control of blood flow

- Peripheral blood flow:
  - Beta-2 receptors cause vasodilatation of the peripheral vascular system
  - Alpha-1 receptor activation causes vasoconstriction of the peripheral vascular system
  - Alpha-2 receptor activation causes contraction of vascular smooth muscle
  - Mean arterial pressure is a product of CO and total peripheral resistance as stated previously:
    - With vasoconstriction, mean arterial pressure increases
    - With peripheral vasodilatation, mean arterial pressure decreases
- Renal blood flow:
  - 20–25% of the CO passes through the kidneys per minute
  - A special feature of renal blood flow is autoregulation:
    - The afferent arterioles have an intrinsic capacity to vary their resistance in response to arterial BP
    - This maintains renal blood flow and filtration at a constant level
    - Disturbance in autoregulation can cause acute kidney injury
- Cerebral blood flow:
  - Normal cerebral blood flow (CBF) is 700mL/min, representing about 14% of the CO
  - Cerebral blood flow is influenced by the following factors (see Figure F.2.2):
    - Arterial PCO_2: hypercapnia increases CBF by vasodilatation; a reduction of PCO_2 from 5.3 to 4.0kPa decreases CBF by 30%
    - Arterial PO_2: hypoxia reduces CBF (minimal effect until <6.7kPa)
    - Cerebral metabolic rate for oxygen ($CMRO_2$)
    - Cerebral perfusion pressure (CPP): autoregulation at MAP of 60–160mmHg
    - Intracranial pressure (ICP): relationship CPP = MAP − ICP
    - Autoregulation is impaired with cerebral disease or trauma

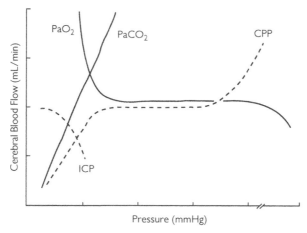

Figure F.2.2 Influence of various factors on cerebral blood flow

- • Sympathetic and parasympathetic activity appear to have little effect
- • Hypothermia reduces CBF by 5% per 1°C drop from normal
- • Various drugs, especially anaesthetic agents: ketamine will increase CBF; benzodiazepines, thiopentone, and propofol will reduce CBF
- ■ The Cushing reflex occurs in response to an increase in ICP and involves systemic vasoconstriction to increase arterial pressure in order to maintain blood flow to the brain. Compensatory bradycardia is also noted
- ■ See Chapter F3, Section 3.1
- • Coronary blood flow:
  - ■ Consists of the left and right coronary arteries:
    - • Left ventricular coronary flow only occurs during diastole, as ventricular pressure is greater than aortic pressure during systole
    - • Coronary flow to the right ventricle and atrium occurs during both systole and diastole
  - ■ Right coronary artery (RCA) arises from the right coronary sinus:
    - • The RCA supplies the right atrium and right ventricle
  - ■ The left main coronary divides into the left anterior descending (LAD) and circumflex:
    - • The LAD supplies the anterior septum and the anterior left ventricular wall
    - • The majority of the left ventricle is supplied by the left coronary artery
    - • Stenosis in the left main artery can cause severe myocardial compromise
  - ■ The sinus node and the AV node are supplied by the right coronary artery in the majority of people
  - ■ Disease in this artery can cause sinus bradycardia and AV nodal block
  - ■ Blood flow from the coronaries returns to the right atrium via accompanying veins
- • Pulmonary blood flow:
  - ■ The lungs are unusual in having a dual blood supply:
    - • Receive deoxygenated blood from the right ventricle via the pulmonary artery
    - • Also have a systemic supply
  - ■ The bronchial circulation arises from the descending aorta
  - ■ The bronchial veins drain into the pulmonary vein
  - ■ Lymphatic channels lie in the potential interstitial space

2.6 The cardiac cycle

- A single cardiac cycle consists of a synchronized electrical event followed by a muscular response by the heart.
- Wave of electrical activity from the SAN through the conduction system and finally to the myocardium—*depolarization*.
- Stimulates muscular contraction.
- Followed by electrical recovery—*repolarization*.
- Mechanical response by the heart is muscular contraction—*systole*.
- Then muscular relaxation—*diastole*.

2.6.1 Electrophysiology

- Electrical activity is a result of cell membrane permeability.
- Movement of ions across the cell membrane changes the charge of the membrane.
- Involves slow and fast ion channels.
- Potassium (K^+), sodium (Na^+), and calcium (Ca^{2+}) are of particular importance:
  - K^+ is a dominant intracellular cation
  - Na^+ and Ca^{2+} are dominant extracellular cations

2.6.2 Action potential—5 phases

See Figure F.2.3.

- *Resting phase*—phase 4:
  - At rest the cardiac cell exhibits a difference in electrical potential over the membrane:
    - Inside the cell—relatively negative
    - Outside the cell—relatively positive
  - Therefore the cell is polarized
  - Difference is due to relative permeability of the membrane to ions:
    - At rest the membrane is more permeable to K^+ then Na^+
    - Therefore small amounts of K^+ diffuse from inside the membrane to outside
    - Diffuse from a high concentration to a low concentration
    - This loss of K^+ leaves the internal cell relatively negative in charge
- *Rapid depolarization*—phase 0:
  - Depolarization is due to greatly increased membrane permeability to Na^+—extracellular Na^+ rushes into the cell via fast channels
  - Augmented by sodium concentration gradient

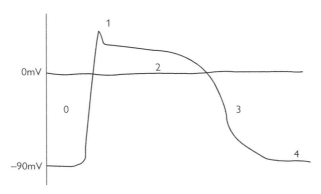

Figure F.2.3 Cardiac action potential

- This influx of +ve charge reverses the relative charge across the membrane:
  - Cell exterior becomes negative
  - Cell interior becomes positive
- *Partial repolarization*—phase 1:
  - On reversal of charge:
    - Fast Na⁺ channels close and K⁺ channels open
    - Less Na⁺ enters the cell
    - More K⁺ leaves it
  - Result is a net flux of +ve charge out of the cell
- *Plateau phase*—phase 2:
  - Sustained plateau corresponding to the refractory period of myocardium
  - No net change in electrical charge occurs during this period
  - A balance is maintained between influx and efflux of +ve ions:
    - Slow inward flow of Ca^{2+} is primarily responsible
    - Some inward flow of Na⁺ ions through slow channels also occurs
    - Inward movement of +ve charge is countered by outward movement of K⁺
- *Rapid repolarization*—phase 3:
  - Slow inward flow of Ca^{2+} and Na⁺ stops
  - Membrane permeability to K⁺ markedly increases
  - K⁺ moves out of the cell, reducing +ve charge inside the cell
  - Inside of the cell regains its relative negativity
  - Outside of the cell returns to its relative positivity
  - At rest, the Na⁺/K⁺ pump maintains the distribution of ions—active transport of Na⁺ out of the cell and K⁺ into it

2.6.3 The fast and slow response

- The earlier given description of action potential (see Chapter F, Section 2.6.2) is found in non-specialized fibres:
  - Known as the fast response
  - Found in fibres located in the atria, ventricles, and His–Purkinje system
- The slow response is found in specialized fibres:
  - Sinoatrial and atrioventricular nodes
- Slow response is more gradual than the fast response.
- Fast response depends on Na⁺ ions.
- Slow channel depolarization depends on Ca^{2+} ions.

2.6.4 Physiological properties of the action potential

- Specialized cell physiology differs from non-specialized:
  - Due to difference in fast and slow action potentials
- Automaticity—ability to generate impulses independently:
  - Due to automatic changes in resting phase of slow response action potential
  - Cells depolarize towards threshold
  - When threshold reached, cell automatically fires
- Known as the 'all-or-nothing phenomenon'.
- Depolarization will not generate an action potential until threshold is reached.
- The SAN spontaneously depolarizes at 60–100bpm—thereby known as the natural pacemaker of the heart.

2.6.5 Conduction velocity

- Conduction velocity related to type of action potential.
- Slow conduction through AV node vs rapid conduction through Purkinje fibres.
- Due to differences in fast and slow response action potentials.

- This delay in conduction allows for ventricular filling during atrial contraction.
- This property also protects the ventricles from atrial tachyarrhythmias.

2.6.6 Excitability

- Immediately after depolarization—absolute refractory period.
- Myocardium is incapable of producing a response to stimulus at this point.
- Relative refractory period follows.
- Here myocardium only responds when a stimulus is larger than normal.
- Repetitive stimulation does not cause tetany due to the refractory period.

2.6.7 Muscle ultrastructure

- Sarcomere is the basic contractile unit of the myocardium.
- Made up of 2 overlapping myofilaments:
  - Thick myosin filament and thin actin filament
  - Linked by cross-bridging
- Sarcomere also contains troponin and tropomyosin proteins.
- At rest the troponin–tropomyosin complex inhibits cross-bridge formation.
- Electrical excitation and mechanical response is known as excitation contraction coupling.
- Action potential is conducted over the cell membrane, or sarcolemma.
- Propagated into the T-tubules, which are depressions in the cell membrane.
- Action potential is conducted cell to cell through intercalated discs.
- Electrical excitation initiates muscular contraction.
- Ca^{2+} released from sarcoplasmic reticulum and other cellular sources.
- Calcium binds to the troponin protein, inactivating the inhibitory effect of the troponin–tropomyosin system.
- Actin and myosin are then free to form cross-bridges.
- Generate mechanical force to shorten the sarcomere.
- Shortening of multiple sarcomeres causes muscular contraction.
- Relaxation is due to Ca^{2+} resorption into the sarcoplasmic reticulum.
- This dissociates the actin–myosin cross-bridges.
- Return of inhibitory effect of the troponin–tropomyosin complex.
- Force of contraction is related to interaction between sarcomeres.
- Addition of calcium increases contractile force.
- Overstretching the sarcomere decreases contractile force by reducing overlap.

2.6.8 Phases of the cardiac cycle

- Mid diastole:
  - Slow ventricular filling
  - Atria and ventricles are relaxed
  - Blood flows passively from atria to ventricles
- Late diastole:
  - The atria contract
  - Contributing 20–30% of ventricular filling
- Early systole:
  - Depolarization spreads to the ventricles
  - Ventricular contraction begins
  - Pressure of ventricles rises above atria
  - Tricuspid and mitral valves closing generate 1st heart sound
  - Ventricular pressure rises
  - Semilunar valves are closed—isovolumetric contraction

- Late systole:
  - Pressure in ventricles exceeds pressure in blood vessels
  - Blood flow into the pulmonary and systemic circulation occurs
  - Initial phase or rapid ejection
  - Followed by a more sustained phase and reduced ejection
- Early diastole:
  - Ventricular chambers relax
  - Ventricular pressure drops below arterial pressure
  - Semilunar valves close, creating the 2nd heart sound
  - Relaxation continues until pressure drops below that of the atria
  - AV valves open
  - Period between semilunar valves closing and opening of AV valves is known as isovolumetric relaxation
  - As AV valves open, passive filling of ventricles occurs
  - 70–80% of filling of the ventricles occurs here

2.7 ECG

- A recording of the electrical activity of the heart.
- Recorded from 2 or more simultaneous points of skin contact.
- When cardiac activity moves towards the positive electrode, an upward deflection occurs.
- When cardiac activity moves away from the positive electrode, a downward deflection occurs.

2.7.1 Waveform

See Figure F.2.4.

- The first deflection is caused by atrial depolarization—the P wave.
- The QRS complex represents ventricular depolarization.
- The T wave represents ventricular repolarization.
- The PR interval is the length of time from the start of the P wave to the start of the QRS complex—the time taken for activation to pass from the sinus node through to the ventricles.
- The QT interval extends from the start of the QRS to the end of the T wave:
  - QT represents the time taken to depolarize and repolarize the myocardium
  - QT segment corresponds to the period between the end of the QRS complex and the start of the T wave—representing ventricular repolarization

2.7.2 Vectors and axis

- Repolarization and depolarization are propagated in different directions.
- The net force is known as the cardiac vector.
- The mean QRS vector lies between −30 degrees and +90 degrees.
- Left axis deviation lies between −30 degrees and −90 degrees.
- Right axis deviation lies between +90 and +150 degrees.

2.8 Pharmacological manipulation of the heart and peripheral circulation

- Myocardial contractility can be impaired by factors such as hypoxaemia and hypocalcaemia.
- If signs of shock persist despite volume replacement, pressor agents can be used to improve CO and BP.

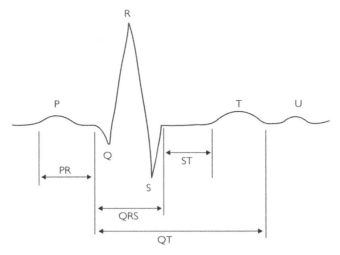

Figure F.2.4 ECG waveform

- Patients can become resistant to the effects of pressor agents—a phenomenon known as 'downregulation'.
- Pressors should be used with caution so that an imbalance between myocardial oxygen supply and demand does not occur.

2.8.1 Epinephrine (adrenaline)

- Stimulates alpha- and beta-adrenergic receptors.
- At low doses, beta effects predominate.
- Produces a tachycardia and a fall in peripheral resistance.
- At higher doses, alpha-mediated vasoconstriction occurs, which increases end-organ perfusion pressure.
- Epinephrine can cause excessive vasoconstriction in some circumstances.
- Minimum effective dose should be used for as short a time as possible.

2.8.2 Norepinephrine (noradrenaline)

- An alpha-adrenergic agonist.
- Useful for patients with severe hypotension associated with low systemic vascular resistance.

2.8.3 Dopamine

- Natural precursor of epinephrine.
- Acts on beta and alpha receptors as well as dopaminergic D1 and D2 receptors.
- In low doses, vasodilatory receptors in the renal, mesenteric, cerebral, and coronary circulation are activated.
- D1 receptors are postsynaptic and mediate vasodilatation.
- D2 receptors are presynaptic and augment vasodilatation by preventing release of epinephrine.
- End-organ failure can therefore be potentially prevented.
- In moderate doses, dopamine increases heart rate, myocardial contractility, and CO.
- In higher doses, the increased epinephrine produced is associated with vasoconstriction.
- This increases afterload and raises ventricular filling pressures.

2.8.4 Dobutamine

- Closely related to dopamine.
- Predominantly beta-1 activity.
- No specific effect on renal vasculature.
- Urine output can increase due to increased CO.
- Reduces systemic vascular resistance.
- Useful in patients with cardiogenic shock and failure.

2.9 Shock

- A complex clinical syndrome with variable haemodynamic manifestations.
- Common denominator is the inadequacy of tissue perfusion.
- This state of hypoperfusion comprises oxygen and nutrient delivery to tissues.
- Tissue hypoxia shifts metabolism from oxidative pathways to anaerobic pathways.
- Consequent production of lactic acid.
- Culminates in cellular destruction and multisystem failure.
- Shock is progressive and self-perpetuating.
- Separated into:
  - Compensated stage:
    - Compensatory responses as described earlier stabilize circulation
  - Progressive stage:
    - Systemic manifestations of hypoperfusion and worsening organ function
  - Refractory stage:
    - Profound cellular abnormalities inevitably lead to death
- Most shock states are characterized by low CO and increased SVR
- However, shock can also occur with a normal or even elevated CO.

2.9.1 Causes of shock

- Can result from a variety of conditions.
- 4 basic aetiological mechanisms:
  - Cardiogenic mechanisms:
    - Secondary to dysrhythmias
    - Secondary to valvular lesions
    - Secondary to myopathy
  - Obstructive mechanisms:
    - Pericardial tamponade
    - Coarctation of aorta
    - Pulmonary embolism
    - Primary pulmonary hypertension
  - Alteration in circulating volume:
    - Haemorrhage
    - Fluid depletion/sequestration
  - Alteration in circulatory distribution:
    - Septicaemia
    - Metabolic/toxic causes
    - Endocrinological (e.g. ketoacidosis)
    - Neurogenic shock
    - Anaphylactic shock
    - Microcirculatory pathology (e.g. polycythaemia, sickle-cell anaemia, fat embolus)

2.9.2 Cardiogenic shock

- This section focuses on cardiogenic shock post-MI.
- Characterized by left ventricular dysfunction.
- Associated with a loss of ~40% of the myocardium.
- As a result of MI, left ventricular contractility and output are impaired.
- Failure of the heart to act as a pump.
- Reduced CO leads to increased arterial hypotension.
- Metabolic acidosis and reduced coronary perfusion occur.
- This further impairs the ventricular function.
- A self-perpetuating cycle occurs.

2.9.3 Pathophysiology of cardiogenic shock

- Can be viewed as a severe form of left ventricular failure (LVF).
- Pathophysiology is similar to LVF; however, there is progression to a greater severity.
- Reduced contractility reduces CO:
  - Increase in left ventricular end-diastolic volume
  - This leads to pulmonary congestion and oedema
- As systemic arterial pressure falls, baroreceptors at the carotid sinus and aorta are stimulated.
- Sympathetic adrenal stimulation produces reflex vasoconstriction, tachycardia, and increased contractility—all act to stabilize CO.
- Contractility is improved further by renal retention of sodium and water—results in increased afterload and preload.
- This causes an increase in cardiac work and oxygen demand by the myocardium.
- Further myocardial dysfunction occurs secondary to ischaemia, causing a vicious cycle of myocardial compromise.
- Shock state progresses until multisystem failure occurs:
  - Respiratory failure:
    - Respiratory compromise develops due to pulmonary congestion and alveolar oedema
    - Can result in adult respiratory distress syndrome (ARDS)
  - Renal failure:
    - Reduced renal perfusion leads to oliguria
    - Urine sodium levels are reduced
    - Acute tubular necrosis can cause acute kidney injury
  - Hepatic failure:
    - Hepatic cellular dysfunction can occur
    - Marked derangements of hepatic function are made manifest
  - GI compromise:
    - Ischaemia of the GI tract can cause bowel ischaemia
    - Bacteria and endotoxins may be absorbed into the circulation, further exacerbating the clinical picture
    - GI motility is almost always present in the shock state
  - Neurological deficit:
    - Cerebral blood flow is autoregulated
    - In pronounced shock, autoregulation is inadequate
    - Symptoms of neurological deficit can occur
  - Haematological deficit:
    - Intravascular aggregation of cellular components occurs
    - Can increase peripheral vascular resistance further
    - Disseminated intravascular coagulation (DIC) can occur

2.10 Oxygen delivery and oxygen consumption (DO_2/VO_2)

- Oxygen delivery is the quantity of oxygen made available to the body in 1 minute.
- It is equal to the CO multiplied by the arterial oxygen content = 850–1200mL/min.
- In general, there is more oxygen delivered to cells than they actually use (240–270mL/min).
- When oxygen consumption is high (during exercise), the increased oxygen requirement is provided by an increase in the CO.
- However, a low CO, a low haemoglobin concentration (anaemia), or low haemoglobin O_2 saturation will result in an inadequate delivery of oxygen, unless a compensatory change occurs in one of the other factors.
- Alternatively, if oxygen delivery falls relative to oxygen consumption, the tissues extract more oxygen from the haemoglobin.
- This can ultimately result in anaerobic metabolism and lactic acidosis.
- Please also see Chapter F1, Section 1.12.

2.11 Body fluid homeostasis

- A number of homeostatic mechanisms operate to maintain electrolyte and osmotic concentration and total body fluid volume.
- These mechanisms include:
  - Water intake regulated by thirst, which is increased by:
    - Hypovolaemia
    - Hyperosmolality
  - Urinary output regulated by:
    - Vasopressin
    - Atrial natriuretic peptide
    - Renin–angiotensin system
- The kidney mediates the majority of control over fluid and electrolyte levels.
- Please see Chapter F4, Section 4.5 for further details.

2.12 Crystalloid solutions

- Crystalloid solutions contain relatively small molecules that may readily pass through capillary and glomerular membranes, but not cell membranes.
- Cell membrane pumps subsequently alter the ion distribution, with water following salt into tissues or cells.
- As a result, electrolyte solutions usually remain within the intravascular space for only about 30 minutes, after which only around 25% of the infused solution is left.
- Fluid shift into the interstitial space is further promoted by increased capillary protein permeability and decreased intravascular colloid oncotic pressure seen as a result of normal physiological responses to trauma.
- Advantages of crystalloids over colloids:
  - Absence of allergenicity or coagulation dysfunction
  - Useful for electrolyte supplementation (e.g. hypokalaemia)
  - Extracellular fluid depletion is thought to be better restored
  - Less increase of interstitial oncotic pressure so large volume administration in the critically ill should be avoided
  - Cost

- Crystalloid fluids include:
  - Sodium chloride 0.9%
  - Glucose (5% or 10% usually)
  - Hartmann's/Ringer lactate solution
  - Sodium bicarbonate (1.26% or 8.4%)

2.13 Colloidal solutions

- Greater and more sustained increase in circulating volume.
- Associated improvements in cardiovascular function and oxygen transport.
- Increased colloid osmotic pressure.
- Solutions include Gelofusine® and Haemaccel®.

2.14 Exudates and transudates

- Important distinction between exudates and transudates.
- Exudates and transudates are caused by different phenomena.

2.14.1 Exudates

- Exudates are caused by inflammatory processes.
- Composition includes water and the dissolved solutes of blood.
- Have a characteristically high protein content, with cell debris content and high specific gravity.
- Usually contains some or all plasma proteins, white blood cells, platelets, and (in the case of local vascular damage) red blood cells
- Specific types of exudates are:
  - Pus—contains bacteria and high concentrations of white blood cells
  - Purulent or suppurative—plasma with both active and dead neutrophils, fibrinogen, and necrotic parenchymal cells
  - Fibrinous—composed mainly of fibrinogen and fibrin; characteristic of rheumatic carditis
- Causes of pleural exudative effusions are:
  - Bacterial pneumonia
  - Pulmonary embolism
  - Cancer

2.14.2 Transudates

- Transudate is extravascular fluid with a characteristically low protein content and a low specific gravity.
- Transudates are typically caused by disturbances of hydrostatic or colloid osmotic pressure, rather than by inflammatory processes.
- Common causes of pleural transudative effusions are:
  - Left ventricular heart failure
  - Cirrhosis
  - Nephrotic syndrome

2.14.3 Definition of pleural effusions

- A pleural effusion is exudative if it meets at least 1 of the following criteria:
  - Protein >2.9g/dL (29g/L)

- Cholesterol >45mg/dL (1.16mmol/L)
- LDH >60% of upper limit for serum
- Light's criteria for an exudative pleural effusion are:
  - Ratio of pleural fluid protein to serum protein >0.5
  - Ratio of pleural fluid LDH and serum LDH >0.6
  - LDH > two-thirds normal upper limit for serum

Neurology

CONTENTS

3.1 Intracranial pressure

- The Munro–Kelly doctrine describes the skull as a rigid cavity of fixed volume.
- It has 3 primary contents:
  - Brain parenchyma (1200–1600mL)
  - CSF (100–150mL)
  - Blood (100–150mL)
- As the volume of their container is fixed, any change in volume of 1 component must be compensated for by the other 2.
- Normal ICP ranges from 0 to 10mmHg (lower in children); when monitored a waveform is visible:
  - This is caused by the systolic pulse transmitted to cerebral vasculature and by respiration
  - Slower, intermittent pressure waves are pathological and associated with states of elevated ICP
- Autoregulation is the mechanism by which cerebral blood flow (CBF) is maintained at a constant despite fluctuations in cerebral perfusion pressure (CPP).
- This mechanism is reliable with a CPP of 60–160mmHg in an uninjured brain.
- Extremes of perfusion or a damaged control mechanism can cause a decoupling.

3.1.1 Raised ICP

- Raised ICP is not in itself a damaging state if CBF is maintained.
- Damage arises from spatial changes in the brain leading to herniation, which can be:
  - Lateral tentorial (unilateral mass effect)
  - Central tentorial (due to diffuse swelling, or can follow initial lateral herniation)
  - Tonsillar (subtentorial mass causes herniation downwards through foramen magnum and sometimes upwards through tentorial hiatus)
- Clinical features of raised ICP:
  - Headache (positional, worse in mornings)
  - Papilloedema (not always present as depends on degree of CSF obstruction)
  - Vomiting (in acute rises)

3.1.2 Measurement of ICP

- Measurement of ICP is important as it enables targeting of BP in neurocritical care to preserve CPP.
- Ventricular catheter technique:
  - A saline-filled catheter is introduced into the frontal horn of the lateral ventricle and connected to a transducer via a 3-way tap
  - Gold standard of measurement but relatively high risk of infection
  - One device permits simultaneous measurement and drainage of CSF
- Parenchymal measurement devices:
  - Can be 'bolted' or tunnelled
  - These use either miniature strain gauges or fibre-optic beam reflection at the device tip to provide an estimate of ICP
  - They are less invasive but are significantly colonized within 5 days of introduction
  - Can only be calibrated before insertion and suffer from 'zero drift' whereby calibration becomes increasingly unreliable
- Subdural catheters:
  - Can be inserted at time of craniotomy but under-read in presence of high ICP and tend to block
- Epidural catheters:
  - Easily placed but there is little understanding of relationship between pressure in epidural space and ICP

3.2 Sensory pathways

3.2.1 Transduction

- Process by which environmental change (stimulus) brings about transmission of electrical impulse in the nervous system.
- Multiple sensory receptors:
  - Photoreceptors (sight)
  - Olfactory receptors (smell)
  - Mechanoelectrical receptors (hearing, fine discriminative touch, vibration, and proprioception)
- Relies on a variety of chemical processes and messengers, including cyclic adenosine monophosphate (cAMP), adenosine triphosphate (ATP), and Ca^{2+}.

3.2.2 Somatosensation

- 2 types of receptor, each with fast and slow subtypes:
  - Type I (sharp sensation, high density of endings near surface of skin, localized sensation):
    - Rapidly adapting Meissner's corpuscle (RA^I)
    - Slowly adapting Merkel's disc (SA^I)
  - Type II (convey information on tissue tension and vibration, deeper, less well localized):
    - Rapidly adapting Pacinian corpuscle (RA^{II})
    - Slowly adapting Ruffini endings (SA^{II})
- Project via peripheral nerves (large and fast axons) to dorsal root ganglia.
- Different somatosensory modalities organize into the dorsal column.
- Somatotopic organization in spinal cord.
- Fixed portions in the cord correspond to anatomical regions of innervation.
- Ipsilateral passage into the spinal cord.

- Synapse at nucleus gracilis and nucleus cuneatus.
- Decussate to medial leminiscus, which projects to ventroposterior nucleus of thalamus.
- Thalamic rod projects to primary somatosensory cortex (SmI):
  - Brodmann's areas 1, 2, 3a, and 3b
  - Contralateral representation of body surface
  - Homunculus proportions in cortex according to receptor density
- Secondary somatosensory cortex (SmII) receives input from SmI and has higher function in object recognition.

3.3 Motor pathways

- Division of systems into motor and sensory is to some extent arbitrary, but areas listed are those where majority of function is dedicated to one task.

3.3.1 Planning and initiation

- Origination of movement is from limbic system and posterior parietal cortex, where intention to move begins.
- This desire to move is converted into motor instructions, in conjunction with basal ganglia, by the working of:
  - Primary motor cortex (MsI, Brodmann's area 4)
  - Supplementary motor area (SMA, medial portion of Brodmann's area 6)
  - Premotor cortex (PMC, lateral portion of Brodmann's area 6)
- Motor homunculus maps cortical areas to motor regions.
- Complex motor requirements (e.g. the hand) require significant cortical area.
- Cortex remains plastic—damage in later life can be compensated for.

3.3.2 Comparison

- Cerebellum (CBM) compares current movement (information from spinal interneurons and muscle receptors) with planned movement to coordinate the two.
- This coordination role is why cerebellar dysfunction causes ataxia rather than weakness.
- 3 functionally discrete systems:
  - VestibuloCBM: eye movements and posture
  - SpinoCBM: posture and axial musculoskeletal function
  - PontoCBM: planning and coordination
- Purkinje cells give rise to muscle memory phenomenon.
- The amount of inhibition required to make actual movements correspond to planned ones is adjusted for in the biochemical makeup of the synapse.

3.3.3 Cortical control of motor neurons (MNs)

- Corticospinal tract largely as described; direct cortical control of spinal MNs (as well as cranial nerves and brainstem, also known as pyramidal tracts).
- Vestibulospinal, reticulospinal, tectospinal, and rubrospinal tracts are all ones that are less directly connected to the motor cortex (extrapyramidal tracts) and have complicated systems interfacing with them.
- This is the 1st point in descending motor pathways at which damage causes outright weakness.

3.3.4 Spinal cord

- Descending pathways synapse with interneurons (INs) in addition to MNs.
- Central pattern generation aids walking:
  - Compound movement is a step

- Comprises swing and stance phase
- CPG centres work in opposition—one for flexion, other for extension

3.3.5 Lower motor neuron (LMN)

- Higher information from brain and INs
- Sequential recruitment of MNs means that muscle fibres work in a logical sequence:
  - Slow contracting fibres
  - Fast contracting, slowly tiring fibres
  - Fast contracting, fast tiring fibres
- Also local information from muscle spindles (important in reflexes for neurological examination) and Golgi tendon organs
- Characteristic LMN lesion of flaccidity, wasting, and areflexia

3.4 Nerve conduction

3.4.1 Resting membrane potential

- Cell membrane nearly impermeable to Na^+ at rest but K^+ can move more freely.
- Intracellular K^+ concentration derived from balance between chemical gradient drawing K^+ out of cell and potential difference this creates, causing some K^+ to be drawn back.
- The equilibrium potential at which these processes are all at steady state can be calculated with the Nernst equation.
- Na^+/K^+-ATPase contributes only small amount, mainly to pump out the small amount of Na^+ leaking into cell.

3.4.2 Action potential (AP)

- Electrical impulse by which transmission occurs in nervous system.
- 'All or nothing' so there is no information from amplitude.
- Frequency of impulses carries information (a digital rather than analogue system).
- AP fires when current coming into cell (due to Na^+) exceeds net current going out.
- This is usually −55mV (critical firing threshold).
- If the threshold is not reached, the AP is not fired and there is no propagation along axon.
- Sequence of events:
  - Incoming depolarizing voltage opens voltage-dependent Na^+ channels
  - Incoming Na^+ opens more Na^+ channels (+ve feedback loop)
  - When net incoming current exceeds outgoing current, mass opening of Na^+ channels occurs
  - Depolarization of membrane occurs and AP spike is generated
  - Falling phase now occurs
  - Voltage-dependent Na^+ channels close
  - Repolarization by Na^+/K^+-ATPase
  - Between spike of AP and point at which cell membrane reaches equilibrium again, cell is refractory:
    - Absolute refractory phase occurs when cell cannot be depolarized
    - Relative refractory phase is when the cell can be depolarized, but only by voltage above normal threshold

3.4.3 Conduction

- Uses principle of local current spread to transmit signals in nervous system.
- This places restrictions on speed of transmission and on signal quality.

- To prevent this, fibres are myelinated if they have a diameter greater than ~1μm.
- The myelin acts as an electrical insulator.
- Gaps between myelinated portions are nodes of Ranvier and have high density of Na^+ channels.
- Conduction in unmyelinated fibres is simply by an advancing front of depolarization.
- Current direction is maintained by the fact that membrane behind is still repolarizing and therefore cannot depolarize, which prevents backflow.
- Conduction in myelinated fibres is similar but relies on nodes of Ranvier:
  - These areas of high density of Na^+ channels are where APs are generated
  - This is known as *saltatory conduction*; it is both quicker and less demanding on cellular metabolism
- Excitatory postsynaptic potentials are the voltages caused in postsynaptic cells by incoming information. They do not result in AP propagation unless the threshold is reached by summation:
  - Temporal summation is serial impulses that eventually cause enough depolarization to fire the AP
  - Spatial summation is the coalescence of several presynaptic neurons firing simultaneously onto one postsynaptic cell, so that the sum of multiple smaller signals fires an AP
- Inhibitory neurons tend to work on conduction pathway by hyperpolarizing the neuron, thereby raising threshold for depolarization.

3.5 Pain

- Nociceptors respond to mechanical, chemical, or thermal insult and derive from neural crest tissue.
- Can have fast or slow axons:
  - Slow pain:
    - Dull or burning
    - Carried by C fibres (smaller diameter therefore slower maximum rate of conduction)
    - Run in lateral spinothalamic tract (LSTT) to reticular formation of brainstem
    - Connections from reticular formation to thalamus and hypothalamus
    - Much less specific localization than fast pain
  - Fast pain:
    - Sharp
    - Alpha delta fibres (large diameter, fast)
    - Runs in LSTT to ventral posterior lateral nucleus of hypothalamus
    - Somatotopic projection to sensory cortex (specific region of cortex corresponds to region of body)
    - Very precisely localized
  - Common to both is synapse at or near segmental level and ascent in contralateral LSTT
- Gate control theory of pain (Melzack and Wall, 1962) states that:
  - Non-nociceptive fibres (alpha beta) can modulate transmission in nociceptive fibres
  - Inhibition of nociceptive fibres can reduce transmission of pain
  - This is the mechanism behind pain relief derived from rubbing briskly at injured region, as well as the basis for transcutaneous electronic nerve stimulation (TENS)
- Pain also modulated directly by brain:
  - Periaqueductal grey matter stimulation activates descending pathways, which modulate nociceptive transmission
  - Pain control sufficient to permit awake abdominal surgery on rats in experiment

3.5.1 Therapeutic control of pain

- Analgesia:
  - Typical (NSAIDs etc.)
  - Atypical (anticonvulsants etc.)
- Blockade of transmission:
  - Local anaesthesia (reversible)
  - Surgical division of nerves (irreversible)
- Other:
  - Modulation via TENS
  - Capsaicin cream

3.6 Sight

3.6.1 The retina

- 2 types of photoreceptor and 1 specialized cell line:
  - Rods:
    - Scotopic vision (better at night)
    - Distributed around retina except the fovea
    - Poor discriminative ability due to the innervation of rods
  - Cones:
    - Photopic (day) vision
    - High density in the fovea
    - 3 different subtypes of pigmentation (imbalance of which leads to colour blindness)
  - Amacrine cells:
    - Receive inputs from bipolar cells (see later bullet point) and other amacrine cells
- Synapse with 2 cell types:
  - Horizontal cells:
    - Control cells for bipolar cells
    - Govern whether cells become more or less polarized when their afferent receptor is struck by light
  - Bipolar cells:
    - Hyperpolarize or depolarize in response to light activation of their afferent
- Ganglion cells receive inputs from bipolar and amacrine cells and provide optical information to the brain via the optic nerve

3.6.2 Optical pathways

- Optic nerves form optic tracts at optic chiasm (anatomically related to pituitary gland).
- Optic radiations project through parietal and temporal lobes via lateral geniculate nucleus (LGN) to primary visual cortex (V1).
- LGN has discrete regions dealing with colour perception and motion detection.
- Contributions from optic tract in midbrain to:
  - Pretectal nucleus: responsible with Edinger Westphal nucleus for consensual pupillary response
  - Superior colliculus
  - Suprachiasmatic nucleus of hypothalamus

3.6.3 Optical cortex

- Primarily V1 in occipital lobe, afferents from LGN.

- Retinotopic mapping based around high-density afferents from fovea.
- Extrastriate areas (in frontal and posterior parietal cortex) are those outside V1 dealing with visual processing.

3.7 Auditory system

- 2 main properties of sound are amplitude and frequency.
- Ear employs a system of mechanotransduction:
  - Sound arrives at outer ear and wave strikes tympanic membrane, making it vibrate
  - Vibration transmitted through middle ear by ossicles
  - Oval window vibrates, causing wave to pass through fluid of cochlea in inner ear
  - Decoupled system provides potential for dampening if pressure too high (ossicles can decouple from oval window)
  - Cochlea contains organ of Corti, lined with hair cells, which is where transduction takes place
  - Inner hair cells transduce signal to cranial nerve (CN) VIII
  - Outer hair cells modulate properties of inner hair cells and have afferents from brainstem structures further up auditory pathway
  - Frequency responsiveness in cochlea governed by seashell shape of organ and infinitesimal differences in structure of hair cells themselves

3.7.1 Auditory pathways

- Organized tonotopically, with specific fibres in pathway receiving inputs from individual hair cells in organ of Corti.
- Therefore have a specific frequency response.
- Cochlear nucleus has dorsal and ventral parts with numerous onward connections.
- Most significant nucleus is the superior olivary complex:
  - Afferents from both ears, so sound perception at this point is bilateral (binaural)
  - Efferents innervate outer hair cells, modulating mechanotransduction

3.7.2 Auditory cortex

- The primary auditory cortex is Brodmann's areas 41 and 42.
- Secondary auditory cortex is significantly more complex, containing Wernicke's area and projecting in turn to Broca's area.
- Interactions between reception and generation of speech are more complex than originally thought, but much of the work is done in this area of the cortex.

3.8 Brainstem reflexes and death

- UK criteria validated by Academy of Medical Royal Colleges.
- Based on rationale that without functioning brainstem, spontaneous ventilation and consciousness are impossible.
- Must be ventilator dependent and in a deep coma.
- Must have excluded all reversible causes.
- Reflexes tested:
  - Pupillary light: pupils must be fixed and dilated
  - Corneal: no response to corneal irritation
  - Vestibulo-occular: injection of iced water into external ear causes nystagmus to contralateral side when intact

- Gag reflex
- Bronchial stimulation: can use suction catheter in ICU environment to stimulate carina
- Hypercapnia: when disconnected from ventilator, allowing increase in PCO_2 (confirmed as >6.5mmol/L on ABG) there is still no respiratory effort
- Note that the situation in USA is radically different, where total failure of the brain must be diagnosed and so higher function is assessed

3.9 Temperature

3.9.1 Thermoregulation

- Thermoregulatory centre in hypothalamus:
  - Central thermoreceptors in hypothalamus
  - Peripheral thermoreceptors in skin
- Negative feedback mechanism:
  - Homeostasis dictates a temperature 'set point'
  - Any deviation causes action to return towards the set point
  - The bigger the deviation, the bigger the corrective action
  - Like a central heating system, with thermoregulatory centre acting as thermostat
- When temperature is too high:
  - Peripheral vasodilatation occurs to divert blood to skin, allowing maximal loss of heat
  - Sweat glands stimulated, promoting evaporative cooling
  - Erector pili muscles relax, collapsing hair layer
  - Metabolic rate is slowed
- When temperature is too low:
  - Peripheral vasoconstriction diverts blood to core—a heat conservation measure
  - Skeletal muscle starts shivering—a heat production measure
  - Erector pili muscles contract, producing a layer of erect body hair to trap heat lost through convection—this is largely vestigial and of little effect in humans
  - Metabolic rate increased

3.9.2 Fever

- The effect of circulating pyrogens results in the resetting of the temperature set point in the hypothalamus.
- Thus fever is not a loss of control of the temperature but its upregulation.
- Pyrogens may be inflammatory mediators or bacterial toxins.
- There is much suggestion that fever is of benefit in fighting infection, but little concrete evidence.

3.9.3 Measurement of temperature

- Core temperature is most valid clinical reading.
- Probes can be used in oesophagus, bladder, rectum, ear, or mouth.
- Ensure equipment is appropriate and calibrated—low reading devices required in hypothermic patients.

3.9.4 Hypothermia

- Classified by core temperature:
  - 32–35° mild
  - 28–32° moderate
  - 20–28° severe

- Clinical features:
  - Early:
    - Tachypnoea
    - Goosebumps
    - Numbness and loss of ability to perform complex tasks
    - Peripheral vasoconstriction
    - Nausea
    - Shivering
    - At later stages may feel paradoxically warm
  - Late:
    - Shivering increasingly marked
    - Gross impairment of coordination
    - Pallor and cyanosis
    - Slow movements and confusion
  - Pre-terminal:
    - No longer shivering
    - Amnesia and dysarthria
    - Irrational urge to get undressed
    - Skin becomes oedematous
    - Organ failure and arrhythmia
- Causes:
  - Decreased heat production—largely metabolic (e.g. hypothyroidism)
  - Increased heat loss—immersion, exposure, etc.
  - Disordered thermoregulation—Wernicke's, MS, stroke

3.9.5 Hyperthermia

- High core temperature (>38.5°C) that is not due to fever.
- Spectrum of clinical presentation from heat cramps to heatstroke.
- Features:
  - Early heat illness:
    - Lethargy and malaise
    - Core temperature can be normal
    - Clinical signs of dehydration, turgor
    - Tachycardia and postural hypotension
    - Responds to cooling and rehydration
  - Later heat illness (heatstroke):
    - Often non-specific precursors of vomiting, nausea, headache
    - Core temperature above 40°C
    - Neurological progression from confusion and ataxia, through delirium, to seizures and eventually coma
    - Biochemical evidence of elevated transaminases, rhabdomyolysis, and acute kidney injury
    - Hyperdynamic CVS; labile cardiovascular function is a sign of impending crisis and should prompt urgent cooling
- Causes:
  - Increased heat production:
    - Overexertion
    - Thyroid storm
    - Phaeochromocytoma
    - Anticholinergics, ecstasy
    - Neuroleptic malignant syndrome (NMS), malignant hyperthermia (MH)
  - Increased environmental temperature

- Decreased cooling:
  - Reduced sweat production
  - Ambient humidity
- NMS can be provoked by any antipsychotic drug and is thought to relate to D2 dopamine receptor blockade
- MH is an autosomal dominant genetic condition causing reaction to inhaled volatile anaesthetics and some muscle relaxants
- Treatment of both NMS and MH is by immediate cessation of causative drug, dantrolene administration, and rapid cooling as per primary hyperthermia

3.10 Effect of altitude and dysbarism

- Please see Chapter F1, Sections 1.15 and 1.16.

Renal

CONTENTS

- Principal role of the kidney is elimination of waste and regulation of the volume and composition of body fluid.
- The glomerular filtration rate (GFR) remains constant in health due to intrarenal regulatory mechanisms.
- In disease, GFR can fall.
- This can be due to reduced intrarenal blood flow, damage to the glomeruli, or obstruction to the ultrafiltrate.
- Decreased GFR is manifest as a rise in urea and creatinine with a measurable decrease in GFR also.

4.1 Uraemia

- The concentration of urea and creatinine is in a state of equilibrium between production and elimination.
- In health, there is a large reserve for renal function.
- Serum urea and creatinine do not rise above the normal range until there is a reduction of 50–60% of the GFR.
- The urea at this point is dependent on the production of urea and on the GFR.
- The level of urea is heavily dependent on protein intake and tissue catabolism.
- Creatinine is less dependent on diet and more dependent on age, sex, and muscle mass.
- Creatinine is used as a guide to the GFR.
- In general, the measurement of serum creatinine is a good way to monitor further deterioration in the GFR.
- A normal serum urea and creatinine does not necessarily mean a normal GFR.

4.2 Measurement of the glomerular filtration rate (GFR)

- GFR is an exact measure of renal function.
- GFR is largely dependent on muscle creatinine production.
- This remains remarkably constant with little effect from protein intake.
- Therefore serum creatinine levels vary little throughout the day.
- 24-hour urine measurements can then be taken, which gives a single serum creatinine value over a 24-hour period.
- Creatinine clearance is a product of urine flow (V) and the urine creatinine concentration (U) divided by the plasma concentrations of creatinine (C) expressed in mL/min.

4.3 Tubular function

- Major function of the kidney is the selective re-absorption or excretion of water.
- Absorption and excretion of certain cations and anions is another important role.
- Active re-absorption from the glomerular filtrate occurs for glucose and amino acids.
- These substances are completely reabsorbed in normality.
- If blood levels of the substrate are sufficiently high then renal threshold is reached where the substrate is not reabsorbed to completion.

4.4 Endocrine function

4.4.1 Renin–angiotensin–aldosterone system (RAAS)

- Juxtaglomerular apparatus are made up of arteriolar smooth muscle cells.
- Sited at the afferent glomerular arteriole.
- These cells secrete renin as a response to certain stimuli.
- Renin converts angiotensinogen to angiotensin I in blood.
- Angiotensin II is generated from angiotensin I by angiotensin-converting enzyme (ACE).
- Angiotensin II is both a vasoconstrictor and a stimulator of the aldosterone hormone.
- It also modifies intrarenal blood flow.

4.4.2 Renin-releasing factors

- Pressure changes in the afferent arteriole.
- Sympathetic tone.
- Chloride and osmotic concentration in the distal tubule via the macula densa.
- Local prostaglandin release.

4.4.3 Endothelins

- Potent vasoactive peptides.
- Also influence cell proliferation and epithelial solute transport.
- Act locally.

4.4.4 Erythropoietin

- Glycoprotein produced by fibroblast cells in the renal interstitium.
- Major stimulus for erythropoiesis.
- Decreased erythropoietin release causes a normochromic, normocytic anaemia.
- Excess erythropoietin can cause a polycythaemia in patients with polycystic kidneys, benign renal cysts, or renal cell carcinoma.

4.4.5 Prostaglandins

- Unsaturated fatty acid compounds.
- Synthesized from cell membrane phospholipids.
- Important in the maintenance of renal blood flow and GFR.
- Have a natriuretic effect.

4.4.6 Natriuretic peptide family

- Found in many tissues but most abundantly in the cardiac atria.
- Have mainly natriuretic and vasorelaxant properties.
- Counterbalance the effects of the RAAS.

4.4.7 Vitamin D metabolism

- Naturally occurring vitamin D requires hydroxylation in the liver.
- Further hydroxylation occurs via the 1-alpha hydroxylase enzyme in the kidney.
- Produce 1,25-dihydroxycholecalciferol (1,25-$(OH)_2$D3).
- Reduced 1-alpha hydroxylase activity in diseased activity results in a relative deficiency in 1,25-$(OH)_2$D3.
- As a result, GI calcium resorption is reduced causing bone demineralization.

4.4.8 Protein and polypeptide metabolism

- The kidney is a major site for catabolism of small molecular weight proteins.
- This includes many hormones such as insulin, PTH, and calcitonin.

4.5 Water balance

- An average man weighing 70kg is composed of about 45L of water.
- Of this 45L, 30L is intracellular.
- The remaining 15L (the extracellular fluid) is made up of the interstitial fluid and plasma.
- In addition, small amounts of fluid are contained in bone, connective tissue, secretions, and CSF.
- Intracellular and interstitial fluids are separated by the cell membrane.
- The interstitial fluid and plasma are separated by the capillary wall.
- Movement at this level is dependent on diffusion.
- The ability to hold water in the compartment is measured as the osmotic pressure.

4.5.1 Osmotic pressure

- Osmotic pressure is the primary determinant of water distribution between the major compartments.
- Concentrations of solute differ in each of the fluid compartments.
- This therefore determines the osmotic pressure.
- K^+ salts are mainly found in the intracellular fluid.
- Na^+ salts are mostly found in the interstitial fluid.
- Proteins are found in the plasma.
- Plasma proteins hold water in the vascular space by an oncotic effect.
- This oncotic effect is counterbalanced by the hydrostatic pressure in the capillary.
- Osmotically active solutes cannot freely leave their compartments.
- This is exemplified by the relative impermeability of the cell wall to certain solutes due to the Na^+/K^+-ATPase. Na^+ is restricted to the extracellular fluid and K^+ to the intracellular fluid.
- Body Na^+ stores are the primary determinant of the extracellular fluid volume.
- Extracellular volume and tissue perfusion are maintained by changes in Na^+ excretion.

4.5.2 Extracellular volume regulation

- Extracellular volume is determined by the Na^+ concentration.
- Regulated by Na^+ balance at the kidney.
- Renal Na^+ excretion varies with circulating volume.
- The effective arterial blood volume (EABV) is the primary determinant of renal Na^+ and water excretion.
- EABV constitutes effective circulatory volume for the purpose of fluid homeostasis.
- This is dependent on a normal ratio between CO and peripheral arterial resistance.
- A decrease in EABV is initiated by a fall in CO or a fall in peripheral arterial resistance.
- When EABV is expanded, urinary Na^+ excretion increases.
- On the other hand, Na^+ excretion is low in the presence of a low EABV and normal renal function.
- Changes in Na^+ excretion can result from alterations in the filtered load and tubular re-absorption.
- The loop of Henle and the distal tubule make a major contribution to body Na^+.

4.5.3 Regulating water excretion

- Affected by thirst and kidney function.
- Some control by intracellular osmoreceptors in the hypothalamus and volume receptors in the capacitance vessels.
- The RAAS also has a direct effect.
- Major control is via osmoreceptors.
- Changes in plasma Na^+ and osmolality are sensed by the osmoreceptors.
- The osmoreceptors are directly responsible for thirst and ADH release.
- Released from supraoptic and paraventricular nuclei.

4.5.4 ADH

- Increases the water permeability of the normally impermeable cortical and medullary collecting tubes in the kidney.
- ADH directly affects the ascending limb of the loop of Henle, reabsorbing NaCl without water.
- This causes the tubular fluid to become dilute and the medullary area becomes concentrated, therefore promoting water re-absorption.
- In the absence of ADH, little fluid is reabsorbed as no NaCl is reabsorbed in the ascending limb.
- ADH effects are via the V2 (vasopressin) receptor.
- This causes the migration of aquaporins to the luminal membrane.
- Re-absorption of water occurs over a favourable osmotic gradient.
- The reabsorbed water is returned to the systemic circulation.
- In the absence of ADH, water channels are returned to the cytoplasm.

4.5.5 Plasma osmolality

- ADH plays a central role in osmoregulation.
- ADH release is directly affected by plasma osmolality.
- As plasma osmolality rises, so too does the circulating ADH level.
- As plasma osmolality falls, the circulating ADH falls also.
- The renal effects of ADH essentially keep any further water loss to a minimum.
- Renal effects of ADH do not replace the existing water deficit.
- Osmoregulation requires an increase in the body water intake.

- This is mediated by the stimulation of thirst.
- Thirst is therefore an important component in osmoregulation.

4.6 Increased extracellular volume

- Occurs in numerous disease states.
- Physical signs depend on the distribution of the volume.
- Depending on the Starling principle (see Chapter F4, Section 4.6.1), fluid accumulation can cause an expansion of interstitial volume, blood volume, or both.

4.6.1 Starling principle

- Distribution depends on venous tone and therefore hydrostatic pressures.
- Distribution is also dependent on capillary permeability, oncotic pressure, and lymphatic drainage.

4.6.2 Clinical signs of increased extracellular volume

- Peripheral oedema.
- Pulmonary oedema.
- Pleural effusion.
- Pericardial effusion.
- Ascites.
- Expansion of circulating volume can cause a raised JVP, cardiomegaly, basal crackles, and added heart sounds.

4.6.3 Causes of increased extracellular volume

- Heart failure—due to the activation of the RAAS in low CO states.
- Hypoalbuminaemia—due to loss of plasma oncotic pressure.
- Hepatic cirrhosis.
- Sodium retention.

4.7 Decreased extracellular volume

- Deficiency of Na^+ and water cause shrinkage of the interstitial space.

4.7.1 Symptoms of decreased extracellular volume

- Thirst.
- Muscle cramps.
- Postural hypotension.
- Loss of skin turgor.
- Lowering of the JVP.
- Peripheral vasoconstriction.
- Tachycardia.

4.7.2 Causes of decreased extracellular volume

- Haemorrhage.
- Burns.
- GI losses.
- Renal loss.

4.8 Disorders of sodium: hyponatraemia/hypernatraemia

- Disorders of Na⁺ concentration are caused by disturbances of water balance.
- Na⁺ content is regulated by volume receptors.
- Water content is adjusted to maintain a normal osmolality and a normal sodium concentration.

4.8.1 Hyponatraemia

- Hyponatraemia—serum sodium is below 135mmol/L.
- A common abnormality.
- Differential diagnosis depends on an assessment of extracellular volume.
- Can be a pseudo-hyponatraemia:
  - Pseudo-hyponatraemia occurs in states of high lipids and protein
  - Can also be caused by taking blood from an arm receiving fluid therapy in the clinical setting

4.8.2 Causes of hyponatraemia

- Salt-deficient hyponatraemia:
  - Due to salt loss in excess of water
  - ADH secretion is initially suppressed via osmoreceptors
  - As fluid is lost, volume receptors override osmoreceptors
  - This stimulates thirst and release of ADH
  - The body tries to retain circulating volume at the expense of osmolality
  - Urinary excretion of Na⁺ falls, creating concentrated urine with low Na⁺ content
- Hyponatraemia due to water excess:
  - Due to an intake of water in excess of the kidneys' ability to excrete water
  - In normal kidneys this is rare
  - Copious fluid administration to a patient is a common cause
  - Clinical features are principally neurological—headache, confusion, generalized convulsion, coma
  - Due to movement of water into brain cells in response to a fall in extracellular osmolality
- Syndrome of inappropriate antidiuretic hormone (SIADH):
  - Important cause of hyponatraemia but often over-diagnosed
  - Diagnosis requires concentrated urine in the presence of hyponatraemia
  - Causes include malignancy (such as small cell lung cancer), CNS disorders, and chest disease such as TB

4.8.3 Hypernatraemia

- Much rarer then hyponatraemia.
- Almost always caused by a water deficit.
- Always associated with increased plasma osmolality—a potent stimulus for thirst.

4.8.4 Causes of hypernatraemia

- ADH deficiency: diabetes insipidus (DI).
- Iatrogenic: administration of sodium infusions.
- Insensitivity to ADH: nephrogenic diabetes insipidus.
- Osmotic diuresis: in hyperosmolar non-ketotic acidosis in diabetics.
- Dehydration.

4.8.5 Symptoms of hypernatraemia

- Non-specific.

- Nausea, vomiting, and confusion can all occur.
- Polyuria, polydipsia, and thirst point towards a diagnosis of DI.

4.9 Disorders of potassium: hypokalaemia/hyperkalaemia

- K^+ mostly intracellular.
- Potassium levels are controlled by uptake of K^+ into cells, renal excretion, and GI losses.
- Na^+/K^+-ATPase controls uptake of K^+ into cells; this uptake is stimulated by insulin, beta-adrenergic stimulation, and theophylline.
- Uptake is decreased by alpha-adrenergic stimulation, acidotic states, and cell death.
- Aldosterone increases renal excretion of K^+.
- Conservation of potassium is relatively inefficient and low dietary intake can result in hypokalaemia.
- A number of drugs can affect aldosterone release and consequently the body's potassium level.
- Heparin and NSAIDs decrease aldosterone release.
- Drugs such as diuretics directly affect renal potassium handling.

4.9.1 Hypokalaemia

- Serum potassium content below 3.5mmol/L.

4.9.2 Causes of hypokalaemia

- Common causes include chronic diuretic treatment and hyperaldosteronism.
- GI losses such as vomiting and diarrhoea can cause hypokalaemia.
- Rarer causes include:
  - Bartter syndrome—impairment of Na^+ and Cl^- re-absorption in the ascending limb
  - Gitelman syndrome—a phenotype variant of Bartter syndrome
  - Liddle syndrome—low renin and aldosterone production

4.9.3 Symptoms of hypokalaemia

- Usually asymptomatic.
- Severe hypokalaemia can cause muscle weakness.
- Atrial and ventricular ectopic beats—felt as palpitations.

4.9.4 Hyperkalaemia

- Serum K^+ levels >5.5mmol/L.
- K^+ levels >6.5mmol/L require urgent treatment.

4.9.5 Causes of hyperkalaemia

- Self-limiting hyperkalaemia occurs after strenuous exercise.
- Other causes involve increased release from cells or failure of excretion.
- Increased K^+ release from cells occurs with tissue damage, tumour lysis, and acidosis.
- Decreased excretion occurs in renal failure, aldosterone deficiency, ACE inhibitor therapy, and Addison's disease.

4.9.6 Symptoms of hyperkalaemia

- Serum K^+ level >7.0mmol/L is a medical emergency associated with ECG changes.
- Usually asymptomatic.
- Can predispose to sudden death.

4.10 Calcium disorders: hypocalcaemia/hypercalcaemia

- 40% of plasma calcium is bound to serum albumin.
- The unbound, ionized component of calcium is physiologically important.
- Many factors affect Ca^{2+} binding to albumin (e.g. myeloma and cirrhosis).

4.10.1 The control of calcium metabolism

- Involves:
  - Parathyroid hormone (PTH)
  - Vitamin D
  - Thyroxine
  - Calcitonin
  - Magnesium

4.10.2 PTH

- Controlled by ionized plasma calcium levels.
- A rise in PTH causes a rise in Ca^{2+}.
- Causes a decrease in phosphate due to re-absorption from bone and increased loss of phosphate at the kidney.
- PTH secretion increases active vitamin D formation at the kidney.

4.10.3 Vitamin D

- Vitamin D3 and vitamin D2 are biologically identical in their actions.
- 1,25-dihydroxy vitamin D (also known as calcitriol) is created in the kidney.
- Calcitriol production is stimulated by a low Ca^{2+} and a drop in phosphate.
- Its main action leads to increased absorption of Ca^{2+} and phosphate from the gut, increased re-absorption of phosphate and Ca^{2+} in the kidney, and increased bone turnover and inhibition of PTH release.

4.10.4 Thyroxine

- Can increase serum Ca^{2+} but this is rare.

4.10.5 Calcitonin

- Made in the C cells of the thyroid.
- Causes a decrease in plasma Ca^{2+} and phosphate.
- Also acts as a marker in medullary carcinoma of the thyroid.

4.10.6 Magnesium

- Low magnesium levels can prevent PTH release and may cause hypocalcaemia.

4.11 Control of micturition

- Changes in the pattern of micturition can be caused by sacral, spinal cord, and cortical disease.

4.11.1 Function: efferent lower motor neuron pathways

- Sympathetic nerves (T12–L2) control bladder wall relaxation, internal sphincter contraction, and ejaculation.

- Parasympathetic nerves (S2–4) supply bladder wall contraction, internal sphincter contraction, and penis/clitoral erection/engorgement.
- Pudendal nerves (somatic) control the external sphincter.

4.11.2 Function: afferent pathways

- Afferent fibres: T12–S4 record changes in pressure within the bladder and tactile sensation of the genitalia.
- On bladder distension, continence is maintained by reflex suppression of the parasympathetic outflow and sympathetic activation.
- This is under voluntary control.

4.11.3 Disorders of micturition: location of lesions

- Cortical.
- Spinal cord.
- Lower motor neuron.

4.11.4 Cortical lesions

- Can cause socially inappropriate micturition—frontal lesions.
- Cause difficulty initiating micturition—precentral lesions.
- Cause loss of sense of bladder function—postcentral lesions.

4.11.5 Spinal cord lesions

- Bilateral pyramidal tract lesions cause frequency of micturition and incontinence.
- Can cause a hypertonic bladder.

4.11.6 Lower motor neuron lesions

- Sacral lesions cause a flaccid, atonic bladder.
- Can cause overflow without warning.

Haematological system

CONTENTS

5.1 Erythropoiesis

- Several precursor stages.
- Occurs in the bone marrow.
- Earliest recognizable cells are pronormoblasts.
- Progressive decrease in cell content of RNA during differentiation.
- Progressive increase in haemoglobin.
- Loss of nucleus between normoblast and reticulocyte stage.

5.1.1 Reticulocytes

- Contain ribosomal RNA.
- Able to synthesize Hb.
- Lose their RNA on release into the circulation, becoming erythrocytes.
- Mature red cells are biconcave, non-nucleated discs.

5.1.2 Normoblasts

- Not normally present in peripheral blood.
- Present in some disease states such as erythroblastic anaemias.

5.1.3 Control of erythropoiesis

- Controlled by erythropoietin (EPO).
- Produced by peritubular cells of the kidney with some production in the liver also.
- Regulated by tissue oxygen tension.
- Production is increased in a hypoxic state.
- EPO increases the number of precursor cells in the marrow dedicated to erythropoiesis.
- Inappropriate production of EPO is seen in certain neoplastic disorders, which result in polycythaemia.

5.1.4 Synthesis of haemoglobin (Hb)

- Hb carries oxygen to tissues and returns carbon dioxide to the lungs.

- Consists of 2 alpha and 2 beta chains.
- Hb-A comprises about 97% of Hb in adults.
- Hb synthesis occurs in the mitochondria of the developing red cell.
- Vitamin B6 is an important coenzyme for Hb synthesis.
- Iron is a major molecule in the Hb complex.

5.1.5 Function of haemoglobin

- The biconcave shape of the red cell markedly increases the surface area for transfer of carbon dioxide and oxygen.
- Hb saturation occurs in the pulmonary capillaries where oxygen partial pressure is high.
- Oxygen is released in the tissues where partial pressure of oxygen is low and Hb has a low affinity for oxygen.
- Binding of 1 oxygen molecule to Hb increases the oxygen affinity of the remaining binding sites—'cooperativity'.
- Cooperativity is the reason why the oxygen dissociation curve is sigmoidal.
- Oxygen binding can be affected by hydrogen ions, carbon dioxide levels, and 2,3-diphosphoglycerate (2,3-DPG).
- Hydrogen ions and carbon dioxide cause a reduction in the oxygen binding affinity of Hb—the Bohr effect.
- Oxygenation of Hb reduces its affinity for carbon dioxide—the Haldane effect.
- These effects help the exchange of carbon dioxide and oxygen at the tissues.
- Red cell metabolism produces 2,3-DPG from glycolysis.
- 2,3-DPG reduces Hb affinity for oxygen.

5.2 Blood groups

- Determined by antigens on the surface of red blood cells.
- ABO and rhesus blood groups are clinically important.
- Other blood groups are present and can cause transfusion reactions.

5.2.1 ABO system

- Involves IgM anti-A and anti-B antibodies.
- These groups can cause rapid haemolysis of incompatible cells.
- Under control of 3 allelic genes—A, B, and O.
- A and B control specific enzymes.
- The O gene is amorphic and therefore not antigenic.

5.2.2 Rh system

- High frequency of development of IgG RhD antibodies in RhD-negative people.
- This occurs after exposure to RhD-positive red cells.
- The antibodies created are responsible for haemolytic disease of the newborn (HDN) and haemolytic transfusion reactions.
- System is coded by allelic genes.

5.2.3 Other blood group systems

- Incompatibilities involving other blood groups, such as Kell, Duffy, and Kidd, can occur, causing transfusion reactions and HDN.

5.2.4 Blood transfusion

- Blood transfusions can immunize the recipient against donor antigens.

- This is known as alloimmunization.
- Repeated transfusions can increase the risk of alloimmunization.

5.3 Coagulation

- The coagulation cascade involves a series of enzyme-mediated reactions.
- Ultimately leads to the conversion of soluble plasma fibrinogen into fibrin clot.
- Coagulation factors are synthesized in the liver.

5.3.1 The coagulation pathway

- Traditionally divided into extrinsic and intrinsic pathways.
- Initiated by binding of activated factor VII in plasma to tissue factor (TF).
- TF is a glycoprotein expressed by injured cells.
- The complex of TF and VII activates factor IX.
- Activated IX then works with factor VIII to activate factor X.
- Factor X amplifies the generation of thrombin by converting prothrombin to thrombin.
- Factor XI is activated by thrombin making a limited contribution to haemostasis.
- Thrombin in the presence of calcium ions activates factor XIII.
- Factor XIII stabilizes the fibrin clot.
- Thrombin helps the activation of XI, V, VIII, and XIII, as well as protein C.
- Ultimately, plasma fibrinogen is converted into fibrin clot.
- Coagulation is limited to the site of injury.

5.4 Thrombolysis

- Medications given in certain clinical scenarios with an aim to prevent and treat thrombosis.
- Common drugs used include streptokinase and tissue type plasminogen activator.
- Urokinase synthesized naturally in the kidney produces plasmin directly.

5.4.1 Streptokinase

- Obtained from haemolytic *Streptococci*.
- Forms a complex with plasminogen, which forms plasmin.
- Streptokinase is antigenic causing development of streptococcal antibodies.
- Activation of plasminogen causes lysis of fibrin in clots and free fibrinogen.
- This can cause low fibrinogen levels, increasing the risk of haemorrhage.

5.4.2 Tissue-type plasminogen activator (TPA)

- Produced using recombinant gene technology.
- Alteplase and reteplase are both TPA.
- Similar side effect profile to streptokinase.

Metabolic response to insult

CONTENTS

6.1 Control of energy production

- Initial hyperglycaemia resulting from increased glucose production and reduced uptake in peripheral tissues.
- Peripherally reduced uptake due to an injury—proportionate insulin resistance, postulated to be due to action of cytokines and dysfunction of glucose transporter proteins.
- This dysfunction persists for several weeks after insult.
- Good evidence that tight glycaemic control reduces both morbidity and mortality in ICU patients.

6.1.1 Clinical considerations

- Analgesia, particularly regional blocks, decreases neurological drive of stress response—a patient in less pain has better homeostasis.
- Volume replacement improves outcome.
- Keeping patient warm reduces catecholamine drive.
- Treating endothelial dysfunction (i.e. SIRS with agents such as activated protein C) limits degree of end-organ dysfunction:
  - Presumed to be due to maintaining the integrity of microcirculation
- Glucose regulation:
  - Conservative: aims to keep glucose below certain value (PRN insulin)
  - Intensive: keeps it within a range of values (sliding scale)

6.2 Metabolic responses to stress including injury, infection, infarction, temperature, and burns

- Response to injury, infection, burns, and infarction is broadly similar.
- Specific aspects alter depending on stimulus—for example, burns cause large amount of tissue damage and subsequent hypovolaemia, so fluid balance disturbances are the most manifest complication.

6.2.1 Cuthbertson's ebb and flow

- Ebb phase is the acute period of suppression within hours of injury:
  - Acidotic
  - Cold
  - Reduced CO, relative hypoxaemia
  - Mediated by catecholamine and cortisol secretion
- Flow phase divided into early (hours to 1st day post-injury), catabolic, and late anabolic stages:
  - 1st part of phase sees mobilization of energy from fat and skeletal muscle stores, increased nitrogen excretion, and high CO
  - Later stages see regeneration of muscle, deposition of fat stores, and a gradual return to normal metabolic state

6.2.2 Activation of response

- Important to treat underlying causes as vigorously as possible, as the response is very proportional to the degree of activation by insult.
- Several groups of factors:
  - Hypovolaemia (believed to be most profound stimulus):
    - Bleeding
    - Gut loss
    - Fluid shift
  - Neurological:
    - Somatic afferents
    - Autonomic
  - Wound factors (largely derived from endothelium, macrophages, and PMNs):
    - Interleukin 1
    - Platelet-activating factor
    - Leukotrienes
  - Free radicals
  - Toxins

6.2.3 If the response goes unchecked

- Systemic inflammatory response syndrome (SIRS):
  - HR >90 or RR >20
  - T <36°C or >38°C
  - WCC <4 × 10^9 or >12 × 10^9
  - Global manifestation involving membrane dysfunction and fluid shift, and often contributing to ventilatory problems
- Multiorgan dysfunction syndrome:
  - The manifestation of the above-mentioned problems on end-organ function
  - Can be reflected in renal function, LFTs, oxygen exchange, etc.

6.2.4 Counter-inflammatory response syndrome

- Provoked by period of SIRS.
- Extremely dangerous as causes immune damping, rendering patient susceptible to nosocomial infection.

PATHOLOGY

Inflammatory response

CONTENTS

1.1 Normal vs abnormal

1.1.1 Normal

- Initial reaction of tissue to 'injury':
  - Vascular phase: dilatation and increased permeability
  - Exudative phase: fluid and cells escape from the permeable vessels
  - Ends with: resolution, suppuration, organization, and progression to chronic inflammation
- Cardinal signs:
  - Calor: heat
  - Rubor: redness
  - Dolour: pain
  - Tumour: swelling
  - Decreased function
- Causes:
  - Physical injury: trauma, crush
  - Chemical injury: acid, alkali, toxins
  - Infective organisms: bacteria, viruses
  - Radiation
  - Temperature: heat, cold
- Vascular phase:
  - Initial vascular dilatation:
    - May last between 15 minutes and several hours
    - Increases blood flow up to 10-fold
    - Increases hydrostatic pressure
    - Results in transudate (low protein)
  - Increased vascular permeability:
    - Leaking of plasma protein into tissues—leading to reduced intravascular oncotic pressure
    - Together with increased hydrostatic pressure leads to fluid leaving vessels for extravascular space

- Caused by contraction of the endothelial cells—mediated by chemical mediators. For example: histamine—direct vascular injury; trauma—endothelial cell injury; radiation; bacterial toxins
- Exudative phase:
  - Accumulation of neutrophils (polymorphonuclear leucocytes) within the extracellular space is the diagnostic histological feature of acute inflammation
  - 3-stage mechanism: margination, adhesion, emigration
  - Margination:
    - Loss of intravascular fluid and increase in plasma viscosity lead to slowing of flow at the site of 'injury', allowing neutrophils to flow closer to the epithelium
  - Adhesion:
    - Increased neutrophil adhesion resulting from interaction between adhesion molecules on neutrophil and endothelial surface
    - Increased expression of adhesion molecules in neutrophil (leucocyte surface adhesion molecule) caused by C5a, leukotriene B4, and tumour necrosis factor (TNF)
    - Increased expression of adhesion molecules on endothelium (ELAM-1, ICAM-1) caused by IL-1, endotoxins, TNF
    - Defective adhesion in diabetes, corticosteroid use, acute alcohol intoxication, and inherited adhesion deficiencies
  - Emigration:
    - Migration through endothelial cells and basement membrane by active amoeboid movement
- Later stages of inflammation:
  - Chemotaxis:
    - Neutrophils are attracted towards certain chemicals—components of complement, IL-8, leukotriene B4, and bacterial products
  - Opsonization:
    - Prepares the particle for phagocytosis by coating in immunoglobulins or complement components
    - Bacterial polysaccharides activate complement via the alternative pathway—generating C3b
    - Antibodies bind to bacterial antigens, activating the classical pathway of complement—also leading to C3b production
    - In immune individuals, immunoglobulins bind to microorganisms leaving an exposed Fc component
    - C3b and Fc act as opsonizing agents, marking the particle for destruction
  - Phagocytosis:
    - Neutrophils start to ingest opsonized particles by sending out pseudopodia around them
    - Once these have met and fused, the particle is contained within a phagosome, bounded by cell membrane
    - Lysosomes (membrane-bound packets of toxic compounds) fuse with the phagosome (forming a phagolysosome) to begin the process of intracellular killing
  - Intracellular killing:
    - Oxygen-dependent and oxygen-independent components
    - Oxygen dependent: neutrophils produce hydrogen peroxide, which reacts with myeloperoxidase producing microbicidal agents; oxygen is reduced by NADPH oxidase to produce free radicals
    - Oxygen independent: lysozymes, lactoferrin, acid hydrolase, and defensins all contribute to intracellular killing

- Defective oxygen killing mechanisms in chronic granulomatous disease (deficiency of NADPH oxidase—recurrent bacterial infections) and myeloperoxidase deficiency (frequent candidal infections)
- Chemical mediators in inflammation:
  - Cause vasodilation and increase vascular permeability as well as emigration of neutrophils and chemotaxis
  - Histamine:
    - Made by mast cells, basophils, and platelets
    - Release stimulated by complement components C3a and C5a, IgE, lysosomal proteins, and physical injury
  - Serotonin: made by platelets
  - Lysosomal compounds: released from neutrophils
  - Prostaglandins:
    - Derived from arachidonic acid
    - Inhibited by NSAIDs
    - Thromboxane A2: made by platelets, causes vasoconstriction and platelet aggregation
    - Prostacyclin: made by endothelium, inhibits platelet aggregation
    - Prostaglandin: pain
  - Cytokines:
    - Also derived from arachidonic acid
    - IL-1 and TNF: fever, increase adhesion molecules, activate neutrophils
    - IL-8: chemotactic
  - Complement cascade:
    - A cascading system of enzymatic proteins activating during inflammation
    - C5a: chemotactic
    - C3b, C4b, C2a: opsonin
    - C3a, C5a: stimulate release of histamine
    - C5b–C9: membrane attack complex (MAC)
  - Kinin cascade:
    - Activated by coagulation factor XII
    - Leads to formation of bradykinin
    - Bradykinin causes vasodilation, increased vascular permeability, bronchoconstriction, and pain
- Local effects of inflammation:
  - Beneficial:
    - Entry of antibodies: vasodilation and increased vascular permeability allow the entry of antibodies into the extracellular space, leading to increased breakdown of microorganisms by lysis or phagocytosis
    - Delivery of nutrients and oxygen: increased blood flow delivers increased nutrients and oxygen to the neutrophils
    - Dilution of toxins: by increasing extracellular fluid
    - Stimulation of the immune system: toxins and particles are drained away in the excess fluid exudate via the lymphatics to adjacent lymph nodes
  - Harmful:
    - Damage to normal tissue: release of enzymes during the inflammatory process may result in digestion of normal tissue
    - Swelling: may cause problems in areas of confined space (e.g. epiglottitis, compartment syndrome, intracranially)
- Systemic effects of inflammation:
  - Malaise
  - Anorexia

- Nausea
- Temperature
- Increased ESR
- Leucocytosis:
  - Neutrophilia in pyogenic infections
  - Eosinophilia in allergic disorders and parasitic infections
  - Lymphocytosis in chronic infection and many viral infections
  - Monocytosis in mononucleosis and certain bacterial infections (TB, typhoid)
- Outcomes of inflammation:
  - Resolution:
    - Usual outcome
    - Restoration of the inflamed tissue to normal
    - Regeneration of damaged tissue
    - Favoured where there has been minimal tissue damage, regenerative capacity of the target tissue, rapid destruction/removal of the causative agent, and rapid removal of the breakdown products of inflammation
  - Suppuration:
    - Persistent causative agent, usually bacterial
    - Pus formation (dead white cells, bacteria, and debris from broken-down cells), gets walled off by a pyogenic membrane
    - This abscess is relatively inaccessible to the body's defences
  - Fibrosis/organization:
    - Large areas of tissue destruction or damage to tissues unable to regenerate
    - Fibrous scarring occurs, forming a scar composed mainly of collagen
    - Scar is inflexible and doesn't contain any specialist structures so may impair tissue/organ function
  - Chronic inflammation:
    - Persistent causative agent
    - Inflammation may last months to years
    - Similar process occurs as in fibrosis but accompanying cellular exudate changes
    - Macrophages, lymphocytes, and plasma cells dominate—these are powerful cytotoxic cells but the toxins they release damage the host's tissues as well as the causative agent

1.1.2 Abnormal

- Abnormalities with the normal pathway of inflammation comprise a large heterogenous group of disorders.
- The immune system is closely involved with a large number of inflammatory disorders:
  - Many immune disorders result in abnormal inflammation
  - Non-immune diseases thought to involve abnormal inflammatory processes include some cancers and atherosclerosis
- As noted previously, a large number of chemical mediators and cellular components are involved in the inflammatory pathway and any of these is open to genetic malformation, which may impair its function or render it non-functional.
- Disorders associated with abnormal inflammation include:
  - Allergies
  - Asthma
  - Autoimmune disorders
  - Chronic inflammation
  - Transplant rejection
  - Vasculitis

1.2 Inflammatory markers

1.2.1 C-reactive protein

- An acute-phase reactant whose levels rise dramatically in response to inflammation.
- Rises in response to increased levels of IL-6, released predominantly by macrophages.
- Synthesized and secreted from the liver.
- Thought to bind to phosphocholine, opsonizing damaged/foreign cells for phagocytosis.
- Used as a diagnostic marker of inflammation.
- Bacterial infections tend to give higher levels of CRP compared to viral infections.

1.2.2 Rheumatoid factor

- An autoantibody—an antibody against the Fc portion of IgG (which is itself an antibody).
- High levels of RF are indicative of rheumatoid arthritis (present in 80%) and Sjögren's syndrome (approaching 100%). The higher the levels, the higher the risk of more destructive arthropathies.

1.2.3 Antinuclear factor

- Antinuclear factors (ANFs), or antinuclear antibodies (ANAs), are a group of autoantibodies directed against the components of the cell nucleus.
- Present in high levels in various autoimmune disorders.
- Conditions associated with high levels of ANF (with their specific subtype of ANF):
  - SLE: all ANF
  - Systemic sclerosis: all ANF, Scl-70
  - Limited scleroderma: all ANF, anti-centromere
  - Sjögren's syndrome: all ANF, anti-RO, anti-La

Immune response

CONTENTS

2.1 Normal

- The normal immune response is divided into a layered response:
  - A physical barrier
  - Innate responses
  - Adaptive responses

2.1.1 Physical barriers

- A number of physical and mechanical barriers protect the body from invasion of foreign organisms:
  - Lungs: coughing and sneezing eject pathogens
  - Eyes: tears flush the eyes
  - Urinary tract: flushed by the passage of urine
  - Lungs and GI tract: mucus barriers prevent their infection
  - GI tract: gastric acid secretion neutralizes most bacteria
  - Genitourinary and GI tracts: commensal flora competitively inhibit the overgrowth of pathogenic organisms
  - Skin: acts as a mechanical barrier against organisms

2.1.2 Innate responses

- Initiated when microbes are identified from components conserved amongst broad groups of microbes.
- Initiated when injured cells send out distress signals.
- Non-specific.
- Does not lead to immunity.
- 4 main functions:
  - Recruiting immune cells to the site of infection/injury
  - Activation of the complement cascade
  - Identification and removal of foreign cells/substances
  - Activation of the adaptive responses by antigen presentation

- Inflammation: one of the 1st responses to infection/injury by the innate immune system. See Chapter G1.
- Innate cellular response:
  - Innate white blood cells: identify and eliminate pathogens
  - Includes neutrophils, eosinophils, basophils, and natural killer cells
- Complement cascade:
  - Biochemical cascade
  - Triggers the recruitment of inflammatory cells
  - Opsonizes pathogens for destruction
  - Destroys the membranes of infected/foreign cells leading to cell destruction

2.1.3 Adaptive responses

- Initiated when enough antigen is presented via the innate response.
- 3 main functions:
  - Recognition of 'non-self' antigens
  - Generation of immune responses specifically tailored to eliminate pathogens or infected cells
  - Development of memory—remembering each pathogen encountered allowing easier elimination of subsequent infections
- Lymphocytes:
  - Cellular component of the adaptive response
  - Subdivided into T and B cells
  - Derived from the same stem cells
- Antigen presentation:
  - Adaptive immunity is dependent on the ability to recognize self and non-self
  - Adaptive immunity is initiated on recognition of non-self antigens
  - Antigens are presented to naive T lymphocytes and activate them to become either CD8 (cytotoxic) cells or CD4 (helper) cells
- T cells:
  - Subdivided into CD8 and CD4 cells, respectively killer and helper cells
  - CD8 (cytotoxic T cells, killer T cells, cytotoxic T lymphocytes (CTLs)):
    - Subgroup of T lymphocytes
    - Induce the death of cells infected with viruses and other parasites, or that are otherwise damaged or malfunctioning
    - Activated when they encounter a specific antigen
    - Once activated they undergo rapid clonal expansion—dividing rapidly—and then travel around the body in search of this antigen
    - When they find cells bearing this antigen they release cytotoxins, puncturing the target cell's membrane and lysing it
    - Activation is tightly controlled and requires a strong antigen activation signal or additional prompting from helper (CD4) cells
    - A few T cells remain even after the resolution of the infection, forming immune memory, which can quickly be activated should the same pathogen be encountered again
  - CD4 (helper T cells):
    - Manage the immune response
    - Activation of helper cells leads to release of assorted cytokines, influencing the activity of many other immune cells
- B cells:
  - Create antibodies:
    - Large 'Y'-shaped proteins that identify and neutralize foreign material

- 5 subtypes—IgA, IgD, IgE, IgG, and IgM
- Each has specific actions against different types of antigen
- Upon activation, B cells produce antibodies specific to an antigen and neutralize it
- Activated by encounter with its specific antigen (with additional signals from T helper cells) and then multiplies and matures into a plasma cell
- Plasma cells pump out antibodies over their short lifetime (2–3 days), which bind to their specific antigen, opsonizing them and activating the complement cascade
- ~10% of plasma cells survive, forming further antigen-specific immune memory cells ready to fight off further infection should it occur

2.2 Abnormal

2.2.1 Hypersensitivity

- An immune response that damages the body's own tissues.
- Subdivided into 4 types based on the mechanisms and time course.
- Type I:
  - Allergic reaction—atopy, anaphylaxis, asthma
  - Provoked by re-exposure to a specific antigen
  - Mediated by IgE, released from mast cells and basophils
- Type II:
  - Cytotoxic, antibody-dependent reaction—autoimmune thrombocytopenic purpura, haemolytic disease of the newborn
  - Antibodies bind to antigens on 'self' cells, marking them for destruction
  - Mediated by IgG and IgM
- Type III:
  - Immune complex disease—SLE, polyarteritis nodosum
  - Small antigen–antibody immune complexes not cleared effectively by the macrophages and deposited in various tissues leading to damage
  - IgG or IgM mediated
- Type IV:
  - Delayed hypersensitivity—type 1 DM, MS
  - T-cell mediated (not antibody dependent)
  - T cells targeting specific 'self' cells proliferate, destroying them on contact

2.2.2 Autoimmunity

- Overactive immune response.
- Failure to distinguish 'self' from 'non-self' leading to immune attack of assorted body tissues.
- Examples include autoimmune hepatitis, Goodpasture's syndrome, MS, and rheumatoid arthritis.

2.2.3 Immunodeficiency

- Occurs when one or more components of the immune system are not present or malfunctioning.
- Can be inherited or acquired.
- Malnutrition is one of the leading causes worldwide.
- Inherited: DiGeorge syndrome, Omenn syndrome.
- Acquired: AIDS, many types of cancer.

CHAPTER G3

Infection

CONTENTS

The candidate should know the typical causes, pathological processes, and investigation of the following infections presenting to an ED.

3.1 Upper respiratory tract

- Comprises a spectrum of disease—common cold, rhinitis, laryngitis, epiglottitis, and sinusitis.

3.1.1 Typical causes

- Mainly viral.
- ~15% bacterial, commonly *Streptococcus*.

3.1.2 Pathological processes

- Person-to-person spread.
- Direct invasion of the mucosal lining of the upper respiratory tract.
- Typical incubation period of 1–5 days.

3.1.3 Investigations

- Rarely required other than in certain situations:
  - Mononucleosis—young people with sore throat, marked lymphadenopathy, and hepatosplenomegaly require testing for infectious mononucleosis
  - Immunocompromised individuals

3.2 Lower respiratory tract and pneumonia

- Inflammation of the lung parenchyma.
- Characterized by consolidation of the alveolar air spaces with exudate and inflammatory cells.

3.2.1 Typical causes

- Bacterial, viral, or fungal:
  - Bacterial:
    - *Haemophilus influenzae*
    - *Streptococcus pneumoniae*
    - *Moraxella catarrhalis*
    - More rarely: *Staphylococcus aureus* (usually postviral), *Legionella, Chlamydia psittaci* (exposure to parrots)
  - Viral:
    - Influenza
    - Parainfluenza
    - RSV
  - Fungal:
    - Rare, usually in immunocompromised individuals
    - *Candida* spp. and *Aspergillus* spp.

3.2.2 Pathological processes

- Usually via inhalation of pathogenic organisms.
- Less commonly secondary to bacteraemia from another source.
- Fever, productive cough, pleuritic chest pain.
- Atypical causes have atypical presentations (e.g. extrapulmonary features).
- Acute inflammation leads to migration of neutrophils into the airspaces; these ingest the microbes and kill them. They also exude a chromatin meshwork containing antimicrobial proteins that trap pathogens—known as neutrophil extracellular traps (NETs).

3.2.3 Investigations

- CXR.
- Sputum culture.
- Blood cultures.
- U&E including CRP.
- FBC.
- ABGs.
- If atypical cause is suspected think about LFTs (transiently and mildly raised in psittacosis, Q fever, and *Legionella*), phosphate (hypophosphataemia suggests Legionnaires disease), urinalysis (for *Legionella* antigen and microscopic haematuria—also in Legionnaires disease).

3.3 Meningitis and encephalitis

- Meningitis: inflammation of the meninges characteristically leading to signs of meningism: headache, neck stiffness, and photophobia.
- Encephalitis: inflammation of the brain parenchyma typically presenting with diffuse and/or focal neuropsychological dysfunction.

3.3.1 Typical causes

- Meningitis:
  - Bacterial:
    - Newborns: group B *Streptococcus, E. coli*
    - Children: *Neisseria meningitides, Strep. pneumoniae, Haemophilus influenzae* type B (vaccination has reduced the incidence of this by >90%)
    - Adults: *N. meningitides, Strep. pneumoniae*
  - Viral:
    - Enteroviruses
    - Herpes simplex type 2
    - Varicella zoster
    - Mumps
    - HIV
  - Fungal:
    - *Cryptococcus neoformans*
    - *Candida* spp.
    - *Aspergillus* spp.
  - Non-infectious:
    - Cancer
    - Systemic inflammatory conditions (e.g. SLE, vasculitis)
- Encephalitis:
  - Viral:
    - Herpes simplex
    - Varicella zoster
    - HIV
    - Rabies
  - Bacterial:
    - Spread from meningitis
    - Syphilis

3.3.2 Pathological processes

- Meningitis:
  - Infective agent reaches the meninges either via the bloodstream or direct contact between the meninges and the nasal cavity. May also be direct contamination of cerebrospinal fluid (CSF) via indwelling devices or skull fractures
  - Agents enter the subarachnoid space at weakness in the blood–brain barrier (e.g. choroid plexus)
  - Inflammation in the subarachnoid space due to the immune response to the presence of infective agent
  - Blood–brain barrier becomes progressively more permeable due to cytokine release, leading to cerebral oedema
  - Inflammation of the meninges due to influx of WBCs leading to interstitial oedema
  - Cerebral vasculitis leads to decreased blood flow and oedema secondary to cell death through hypoperfusion
  - Oedema leads to raised intracranial pressure
- Encephalitis:
  - Fever, headache, photophobia, and confusion (occasionally seizures) are manifestations of the condition brought on by the inflammation of the brain parenchyma
  - The body's defence mechanisms cause this inflammation

3.3.3 Investigations

- Meningitis:
  - FBC, CRP, blood cultures, viral serology, meningococcal PCR
  - Lumbar puncture (LP; contraindicated if signs/symptoms of raised intracranial pressure—if present then a CT is required prior to LP):
    - CSF in bacterial meningitis: raised WCC (neutrophils), high protein, low glucose
    - CSF in viral meningitis: raised WCC, normal or high protein, normal glucose
- Encephalitis:
  - FBC, CRP, blood cultures
  - LP: normally raised WCC, normal protein, normal glucose
  - MRI is the most useful imaging modality

3.4 Myocarditis and endocarditis

- Myocarditis—inflammation of the myocardium; presents with a variable picture.
- Endocarditis—inflammation of the endocardium; usually involves the valves and again has a variable presentation.

3.4.1 Typical causes

- Myocarditis:
  - Viral: HIV, coxsackievirus, *Enterovirus, Cytomegalovirus*, rubella, and polio
  - Bacterial: *Brucella, Neisseria gonorrhoeae* (gonococcus), *Haemophilus influenzae*
  - Fungal: *Aspergillus, Candida*
  - Drugs: ethanol, chemotherapeutic agents, antipsychotics, antibiotics (e.g. penicillin, chloramphenicol)
  - Bites/stings: scorpion, snake, black widow spider
  - Toxins: arsenic, lead, mercury
  - Physical agents: radiation, electric shock
  - Systemic inflammatory disorders: SLE, sarcoidosis, RA, systemic vasculitis (e.g. Wegener's granulomatosis)
- Endocarditis:
  - Usually infective: *Streptococcus, Staphylococcus*

3.4.2 Pathological processes

- Myocarditis:
  - Symptoms are related to the inflammation of the myocardium or the weakness that is secondary to it
  - Direct cytotoxic effects of the causative agent
  - Immune response to the causative agent
  - Acute myocardial damage: myocyte destruction as a consequence of the causative agent
  - Chronic myocardial damage: continuing destruction of myocytes is autoimmune in nature due to abnormal expression of human leucocyte antigen (HLA)
- Endocarditis:
  - Generally occurs due to turbulence around the endothelial surface allowing bacteria to adhere to lesions on the endocardium during transient bacteraemia. Lesions/turbulence may be secondary to underlying structural problems, damaged heart valves (e.g. by rheumatic fever), or prosthetic valves
  - New-onset murmur caused by the vegetations on the heart valves
  - Low-grade fever

- Petechiae, splinter haemorrhages, Osler's nodes (tender subcutaneous nodules on pads of digits), Janeway lesions (non-tender maculae on palms and soles), and Roth spots (retinal haemorrhages) are the classic signs of infective endocarditis, though only ~50% of patients present with them
- Signs of systemic infectious emboli in left-sided disease

3.4.3 Investigations

- Myocarditis:
  - ECG: diffuse T-wave inversion, saddle-shaped ST segment elevation
  - FBC, CRP, blood cultures, troponin
  - Viral titres
  - Echocardiography
  - Myocardial biopsy is the gold standard
- Endocarditis:
  - Duke Criteria need to be fulfilled to establish a diagnosis of endocarditis. Either 2 major criteria, 1 major and 3 minor, or 5 minor criteria need to be fulfilled
  - Major criteria:
    - Positive blood cultures (2 separate cultures from 2 separate sites drawn 12 hours apart, positive for typical endocarditis organisms)
    - Evidence of endocardial involvement on echo (e.g. vegetation, abscess, new-onset regurgitation)
  - Minor criteria:
    - Predisposing factor (known lesion, IVDU)
    - Fever >38°C
    - Evidence of embolism
    - Immunological condition
    - Positive blood culture that doesn't meet major criteria
    - Positive echo that doesn't meet major criteria

3.5 Hepatitis

- Injury to the liver characterized by the presence of inflammatory cells within the organ.
- Can be self-limiting or lead to scarring.
- May be acute (<6 months' duration) or chronic.

3.5.1 Typical causes

- Viruses:
  - Hepatitis A:
    - Picornavirus
    - Single-stranded RNA
    - Faeco–oral spread
    - Causes acute hepatitis
    - Self-limiting
    - Vaccine available
  - Hepatitis B:
    - Hepadnavirus
    - DNA virus
    - Blood/body fluid spread
    - Can be acute and self-limiting (less so in children)

- May lead to chronic hepatitis, cirrhosis, and hepatocellular carcinoma
- Vaccine available
- Hepatitis C:
  - Hepacivirus
  - Single-stranded RNA
  - Blood/body fluid spread (usually blood)
  - Acute phase usually asymptomatic
  - Variable chronic course but may progress to cirrhosis
  - No vaccine available
- Hepatitis D:
  - Deltavirus
  - Small, circular, single-stranded RNA virus
  - Occurs only in conjunction with Hep B
  - Transmission mostly associated with IV drug use
  - Mumps, rubella, cytomegalovirus, Epstein–Barr
- Alcohol.
- Toxins/drugs:
  - Amatoxin-containing mushrooms (e.g. death cap)
  - Amiodarone
  - Amitriptyline
  - Halothane
  - Ketoconazole
  - Methotrexate
  - Paracetamol
  - Phenytoin
- Autoimmune.
- Metabolic:
  - Haemochromatosis
  - Wilson's disease

3.5.2 Pathological processes

- Initial features are usually non-specific—aches, fever, nausea, vomiting, diarrhoea.
- More specific signs/symptoms include loss of appetite, dark urine, jaundice, abdominal pain, hepatomegaly.
- Extensive damage to the liver in chronic hepatitis leads to healing with scarring (cirrhosis) and therefore development of the signs/symptoms of cirrhosis (e.g. hepatomegaly, jaundice, palmar erythema, gynaecomastia, ascites, spider naevi).

3.5.3 Investigations

- FBC.
- U&E, including LFTs.
- Clotting studies.
- Hepatitis serology.

3.6 Gastroenteritis

- Inflammation of the GI tract; most often caused by viruses, less so by bacteria.
- Inadequate treatment leads to ~5–8 million deaths per year globally.
- Main symptoms are diarrhoea with or without vomiting.

3.6.1 Typical causes

- Viral:
  - Norovirus (~70% of food-borne cases)
  - Rotavirus (~20% of food-borne cases)
  - Adenovirus
  - Astrovirus
- Bacteria:
  - *Salmonella*
  - *Shigella*
  - *Staphylococcus*
  - *Campylobacter*
  - *E. coli*
  - *Clostridium*

3.6.2 Pathological processes

- Infectious agents adhere to mucous membrane, invade, and produce enterotoxin and/or cytotoxin.
- Leads to increased fluid secretion and/or decreased absorption, giving increased fluid content within the bowel that cannot adequately be reabsorbed. This in turn leads to dehydration and loss of electrolytes.
- Enterotoxins (typically *E. coli* or cholera infections) act directly on secretory mechanisms leading to production of copious amounts of watery diarrhoea.
- Cytotoxins (typically *Shigella* or *C. difficile* infections) destroy mucosal cells leading to a decreased reabsorptive ability.

3.6.3 Investigations

- FBC.
- U&E.
- Stool culture.

3.7 Urinary tract infection (UTI)

- Defined as a significant bacteriuria in the presence of symptoms.
- Much more common in women. In males aged 3 months to 50 years, incidence of UTI is low and the possibility of an anatomical abnormality must be entertained in this age group.

3.7.1 Typical causes

- ~80% of community-acquired UTIs are caused by *E. coli*.
- Other less common pathogens include *Staphylococcus saprophyticus*, *Klebsiella*, and *Proteus*.

3.7.2 Pathological processes

- Bacteria ascend into the bladder via the urethra.
- Sexual intercourse may promote this migration.
- Normally a thin film of urine remains in the bladder after emptying and any bacteria present are removed by mucosal cell production of organic acids.

3.7.3 Investigations

- Mid-stream urine (MSU).

3.8 Sexually transmitted disease (STD)

- STD (or STI—sexually transmitted infection) is an illness with a significant chance of transmission during sexual contact.

3.8.1 Typical causes

- Bacterial:
  - Gonorrhoea
  - Syphilis
  - Non-gonococcal urethritis
  - Chlamydia
- Viral:
  - HIV
  - Hepatitis (B)
  - Herpes simplex
  - Genital warts
  - Cervical cancer (from human papilloma virus—recently introduced vaccination programme should reduce/eradicate this)
- Fungal: tinea cruris.
- Parasites: *Phthirius pubis* (crab louse).

3.8.2 Pathological processes

- Infections are more easily transmitted through mucous membranes as they allow certain pathogens through.
- Some pathogens occur in larger amounts in genital fluids compared to saliva.

3.8.3 Investigations

- Urethral swabs.
- Vaginal swabs.
- MSU.
- Bloods for HIV may be indicated.
- Syphilis serology.

3.9 Pelvic inflammatory disease (PID)

- Inflammation of the female uterus, fallopian tubes, and/or ovaries.
- May progress to scar formation with adhesions to nearby tissues and organs.
- Scarring may lead to fertility problems and increase the chance of ectopic pregnancies.

3.9.1 Typical causes

- Gonorrhoea.
- Chlamydia.

3.9.2 Pathological processes

- Pelvic inflammatory disease is caused by organisms ascending to the upper female genital tract from the vagina and cervix.

3.9.3 Investigations

- FBC.
- CRP.
- Urinalysis.
- High vaginal swabs.

3.10 Cellulitis

- An acute spreading infection of the dermis and subcutaneous tissues.

3.10.1 Typical causes

- Group A *Streptococcus*.
- *Staphylococcus aureus*.
- Facial cellulitis is frequently associated with *Haemophilus influenzae* type B and *Streptococcus pneumoniae*.

3.10.2 Pathological processes

- Skin and subcutaneous tissues are involved when microorganisms invade disrupted skin.
- Cellulitis frequently occurs in areas where no apparent injury exists. This is common in dry and irritated skin where microscopic breaks allow penetration of bacteria.

3.10.3 Investigations

- Not usually required.
- FBC, U&E, and blood cultures, along with wound swabs, may be considered in more severe infections.

3.11 Infection of bones and joints

- Osteomyelitis (bone infection) is an acute or chronic inflammatory process of the bone and its structures secondary to infection with pyogenic organisms.
- Septic arthritis (joint infection) is inflammation of a synovial membrane with purulent effusion into the joint capsule, usually due to bacterial infection.

3.11.1 Typical causes

- Osteomyelitis:
  - *Staphylococcus aureus* is far and away the most common organism
  - Occasionally *Enterobacter* or *Streptococcus* spp.
- Septic arthritis:
  - *Staphylococcus aureus*
  - *Streptococcus* spp.
  - *Haemophilus influenzae*—was the most common cause in children but is now uncommon in areas where vaccination is practised
  - *Neisseria gonorrhoea*—in young adults
  - Tuberculous—typically in the spine

3.11.2 Pathological processes

- Osteomyelitis:
  - The infection may be localized or it may spread through the periosteum, cortex, marrow, and cancellous bone
  - Haematogenous osteomyelitis is an infection caused by bacterial seeding from the blood
  - Direct osteomyelitis is caused by direct contact of the tissue and bacteria during trauma or surgery
  - Once the bone is infected, leucocytes enter the infected area and in their attempt to engulf the infectious organisms they release enzymes that lyse the bone
  - New bone formation around the area of necrosis is called an involucrum
- Septic arthritis:
  - Bacteria are carried by the bloodstream from an infectious focus elsewhere, introduced by a wound that penetrates the joint, or introduced by extension from adjacent tissue
  - The knee accounts for ~40–50% of joint infections; the hip accounts for 20–25% of joint infections
  - In infants and very young children, hip involvement is most common

3.11.3 Investigations

- Osteomyelitis:
  - FBC
  - CRP
  - Blood cultures
  - X-ray (bony changes are not evident for 14–21 days and initially manifest as periosteal elevation followed by cortical or medullary lucencies)
- Septic arthritis:
  - FBC
  - CRP
  - Blood cultures
  - X-ray
  - Joint aspiration for microscopy and culture (should be undertaken in sterile environment, e.g. theatre)

3.12 AIDS

- Disease of the immune system caused by HIV.

3.12.1 Cause

- HIV.

3.12.2 Pathological processes

- Spread by sexual contact; blood or blood products (if not screened) including shared needles in IVDU and needle stick injuries; and mother to child.
- Enters macrophages and CD4 T cells.
- An enzyme called reverse transcriptase liberates the single-stranded RNA genome from the attached viral proteins and copies it into a complementary DNA molecule.
- Viral DNA is then transported into the cell nucleus.
- Integration of the viral DNA into the host cell's genome is carried out by another viral enzyme called integrase.

3.12.3 Investigations

- Serological tests for HIV.

3.13 Pyrexia of unknown origin (PUO)

- An elevated temperature for which no cause has been found despite thorough investigation.

3.13.1 Typical causes

- Infections (e.g. extrapulmonary tuberculosis, endocarditis).
- Neoplasms (e.g. lymphoma).
- Collagen vascular disorders (e.g. temporal arteritis).
- Other causes (e.g. drug reactions).

3.13.2 Pathological processes

- Vary dependent upon the cause.

3.13.3 Investigations

- Repeated, thorough history and examination.
- FBC.
- U&E.
- Cultures: blood, sputum, urine, stool, CSF.
- Vial serology.
- Autoantibodies.
- CRP, ESR.
- CXR.
- Possibly abdominal ultrasound (USS)/CT.

3.14 Malaria

- Malaria is a vector-borne infectious disease.
- Caused by parasitic protozoa species of the genus *Plasmodium*.
- 4 main types that affect humans: *Plasmodium vivax*, *P. ovale*, and *P. malariae* cause milder disease in humans that is not generally fatal; *P. falciparum* causes the most severe morbidity and mortality.
- Most deadly vector-borne disease worldwide.
- 350–500 million cases of malaria worldwide per year, killing 1–3 million people.
- No vaccine available and preventative drugs are not 100% effective.

3.14.1 Causes

- *P. vivax*.
- *P. ovale*.
- *P. malariae*.
- *P. falciparum*.

3.14.2 Pathological processes

- Primary host and vector is female *Anopheles* mosquito.
- When an infected mosquito bites a human, a number of sporozoites from the saliva are injected into the bloodstream.

- These migrate to the liver where they infect hepatocytes (within 30 minutes of injection) and multiply asexually for ~6–15 days.
- Differentiate into merozoites and, following rupture of the hepatocytes, escape into the bloodstream and infect red blood cells (RBCs).
- Multiply asexually within the RBCs, periodically breaking out to infect more RBCs, leading to the classic periodic fever.
- P. vivax and P. ovale may lie dormant in the liver as hypnozoites for periods of up to 3 years (normally 6–12 months).
- The parasite is relatively protected from the immune system due to reproduction within the body's own cells.
- Some merozoites differentiate into gametocytes, which can be picked up by another feeding mosquito and can then reproduce sexually within its gut, producing sporozoites that travel to the salivary glands, thus completing the cycle.

3.14.3 Investigations

- Thick and thin blood films should identify the protozoa but may need to be repeated.
- FBC, U&E, and blood cultures may also be indicated.

3.15 Fungal infection

- May be superficial (e.g. cutaneous tinea infections) or systemic (e.g. *Aspergillus* pneumonia).

3.15.1 Typical causes

- Superficial:
  - Tinea versicolor—caused by *Malassezia globosa*; yeast infection leading to lighter or darker patches of skin
  - Ringworm (tinea)—caused by dermatophytes; classified by region infected:
    - Tinea capitis—scalp
    - Tinea corporis—trunk and extremities
    - Tinea cruris—groin
- Systemic:
  - *Candida*
  - Aspergillosis

3.15.2 Pathological processes

- Superficial fungi thrive in warm, moist conditions.
- May be present on skin without active infection.
- Spread by person-to-person contact.
- Most systemic fungal infections are opportunist infections, affecting those with already compromised immune systems.

3.15.3 Investigations

- Skin/nail scrapings.
- Direct examination with UV (Wood's) light will fluoresce ~50% of ringworm fungi.
- Other investigations as appropriate, dependent on site of infection.

Wound healing

CONTENTS

4.1 General principles

- 5 stages:
  - Haemostasis
  - Inflammation
  - Reconstruction
  - Epithelialization
  - Maturation

4.1.1 Haemostasis

- Primary haemostasis—local vascular contraction and platelet plug formation.
- Activation of the clotting cascade.

4.1.2 Inflammation

- Prepares the wound for healing.
- Serves to remove bacteria, foreign material, and devitalized tissue.
- Prolongation of this stage will lead to proliferation and increased activity of macrophages.
- This leads to increased inflammation and ultimately poor wound healing.

4.1.3 Reconstruction—fibroplasia and contraction

- Fibroblasts begin synthesizing collagen and elastin (takes ~4 days).
- Macrophages release growth factor stimulating new blood vessel formation.
- Contraction (movement of the wound edges toward the centre of the defect) mediated by fibroblasts (which have the ability to contract).

4.1.4 Epithelialization

- In wounds that are closed the surface develops epithelial coverage in ~24–48 hours.
- Surface debris/eschar/devitalized wound edges impair this process.

4.1.5 Maturation

- Amount of scar tissue influenced by forces across the wound.
- Wound gains strength as collagen matures.
- Further remodelling/maturation for up to 2 years.

4.2 Specific tissues

4.2.1 Skin

- Mechanism of injury:
  - Laceration
  - Incised wound
  - Abrasion
  - Bite
  - Burn
  - Crush
  - Chemical injury
  - Puncture wound
- Timing of the wound:
  - Consider need for delayed closure
- Environment:
  - Potential wound contamination
  - Foreign body

4.2.2 Tendon

- Reconstruction stage lasts about 6 weeks.
- Never regains full strength.
- Heals with fibrous tissue scar.
- Controlled movement of tendon during reconstruction stage improves healing.

4.2.3 Peripheral nerve

- 3 categories of injury based on the damage sustained by the nerve components, nerve functionality, and the ability for spontaneous recovery:
  - Neurapraxia:
    - Mildest form of nerve injury
    - Reduction or block of conduction across a segment
    - Nerve conduction is preserved both proximal and distal to the lesion but not across the lesion
    - For example, foot 'going to sleep' after legs have been crossed for too long
  - Axonotmesis:
    - More severe grade of nerve injury
    - Neural tube intact but axons are disrupted
    - These nerves are likely to recover
  - Neurotmesis:
    - Most severe grade of peripheral nerve injury
    - The neural tube is severed
    - These injuries are likely permanent without repair

4.2.4 Bone

- Classically divided into 3 phases:
  - Reactive:
    - Equivalent to haemostatic and inflammatory stages
  - Reparative:
    - Callus formation and lamellar bone deposition—equivalent to reconstruction and epithelialization stages
    - The periosteal cells proximal to the fracture gap and fibroblasts within the granulation tissue at the fracture develop into chondroblasts and form hyaline cartilage
    - The periosteal cells distal to the fracture gap develop into osteoblasts and form woven bone
    - These tissues grow and unite to form a fracture callus
    - The next phase is the replacement of the fracture callus with lamellar bone by osteoblasts
  - Remodelling:
    - The lamellar bone is replaced with compact bone and eventually the remodelled bone closely resembles the original structure
    - Can take up to 18 months
    - Usually about 80% of normal strength by ~3 months

4.2.5 Myocardium

- Usually injured by infarction.
- Coronary arteries are end arteries so blockage leads to cell death.
- No reparative/regenerative capability.
- Leads to collagen scar formation, which may lead to arrhythmias or rupture.

4.2.6 Brain

- No reparative/regenerative function.
- Can lead to permanent disabilities.
- Some degree of compensation/taking over of function from other brain areas.

Haematology

CONTENTS

5.1 Anaemia

- Less than normal number of RBCs or lower than normal concentration of haemoglobin.

5.1.1 Classification

- By size of RBC:
  - Macrocytic: larger than normal
  - Microcytic: smaller than normal
  - Normocytic: normal size

5.1.2 Causes

- Macrocytic:
  - Megaloblastic anaemia:
    - Deficiency of vitamin B12, folate, or both
    - Can be caused by insufficient intake or insufficient absorption
    - Vitamin B12 deficiency can cause neurological symptoms whereas folate deficiency does not
    - Pernicious anaemia is secondary to insufficient absorption of vitamin B12 caused by a lack of intrinsic factor; this is usually a result of autoantibodies targeting parietal cells that produce it or targeting intrinsic factor itself
    - Insufficient absorption can also be secondary to removal of part of the stomach (e.g. gastric bypass surgery)
  - Hypothyroidism
  - Methotrexate and other drugs that inhibit DNA synthesis
  - Alcoholism and other forms of liver disease can cause a macrocytosis but not necessarily anaemia
- Microcytic:
  - Problems with haem synthesis (e.g. iron deficiency)
  - Problems with globin synthesis (e.g. thalassaemia)
  - Lead poisoning

- Normocytic:
  - Acute blood loss
  - Anaemia of chronic disease—the result of the actions of cytokines on iron metabolism
  - Aplastic anaemia
  - Haemolytic anaemia

5.1.3 Investigations

- FBC.
- ESR.
- Ferritin.
- Serum iron.
- Transferrin.
- Serum vitamin B12 and folate.
- In difficult cases, a bone marrow biopsy may be necessary.

5.2 Leukaemia

- Malignant disease of the blood or bone marrow leading to an increase in white blood cells.
- Presents with symptoms related to dysfunction of blood constituents (e.g. excessive bruising, excessive bleeding, petechial haemorrhages, frequent infections, and anaemia). Also fever, chills, night sweats, splenomegaly, and weight loss.

5.2.1 Classification

- Acute leukaemias:
  - Characterized by the rapid increase of immature blood cells
  - Crowding makes the marrow unable to produce healthy cells
  - Immediate treatment required due to rapid progression and accumulation of malignant cells, which spill over into the bloodstream
  - Most common form of leukaemia in children
- Chronic leukaemias:
  - Excessive build-up of more mature, abnormal WBCs
  - Takes months/years to progress
  - May be monitored for some time before treatment is begun
  - Mostly occurs in older people but can affect any age group
- Additionally, each of the earlier mentioned divisions can be subdivided according to the cell line affected:
  - Lymphoblastic leukaemias: affect lymphocytes, usually B cells
  - Myeloid leukaemias: affect the marrow cells that go on to form RBCs, eosinophils, basophils, and neutrophils as well as platelets

5.2.2 Acute lymphoblastic leukaemia

- Most common type of leukaemia in young children.
- Also affects adults, especially those over 65.
- Treatment: usually chemo- and radiotherapy.
- Survival: ~85% in children, ~50% in adults (overall).

5.2.3 Chronic lymphoblastic leukaemia

- Most commonly affects adults over 55.
- Almost never affects children.

- Treatment: incurable but treatments are based on controlling symptoms and are almost always chemotherapy based.

5.2.4 Acute myeloid leukaemia

- Occurs more commonly in adults than children.
- More commonly in men than women.
- Treatment: chemotherapeutic agents.
- Survival: ~40% at 5 years.

5.2.5 Chronic myeloid leukaemia

- Occurs mainly in adults.
- A small number of children affected.
- Treatment: chemotherapeutic agents.
- Survival: ~90% at 5 years.

5.3 Lymphoma and myeloma

5.3.1 Lymphoma

- Heterogenous group of lymphocyte cancers presenting as a solid mass of lymphoid cells.
- Latest classification system is the WHO classification system from 2008 which groups lymphomas by cell type:
  - Mature B-cell neoplasms:
    - Burkitt's lymphoma
    - Follicular lymphoma
  - Mature T-cell and natural killer (NK) cell neoplasms:
    - Aggressive NK cell lymphoma
    - Anaplastic large cell lymphoma
  - Hodgkin's lymphoma:
    - Treated as a separate group but now recognized as being a mature B-cell neoplasm
- Signs and symptoms can include:
  - Night sweats
  - Weight loss
  - Lymph node enlargement
  - Splenomegaly
  - Hepatosplenomegaly
- Investigations:
  - FBC
  - U&E including LFTs and LDH
  - CXR
  - Full diagnosis/staging will require CT and biopsy
- Treatment and prognosis are dependent on the exact classification of the disease but treatment will usually include a combination of radiotherapy and chemotherapy.

5.3.2 Myeloma

- An incurable cancer of plasma cells (the B cells responsible for the production of antibodies).
- Difficult to diagnose due to effects on many body systems.

- Signs and symptoms are varied and are caused by the varying proteins released from the malignant plasma cells or their consequences:
  - Bone pain/fractures:
    - Usually spine and ribs
    - Production of RANKL (receptor activator for nuclear factor κB-ligand) by plasma cells, which binds to receptors on osteoclasts and induces bone resorption
    - The bone lesions are lytic and lead to hypercalcaemia
  - Infections:
    - Decreased production and increased destruction of normal antibodies opens the patient up to an increased risk of infection
  - Anaemia
  - Renal failure:
    - Hypercalcaemia damages the kidneys, as can the deposition of light chains produced by the malignant plasma cells, leading to either acute or chronic renal failure
  - Neurological symptoms:
    - Weakness, confusion, and fatigue secondary to hypercalcaemia
    - Also pathological vertebral fractures may lead to spinal cord syndromes
- Investigations:
  - FBC
  - U&E including calcium
  - Serum and urine electrophoresis:
    - Looking for paraproteins (e.g. Bence–Jones urinary paraproteins)
  - Further investigations may well include a skeletal survey and bone marrow biopsy along with further bloods looking at immunoglobulin levels and β2-microglobulin
- Treatment is usually aimed at inducing remission and is usually based on high-dose chemotherapy.
- Bone marrow transplant may be offered to younger patients.

5.4 Coagulation

5.4.1 Platelet disorders

- Platelets arise from the fragmentation of the cytoplasm of megakaryocytes in the bone marrow.
- Circulate as anuclear cells.
- Platelet disorders lead to problems with primary haemostasis (platelet plug formation) and therefore have different signs and symptoms to secondary haemostatic problems (e.g. coagulation factor deficiencies).
- Broadly divided into 4 categories:
  - Disorders leading to reduced platelet count:
    - Thrombocytopenia (e.g. idiopathic thrombocytopenic purpura (ITP)): an autoimmune disorder with autoantibodies against platelets
    - Aplastic anaemia: can be autoimmune or toxin mediated (e.g. drugs), or secondary to infection (e.g. viral hepatitis). Leads to a pancytopenia as the bone marrow fails to produce enough new cells
    - Gaucher's disease: a lysosomal storage disease leading to the accumulation of lipids within cells and tissues, including the bone marrow, leading to a pancytopenia
  - Disorders leading to raised platelet count:
    - Thrombocytosis: can be primary (or essential thrombocytosis) or reactive

- Primary thrombocytosis is a myeloproliferative disorder of unknown cause, which in some cases may progress into acute myeloid leukaemia or myelofibrosis. May lead to very high platelet counts and increased risk of thrombosis
- Reactive thrombocytosis may be due to inflammation, hyposplenia, or asplenia
- Disorders leading to platelet dysfunction and/or reduced count:
  - HELLP syndrome: a variant of pre-eclampsia consisting of **H**aemolytic anaemia, **E**levated **L**iver enzymes, and **L**ow **P**latelets. Activation of the clotting cascade leads to overconsumption of platelets
  - Haemolytic-uraemic syndrome: mediated by toxins released from enterohaemorrhagic *E. coli*. Causes haemolytic anaemia, acute kidney injury (uraemia), and thrombocytopenia. It predominantly affects children
  - Dengue: a viral haemorrhagic fever caused by the flavivirus, found in the tropics. Headaches, myalgia, arthralgia, fever, and petechial rash are the main symptoms. Causes a thrombocytopenia
- Disorders of platelet adhesion:
  - Von Willebrand disease: a deficiency of von Willebrand factor, which is required for clotting
  - 4 types of inherited disease:
    - 1: heterozygous for defective gene, leads to decreased levels of VWF
    - 2: qualitative defect, bleeding tendency varies dependent on exact defect
    - 3: homozygous for defective gene (most severe form)
    - 4: platelet type, a defect in the VWF receptor on the platelet
- Signs and symptoms:
  - Bleeding from mucous membranes (e.g. epistaxis, bleeding from gums)
  - Bruising
  - Petechial rash
- Investigations:
  - FBC including blood films
  - May require more specialist investigations (e.g. bleeding times, bone marrow biopsy)
- Treatment is dependent on cause.

5.4.2 Inherited and acquired coagulation disorder

- Inherited:
  - Haemophilia:
    - Recessive X-linked disorders affecting clotting factors
    - Haemophilia A (factor VIII deficiency) is the most common
    - Haemophilia B or Christmas disease is a deficiency of factor IX
    - Leads to secondary haemostasis problems: major haemorrhage, re-bleeding, haemarthrosis (traumatic or spontaneous), and large soft tissue haematomas
    - Treated/controlled with regular infusions of the missing factor
    - Some haemophiliacs develop antibodies against the replacement factors, leading to increased requirements of the factor or the need for non-human factors, such as porcine factor VIII
  - Von Willebrand disease (see Section 5.4.1)
- Acquired:
  - Toxins/drugs (e.g. rattlesnake and viper venom, warfarin):
    - Warfarin inhibits the vitamin K-dependent synthesis of clotting factors II, VII, IX, and X, as well as protein C, protein S, and protein Z (regulatory proteins)
  - Infections, such as viral haemorrhagic fevers (VHFs) (e.g. dengue, Ebola, etc.)

- In most VHFs the aetiology of the coagulopathy is most likely multifactorial (e.g. hepatic damage, consumptive coagulopathy, primary marrow dysfunction)
- Liver failure:
  - Liver failure leads to decreased protein synthesis
- DIC:
  - A consumptive coagulopathy leading to depletion of platelets and clotting factors
  - Leads to the formation of microemboli within the vascular system, which can affect end-organ function
  - Many causes: cancer (lung, pancreas, stomach), eclampsia, amniotic fluid embolus, massive trauma, burns, infections (Gram-negative sepsis, *Strep. pneumoniae*, malaria), snake/scorpion venom

5.4.3 Thrombophilia

- Abnormality in the coagulation system leading to hypercoagulability.
- Can be congenital or acquired:
  - Congenital:
    - Factor V Leiden: factor V is a co-factor of factor X leading to activation of thrombin. Normally broken down by protein C to limit the extent of the clotting. Factor V Leiden is a variant that cannot be degraded by protein C
    - Protein C deficiency: anticoagulant that inhibits the effects of factors V and VIII
    - Protein S deficiency: protein S is a vitamin K-dependent anticoagulant that acts as a co-factor to protein C
  - Acquired:
    - Antiphospholipid antibodies: autoimmune disease with antibodies against phospholipid. Various forms that lead to either upregulation of prothrombotic factors, inhibition of antithrombotic factors, or a combination of these
    - Oestrogen-containing contraceptives
    - Smoking
- Signs and symptoms:
  - DVT and PE and their associated signs and symptoms are the most common consequence of thrombophilia, although clots may form in more unusual places (e.g. venous sinus thrombosis, portal vein thrombosis, hepatic vein thrombosis, mesenteric vein thrombosis, and renal vein thrombosis)
  - Recurrent miscarriage
- Investigations:
  - FBC
  - D-dimer
  - Autoantibody screen
  - Further specialist investigations such as bleeding times and genetic screening may be indicated
- Treatment:
  - Treatment of DVT and PE will require a period of anticoagulation dependent on local policies and underlying cause

EVIDENCE-BASED MEDICINE

Types of trials

CONTENTS

1.1 Descriptive terms

- Longitudinal: more than one point in time.
- Cross-sectional: single point in time (snap-shot).
- Prospective: present and future (looks forwards).
- Retrospective: present and past (looks backwards).

1.2 Trial types

1.2.1 Case report

- A single person:
  - Usually anecdotal
  - Prone to chance association and bias
- Can be used to generate a hypothesis.

1.2.2 Case series

- A group of people.
- Useful for studying rare diseases:
  - Symptoms and signs
  - Aetiological factors
  - Associations and prognostic factors
  - Treatment approaches

1.2.3 Cohort study

- Group of subjects exposed to a risk factor are matched to a group not exposed (control group):
  - Both groups followed up for outcomes

- For example, people classified by biochemical marker concentration at the beginning of the study, before any have cancer, and followed up for many years
- Advantages:
  - Ethically safe, cheaper, and easier than RCT
  - Subjects can be matched
  - Timing and directionality of events
- Disadvantages:
  - Difficult to identify controls
  - Hidden confounders
  - Hard to blind
  - No randomization
  - Requires large numbers/long follow-up for rare diseases

1.2.4 Case–control study

- Subjects with an outcome matched with those who don't (control group):
  - Previous exposures explored
  - For example, people with various cancers compared against people without cancer—but matched for age, social class, gender, etc.
- Advantages:
  - Quick and cheap
  - Good for rare disorders, or those with a long gap between disease/exposure
  - Can use small numbers
- Disadvantages:
  - Reliance on recall and records
  - Confounders
  - Selection of control groups difficult
  - Bias: recall and selection

1.2.5 Randomized controlled trial (RCT)

- Gold-standard design for studying treatment effects.
- Subjects given 2 treatments:
  - Treatment under investigation given to experimental group
  - Standard intervention, placebo, or no treatment given to control group
- Differences in outcomes reported.
- Random allocation to treatment groups:
  - Minimizes selection bias
  - Should equally distribute confounding factors
- Reliable measure of efficacy.

1.2.6 Crossover trial

- All subjects receive one treatment then switch to the other treatment half-way through the study.
- Subjects are their own controls:
  - Must ensure no carry-over effects
  - Washout periods
- Advantages:
  - Subjects serve as own controls, so requires only low numbers
  - All patients receive treatment
  - Can use statistical tests which assume randomization
  - Blinding

- Disadvantages:
  - All patients receive placebo or treatment
  - Unknown length of washout periods
  - Cannot be used for treatments with permanent effects

1.2.7 Systematic review

- Review of all pertinent articles in the field.
- Results pooled.
- Overall conclusions: more accurate than individual studies.

1.2.8 Meta-analysis

- Collection of all the results from all the trials on a given subject into quantitative assessment: particularly useful when there are lots of little trials, each too small to give a conclusive answer.
- May show that a treatment previously believed to be ineffective is in fact beneficial, or 'best practices' were flawed.

Blinding

CONTENTS

2.1 Definition

- Aim of blinding is to ensure that no one knows what is really going on:
  - So they can't guess and influence the outcome
  - Everyone only sees the part you want them to see, and don't have the bigger picture
- Need to know whether difference observed is a result of the intervention, not the expectation of the intervention:
  - Avoids interference in results (conscious or not)
  - Decreases observation bias

2.2 Methods

- No blinding:
  - Open-label trial
- Single blinding:
  - Researcher *or* subject blind to allocation
- Double blinding:
  - Researcher *and* subject blind to allocation
- Triple blinding:
  - Researcher *and* subject *and* analyst blind to allocation

Bias

CONTENTS

3.1 Definition

- An error not due to chance:
  - Systematic deviation from the truth
  - May lead to misleading results and wrong conclusions
  - No statistical measure or control
  - Good research design minimizes bias

3.2 Categories of bias

- Reporting:
  - Literature review
  - Reduced by, for example, translation
- Publication:
  - Publication of trials which are positive rather than negative
- Selection:
  - Recruitment
  - Overcome by, for example, randomizing patients
- Performance:
  - Running trial: different care provided in difference arms (e.g. in different centres)
  - Reduced by, for example, blinding
- Observation:
  - Failure to measure or classify the exposure or outcomes correctly:
    - Interviewer bias: change in approach
    - Recall bias: selective memory
    - Response bias: subjects answer questions in the way they believe the researcher wants them to answer
  - Reduced by, for example, blinding
- Attrition:
  - Analysing results: dropouts differ in different arms of study
  - Reduced by, for example, intention-to-treat analysis

Statistical terms

CONTENTS

4.1 Incidence

- Incidence—rate of new cases over a period of time:
  - Number of new cases/population

4.2 Prevalence

- Prevalence—simplest measure of frequency:
  - Point prevalence: proportion of people with disease at a particular time
  - Period prevalence: proportion of people with disease over a specific time period
  - Lifetime prevalence: proportion of people with disease or had disease at any point in time

4.3 Qualitative data

- Categorical data.
- Compared with 'chi-squared test'.
- For example, gender, colour of hair.

4.4 Quantitative data

- Numerical data.
- Compared with 't-test'.
- Discrete data: finite number of possible values and tend to be made of integers (e.g. waiting time in minutes, number of non-attenders).
- Continuous data: infinite possibilities and can include decimal places (e.g. weight of patients, size of abdominal aortic aneurysm).

Normal distribution

CONTENTS

5.1 Bell-shaped curve

- Characteristic bell-shaped curve for parametric data.
- Symmetrical about its mean (peak of curve).
- Mean = median = mode.

5.2 Standard deviation (SD)

- SD = square root of variance:
  - The degree of data spread about the mean
  - A measure of precision
- Key property of the normal distribution is that we know the proportion of observations that will lie between any 2 values of the variable, as long as we know the mean and SD:
  - 68% within range of 1 SD
  - 95% within 2 SDs
  - 99.7% within 3 SDs

5.3 Confidence interval (CI)

- Width of CI indicates the precision of the estimate: 95% = range in which we can be 95% confident that the true value for the population lies.
- Larger sample = narrower CI.
- When quoted alongside a difference between 2 groups, a CI that includes 0 is statistically non-significant.
- When quoted alongside a ratio, a CI that includes 1 is statistically non-significant.

2 × 2 Contingency table

CONTENTS

6.1 Sensitivity

- Proportion of subjects with the disorder (by gold standard) who have a positive result (by new test).
- True positive rate.

6.2 Specificity

- Proportion of subjects who do not have the disorder and who have a negative test.
- True negative rate.

6.3 Positive predictive value (PPV)

- Proportion of subjects who have a positive test result who do have the disorder.

6.4 Negative predictive value (NPV)

- Proportion of subjects with a negative test result who do not have the illness.

6.5 Likelihood ratio for a +ve result (LR+)

- How much more likely a positive test is to be found in a person with, as opposed to without, the condition.

6.6 Likelihood ratio for a −ve result (LR−)

- How much more likely a negative test is to be found in a person with, as opposed to without, the condition.

Table H.6.1 A 2×2 contingency table for tests

		Disease status by gold standard		Totals
		Positive	Negative	
Disease status by new test	Positive	*a*	*b*	*a + b*
	Negative	*c*	*d*	*c + d*
Totals		*a + c*	*b + d*	*a + b + c + d*

6.7 2 × 2 Contingency table for tests

See Table H.6.1 for a 2 × 2 contingency table for tests.

- Sensitivity = a/(a + c).
- Specificity = d/(b + d).
- PPV = a/(a + b).
- NPV = d/(c + d).
- LR+ = sensitivity/(1 − specificity).
- LR− = (1 − sensitivity)/specificity.

Risks

CONTENTS

7.1 2 × 2 Contingency table for risks

See Table H.7.1 for a 2 × 2 contingency table for risks.

7.2 Measures

- Control event rate (CER):
  - c/c + d
- Experimental event rate (EER):
  - a/a + b
- Absolute risk reduction (ARR):
  - CER − EER
- Relative risk (RR):
  - EER/CER
- Relative risk reduction (RRR):
  - ARR/CER
- Number needed to treat (NNT):
  - 1/ARR
  - Number of people needed to be treated for 1 additional person to benefit
  - The lower the better
- Number needed to harm (NNH):

  Opposite of NNT (for adverse outcomes)

Table H.7.1 A 2×2 contingency table for risks

		Outcome event		Totals
		Positive	Negative	
Exposure	Positive	a	b	$a + b$
	Negative	c	d	$c + d$
Totals		$a + c$	$b + d$	$a + b + c + d$

Errors

CONTENTS

8.1 Type 1 error

- Type 1 error = null hypothesis rejected when it is true:
  - False positive:
    - A difference found between groups when no such difference exists
  - The possibility of a type 1 error should be considered with every significant finding:
    - Usually attributable to bias
  - Probability of making a type 1 error = α (typically 0.05):
    - $\alpha = 0.05$ = there is only a 5% chance of erroneously rejecting the null hypothesis

8.2 Type 2 error

- Type 2 error = null hypothesis accepted when it is false:
  - False negative:
    - Failing to uncover a difference between the groups that actually exists
  - The possibility of a type 2 error should be considered with every non-significant finding:
    - Usually because sample size is not large enough
  - Probability of making a type 2 error = β (typically 0.8)
  - Type 2 errors can be avoided by power calculations

Index

Tables and figures are indicated by an italic *t* and *f* following the page/paragraph number.

Printed and bound by CPI Group (UK) Ltd, Croydon, CR0 4YY